Lecture Notes in Computer Science   8498

Commenced Publication in 1973
Founding and Former Series Editors:
Gerhard Goos, Juris Hartmanis, and Jan van Leeuwen

Danail Stoyanov   D. Louis Collins
Ichiro Sakuma   Purang Abolmaesumi
Pierre Jannin (Eds.)

Information Processing in Computer-Assisted Interventions

5th International Conference, IPCAI 2014
Fukuoka, Japan, June 28, 2014
Proceedings

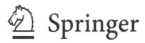

Springer

Volume Editors

Danail Stoyanov
University College London, UK
E-mail: danail.stoyanov@ucl.ac.uk

D. Louis Collins
McGill University, Montreal, QC, Canada
E-mail: louis.collins@mcgill.ca

Ichiro Sakuma
The University of Tokyo, Japan
E-mail: sakuma@bmpe.t.u-tokyo.ac.jp

Purang Abolmaesumi
University of British Columbia, Vancouver, BC, Canada
E-mail: purang@ece.ubc.ca

Pierre Jannin
Inserm/Université de Rennes 1, France
E-mail: pierre.jannin@univ-rennes1.fr

ISSN 0302-9743   e-ISSN 1611-3349
ISBN 978-3-319-07520-4   e-ISBN 978-3-319-07521-1
DOI 10.1007/978-3-319-07521-1
Springer Cham Heidelberg New York Dordrecht London

Library of Congress Control Number: 2014939558

LNCS Sublibrary: SL 6 – Image Processing, Computer Vision, Pattern Recognition, and Graphics

Typesetting: Camera-ready by author, data conversion by Scientific Publishing Services, Chennai, India

Printed on acid-free paper

Springer is part of Springer Science+Business Media (www.springer.com)

Preface

The 5th International Conference on Information Processing in Computer-Assisted Interventions, IPCAI 2014, was held in Fukuoka, Japan, at the Fukuoka Convention Center on June 28, 2014.

The IPCAI series of meetings was created as a forum to present and discuss the latest developments in computer-assisted interventions (CAI). With the paradigm shift towards minimally invasive surgery, computers and advanced surgical assist devices are increasingly present in the modern operating room and have a significant influence on how procedures are performed. Through the use of CAI systems it is possible to carry out surgical interventions that are more precise and less invasive than conventional procedures by providing enhanced surgical planning, instrument dexterity, positioning accuracy, real-time imaging, guidance and visualization. The wealth of added information in a CAI system can be processed in realtime or stored to facilitate quantitative analysis of surgical workflow and ergonomics, tracking of patient outcomes and improvements in treatment. Going beyond procedure-specific or system-specific CAI technologies, it is the synergy between the different CAI concepts and capabilities that gives rise to a new paradigm. To promote and develop these concepts further, the IPCAI series seeks to showcase papers presenting novel technical algorithms and theory, clinical needs and applications, as well as hardware and software systems and their validation.

This year, IPCAI was hosted outside Europe for the first time and we received 58 full paper submissions: 38 from Europe, 11 from North America, and 9 from Asia. Divided by primary topic category, 14 submissions were in Planning, Simulation, and Patient-Specific Models for Computer-Assisted Interventions, 14 in Medical Robotics and Surgical Navigation, 15 in Interventional Imaging and Advanced Intra-op Visualization, 5 in Cognition, Modeling and Context Awareness, and 10 in Clinical Applications, Systems, Software, and Validation. The submissions were coordinated by nine area chairs and reviewed by a total of 114 external reviewers. "Primary" and "secondary" area chairs were assigned to each paper and each paper received at least three external reviews. After the initial review process, the authors were given the opportunity to respond to the reviewers' and the area chairs' comments. Reviewers and area chairs then had the opportunity to revise their review based on the authors' response. After the review process was complete, papers that received unanimous accept recommendations were automatically accepted and papers without a single vote for acceptance were automatically rejected. Finally, an independent body consisting of the five program board members as well as the program and general chairs discussed all remaining papers and made decisions on them. We finally accepted 28 papers for the meeting's program and the program chairs checked the final material to ensure that all reviewers' comments were addressed.

The format of IPCAI is designed to encourage interaction and allows time for constructive discussion and as such all authors of accepted papers were asked to give short five-minute platform presentations. In addition, each paper was presented as a poster during interactive sessions with organized discussion. The conference delegates were then asked to vote for a list of papers that they wanted to see discussed in a longer platform presentation. The papers with the highest number of votes were then presented in detailed podium sessions during the afternoon for questions from the attendees and the committee members.

We would like to take this opportunity to thank the area chairs, program board, and all of the reviewers for their help and efforts to maintain the high quality of the series and select outstanding papers stimulating an exciting discussion at the meeting. Finally, we would also like to thank all the authors who submitted their research to IPCAI and for their subsequent work in revising the papers for final publication.

June 2014

Danail Stoyanov
Louis Collins
Ichiro Sakuma

IPCAI Organization

2014 IPCAI Executive Committee

Program Chairs

Danail Stoyanov   CMIC, UCL, UK
Louis Collins   McGill University, Canada
Ichiro Sakuma   University of Tokyo, Japan

General Chairs

Purang Abolmaesumi   UBC, Canada
Pierre Jannin   INSERM, Rennes, France

Area Chairs

Ken Masamune   University of Tokyo, Japan
Lena Meier-Hein   DKFZ, Germany
Arianna Menciassi   SSSA, Italy
Peter Mountney   Siemens Corporate Research, USA
Ryoichi Nakamura   Chiba University, Japan
David Noonan   Philips Research, USA
Terry Peters   Robarts Research Institute, Canada
Ferdinando Rodriguez   Imperial College London, UK
   y Baena
Ziv Yaniv   Children's National Medical Center, USA

Program Board

Dave Hawkes   CMIC, UCL, UK
Kensaku Mori   Nagoya University, Japan
Nassir Navab   TUM, Germany
Tim Salcudean   UBC, Canada
Russell Taylor   JHU, USA

Local Organization, Web and Administration Chairs

Franziska Schweikert   CARS office, Germany
Ryu Nakadate   Kyushu University, Japan
Max Allan   CMIC, UCL, UK

IPCAI Steering Committee

Kevin Cleary   DC Children's Hospital, USA
Gabor Fichtinger   Queen's University, Canada
Makoto Hashizume   Kyushu University, Japan

Dave Hawkes   CMIC, UCL, UK
Pierre Jannin   INSERM, Rennes, France
Leo Joskowicz   Hebrew University, Israel
Ron Kikinis   Boston, USA
Heinz Lemke   Leipzig, Germany
Kensaku Mori   Nagoya University, Japan
Nassir Navab   CAMP/TUM, Germany
Terry Peters   Robarts Research Institute, Canada
Tim Salcudean   UBC, Canada
Gabor Szekely   ETH, Switzerland
Russell Taylor   JHU, USA
Guang-Zhong Yang   Imperial College, UK

Reviewers

Max Allan   Caroline Essert
Ron Alterovitz   Baowei Fei
Junpei Arata   Aaron Fenster
Mariana Bernardes   Vincenzo Ferrari
Tim Beyl   Bernhard Fuerst
Wolfgang Birkfellner   Stamatia Giannarou
Stuart Bowyer   Petros Giataganas
Chiara Caborni   Ben Glocker
Marina Carbone   Óscar Grasa
Jorge Cardoso   Ozgur Guler
Pietro Cerveri   Ilker Hacihaliloglu
Claire Chalopin   Gregory Hager
Ping-Lin Chang   Noby Hata
Elvis Chen   Yuichiro Hayashi
Kiyoyuki Chinzei   Tobias Heimann
Gastone Ciuti   Jaesung Hong
Neil Clancy   Joachim Hornegger
Matt Clarkson   Yipeng Hu
Kevin Cleary   Leo Joskowicz
Louis Collins   Ankur Kapoor
Mirko Comparetti   Ali Khan
Brian Courtney   Yo Kobayashi
Danilo De Lorenzo   Martin Kochan
Elena De Momi   Alexandre Krupa
Adrien Desjardins   Mirko Kunze
Pierre-Francois d'Haese   Pablo Lamata
Sanja Dogramadzi   Catherine Laporte
Xiaofei Du   Su-Lin Lee
Roy Eagleson   Christian Linte
Dan Elson   Fangde Liu

Hongbin Liu
Gian-Luca Mariottini
Ken Masamune
Yoshitaka Masutani
Michael Miga
Daniel Mirota
José Montiel
Kensaku Mori
Yoshihiro Muragaki
George Mylonas
Nassir Navab
Thomas Neumuth
Stéphane Nicolau
David Noonan
Asli Okur
Nicolas Padoy
Tassanai Parittotokkaporn
Chris Payne
Graeme Penney
Franjo Pernus
Joshua Petersen
Aleksandra Popovic
Philip Pratt
Bharat Ramachandran
Rogério Richa
Christian Rieder

Esther Rodriguez Villegas
Robert Rohling
James Ross
Ofri Sadowsky
Ikuma Sato
Yoshinobu Sato
Christian Schumann
Alexander Seitel
Gregory Slabaugh
Stefanie Speidel
Jan Stuehmer
Takashi Suzuki
Raphael Sznitman
Stephen Thompson
Junichi Toduda
Johannes Totz
Nick Tustisuon
Eranga Ukwatta
Tamas Ungi
Anant Vemuri
Tom Vercauteren
Marco Visentini-Scarzanella
Kirby Vosburgh
Thomas Wendler
Jianhua Yao
Li Zhang

Table of Contents

Medical Robotics and Surgical Navigation

2D-3D Pose Tracking of Rigid Instruments in Minimally Invasive
Surgery.. 1
    Max Allan, Stephen Thompson, Matthew J. Clarkson,
    Sébastien Ourselin, David J. Hawkes, John D. Kelly, and
    Danail Stoyanov

Robust Real-Time Visual Odometry for Stereo Endoscopy Using Dense
Quadrifocal Tracking 11
    Ping-Lin Chang, Ankur Handa, Andrew J. Davison,
    Danail Stoyanov, and Philip "Eddie" Edwards

Comparative Assessment of a Novel Optical Human-Machine Interface
for Laparoscopic Telesurgery 21
    Fabien Despinoy, Alonso Sánchez, Nabil Zemiti, Pierre Jannin, and
    Philippe Poignet

Modelling and Control of an ERF-Based Needle Insertion Training
Platform... 31
    Adrián Graña, Alonso Sánchez, Nabil Zemiti, and Philippe Poignet

Intraoperative Cone Beam CT Guidance for Transoral Robotic
Surgery.. 41
    Wen P. Liu, Jeremy D. Richmon, Mahdi Azizian,
    Jonathan Sorger, and Russell H. Taylor

Robotic Device for Acquisition of Wide and High Resolution MRI
Image Using a Small RF Coil................................... 51
    Kohei Miki and Ken Masamune

Building Surrogate-Driven Motion Models from Cone-Beam CT via
Surrogate-Correlated Optical Flow 61
    James Martin, Jamie McClelland, Benjamin Champion, and
    David J. Hawkes

Clinical Applications, Systems, Software and Validation

Vascular 3D+T Freehand Ultrasound Using Correlation of Doppler and
Pulse-Oximetry Data... 68
    Christoph Hennersperger, Athanasios Karamalis, and Nassir Navab

Semi-automated Quantification of Fibrous Cap Thickness in
Intracoronary Optical Coherence Tomography 78
   Guillaume Zahnd, Antonios Karanasos, Gijs van Soest,
   Evelyn Regar, Wiro J. Niessen, Frank Gijsen, and Theo van Walsum

A System for Ultrasound-Guided Spinal Injections: A Feasibility
Study 90
   Abtin Rasoulian, Jill Osborn, Samira Sojoudi, Saman Nouranian,
   Victoria A. Lessoway, Robert N. Rohling, and Purang Abolmaesumi

The 'Augmented' Circles: A Video-Guided Solution for the
Down-the-Beam Positioning of IM Nail Holes 100
   Roberto Londei, Marco Esposito, Benoit Diotte, Simon Weidert,
   Ekkehard Euler, Peter Thaller, Nassir Navab, and Pascal Fallavollita

CT to US Registration of the Lumbar Spine: A Clinical Feasibility
Study 108
   Simrin Nagpal, Purang Abolmaesumi, Abtin Rasoulian,
   Tamas Ungi, Ilker Hacihaliloglu, Jill Osborn, Dan P. Borschneck,
   Victoria A. Lessoway, Robert N. Rohling, and Parvin Mousavi

A Computer Assisted Planning System for the Placement of sEEG
Electrodes in the Treatment of Epilepsy 118
   G. Zombori, R. Rodionov, M. Nowell, M.A. Zuluaga,
   Matthew J. Clarkson, C. Micallef, B. Diehl,
   T. Wehner, A. Miserochi, Andrew W. McEvoy,
   John S. Duncan, and Sébastien Ourselin

Articulated Statistical Shape Model-Based 2D-3D Reconstruction
of a Hip Joint 128
   S. Balestra, S. Schumann, J. Heverhagen, L. Nolte, and G. Zheng

Workflow Modelling and Surgical Skill Analysis

Pairwise Comparison-Based Objective Score for Automated Skill
Assessment of Segments in a Surgical Task 138
   Anand Malpani, S. Swaroop Vedula, Chi Chiung Grace Chen, and
   Gregory D. Hager

Random Forests for Phase Detection in Surgical Workflow Analysis 148
   Ralf Stauder, Aslı Okur, Loïc Peter, Armin Schneider,
   Michael Kranzfelder, Hubertus Feussner, and Nassir Navab

Knowledge-Driven Formalization of Laparoscopic Surgeries
for Rule-Based Intraoperative Context-Aware Assistance 158
   Darko Katić, Anna-Laura Wekerle, Fabian Gärtner,
   Hannes Kenngott, Beat Peter Müller-Stich, Rüdiger Dillmann, and
   Stefanie Speidel

Temporally Consistent 3D Pose Estimation in the Interventional Room
Using Discrete MRF Optimization over RGBD Sequences   168
    Abdolrahim Kadkhodamohammadi, Afshin Gangi,
    Michel de Mathelin, and Nicolas Padoy

Relevance-Based Visualization to Improve Surgeon Perception   178
    Olivier Pauly, Benoît Diotte, Séverine Habert, Simon Weidert,
    Ekkehard Euler, Pascal Fallavollita, and Nassir Navab

Towards Better Laparoscopic Video Database Organization by
Automatic Surgery Classification   186
    Andru P. Twinanda, Jacques Marescaux, Michel De Mathelin, and
    Nicolas Padoy

Model-Based Identification of Anatomical Boundary Conditions in
Living Tissues   196
    Igor Peterlik, Hadrien Courtecuisse, Christian Duriez, and
    Stéphane Cotin

Interventional Imaging and Advanced Intra-op Visualization

Fast Semi-dense Surface Reconstruction from Stereoscopic Video in
Laparoscopic Surgery   206
    Johannes Totz, Stephen Thompson, Danail Stoyanov,
    Kurinchi Gurusamy, Brian R. Davidson, David J. Hawkes, and
    Matthew J. Clarkson

Deblurring Multispectral Laparoscopic Images   216
    Geoffrey Jones, Neil Clancy, Simon Arridge, Dan Elson, and
    Danail Stoyanov

Simulated Field Maps: Toward Improved Susceptibility Artefact
Correction in Interventional MRI   226
    Martin Kochan, Pankaj Daga, Ninon Burgos, Mark White,
    M. Jorge Cardoso, Laura Mancini, Gavin P. Winston,
    Andrew W. McEvoy, John Thornton, Tarek Yousry,
    John S. Duncan, Danail Stoyanov, and Sébastien Ourselin

Orientation-Driven Ultrasound Compounding Using Uncertainty
Information   236
    Christian Schulte zu Berge, Ankur Kapoor, and Nassir Navab

2D/3D Catheter-Based Registration for Image Guidance in TACE
of Liver Tumors   246
    Pierre Ambrosini, Danny Ruijters, Adriaan Moelker,
    Wiro J. Niessen, and Theo van Walsum

Filter-Based Speckle Tracking for Freehand Prostate Biopsy: Theory,
ex vivo and *in vivo* Results...................................... 256
*Narges Afsham, Siavash Khallaghi, Mohammad Najafi,
Lindsay Machan, Silvia D. Chang, Larry Goldenberg, Peter Black,
Robert N. Rohling, and Purang Abolmaesumi*

Efficient Tissue Discrimination during Surgical Interventions Using
Hyperspectral Imaging... 266
Dorra Nouri, Yves Lucas, and Sylvie Treuillet

Author Index... 277

2D-3D Pose Tracking of Rigid Instruments in Minimally Invasive Surgery

Max Allan[1,2], Steve Thompson[1,3], Matthew J. Clarkson[1,3],
Sébastien Ourselin[1,3], David J. Hawkes[1,3], John Kelly[4], and Danail Stoyanov[1,2]

[1] Centre for Medical Image Computing, UCL, London, UK
[2] Department of Computer Science, UCL, London, UK
[3] Department of Medical Physics and Bioengineering, UCL, London, UK
[4] Division of Surgery and Interventional Science, Medical School, UCL, London, UK
{maximilian.allan.11,s.thompson,m.clarkson,s.ourselin,
d.hawkes,j.d.kelly,d.stoyanov}@ucl.ac.uk

Abstract. Instrument localization and tracking is an important challenge for advanced computer assisted techniques in minimally invasive surgery and image-based solutions to instrument localization can provide a non-invasive, low cost solution. In this study, we present a novel algorithm capable of recovering the 3D pose of laparoscopic surgical instruments combining constraints from a classification algorithm, multiple point features, stereo views (when available) and a linear motion model to robustly track the tool in surgical videos. We demonstrate the improved robustness and performance of our algorithm with optically tracked ground truth and additionally qualitatively demonstrate its performance on *in vivo* images.

1 Introduction

Image-based instrument tracking and localization has important applications in computer assisted interventions (CAI) and in robotic minimally invasive surgery (RMIS). Computing the pose of the instruments is critical for enabling enhanced guidance and navigation where precise knowledge of the sub-surface patient anatomy can assist the surgeon to avoid critical structures and accurately excise tissue. With robotic manipulators, virtual fixtures can be applied if the tools approach delicate regions [1] or alternatively haptic feedback can be used to improve instrument-tissue manipulation [2]. The major challenge with localizing the tools is in developing a system that integrates into the operating room with minimal disruption of the workflow or additional invasion of the patient anatomy. While instrument tracking can be realised by using hardware sensors, encoders or external optical systems, such approaches require extensive hardware integration and still have limitations in accuracy and integration into the operating theatre. A significant advantage of image-based methods [3,4] is that they recover the tool's position and orientation directly in the surgeon's viewing reference and do not require any additional hardware [5,6].

D. Stoyanov et al. (Eds.): IPCAI 2014, LNCS 8498, pp. 1–10, 2014.

For minimally invasive surgery (MIS), instrument detection based purely on images has been investigated for a number years [7]. Recent state-of-the-art methods involve the use of trained classifiers and combine the detection and subsequent tracking of instruments [8,9]. Such algorithms achieve excellent results but from a single image only the 2D image position of the instrument is recovered. The full 3D position and orientation of the instrument can be recovered using specialized fiducial markers machined onto the instruments, however, this approach is restrictive and it interferes with the hardware making it difficult for general theatre use with arbitrary instruments [10]. Naturally appearing features can potentially also be used to localize the instrument. For example, edge information with gradient direction filtering based on the trocar position has been demonstrated [11]. This constraint can cope with significant image noise but estimating the trocar position can be complex in the presence of insufflation and physiological motion such as breathing and heart rate. Gradient based point features can also be combined with color-based features and classification to track articulated robotic instruments [12] or as part of a brute force matching of rendered tool templates [13]. Such methods can be implemented in real-time with GPU processing but they rely heavily on kinematic data from the robotic system and this therefore limits their application to non-robotic procedures. Additionally, the gradient features are focussed around the tip of the articulated instrument which fails to exploit the large constraint provided by the cylindrical instrument shaft. In [14] we demonstrated the use of this constraint for five degrees of freedom (5 DOF) instrument localization.

In this paper we propose combining constraints from feature points with a region based level set segmentation to develop an instrument localization and tracking framework that is more robust than using either individual technique in isolation. We handle challenging data containing occlusions and large reflections by exploiting strong prior knowledge of the instrument appearance and shape though discriminative classification with a Random Forest (RF) and by applying constraints to the level set propagation. We formulate this within a cost function that is simple to optimize and robust to noise in the image. The addition of multi-view constraints to suit an emerging line of stereo laparoscopes add further information and temporal motion is incorporated with a Kalman filter. We show that these modifications provide improvement over previous work by comparison experiments with *ex vivo* tissue and ground truth tracking provided by an optical system. To further illustrate the effectiveness of our algorithm we include qualitative results from MIS videos.

2   Method

2.1   Region Based Alignment

Region based tracking methods using level sets are generally framed as the maximization of an energy functional

$$E = \int_{\Omega_f} r_f(I(\mathbf{x}), C))d\Omega + \int_{\Omega_b} r_b(I(\mathbf{x}), C)d\Omega \qquad (1)$$

where $r_{f|b}$ represent functions which measure the agreement between the information in the pixels $\mathbf{x}$ of image I within a contour C (the foreground) and outside the contour (the background) with learned statistical models. These agreement functions are summed over the foreground and background regions $\Omega_{f|b}$. Normally this energy functional is maximized by finding the set of pose parameters which define the optimal segmentation of the target image into a foreground and background region.

The significant challenges within region based tracking are selecting a function $r(.)$ to measure the region agreement and choosing the parameters which determine the evolution of the contour. By assuming a weak constraint, which can be relaxed, that we are tracking a rigid object we solve the latter problem by following [15] optimizing in the space of the 6 degrees of freedom of a rigid transformation, constraining the contour to belong to the set of image plane projections of our target object at the current estimate of pose.

Selecting the function $r(.)$ is problematic in MIS as the complex lighting and occlusions lead to ambiguous regions for which simple classification models fail. Following [14] we learn the function $r(.)$ with random decision forests trained on the Hue, Saturation, Opponent 2 and Opponent 3 color spaces, which were demonstrated by the authors to have good performance on MIS images.

2.2 Incorporating Stereo Constraints

A significant challenge of 3D pose estimation using a monocular camera is the difficulty in estimating the depth of the target object purely from perspective cues [14]. Incorporating stereo constraints is important for creating a system that is capable of reliably estimating 3D information. Practically, stereo acquisition is also more common now with 3D laparoscope systems recently becoming available from a variety of commercial manufacturers [16]. We incorporate stereo as a special case multi-view constraint [15] by constructing the cost function over both images of the stereo pair before solving for the pose in the reference camera coordinate system.

2.3 Refinement with Point Based Tracking

One of the challenges of region based tracking is that it struggles to refine the pose to highly accurate solutions when there are ambiguous contours or noise around the edge of the target object. However, it is good at providing a reasonably close solution to the global maximum.

Point based tracking methods however can provide highly accurate pose estimation but suffer heavily from data association errors, particularly when working with relatively featureless surfaces such as those found on medical instruments. The robustness of region based tracking can be combined with the high precision of point based tracking by jointly optimizing for both features. We avoid the difficulties of data association errors by searching for matches in a small region around expected locations of feature points (as suggested by the current estimated pose of the target object).

This results in our overall discretized energy functional being represented as

$$E = \sum_{i \in \mathcal{I}_{l|r}} \sum_{\mathbf{x} \in \Omega_i} \left(r_f(\mathbf{x}) H(g(\mathbf{x})) + r_b(\mathbf{x})(1 - H(g(\mathbf{x}))) \right) + \lambda \sum_{\mathbf{y} \in \Gamma} |\mathbf{y}' - P(\mathbf{y})|^2 \quad (2)$$

where $\mathbf{y}'$ is a matched feature in the image (we perform feature matching exclusively in the left image for simplicity) and $P(\mathbf{y})$ is the projection of its corresponding 3D point. λ is a weighting parameter used to modify the contribution of the point alignments. $H(.)$ is the smoothed Heaviside function of the level set embedding function $g(\mathbf{x})$, which is represented as a signed distance function as is typical in the level set formulation of image segmentations [17]. $\mathcal{I}_{l|r}$ are set of the left and right images (although this could represent any number of calibrated images) and $\mathbf{x} \in \Omega_i$ refer to the pixels in a single image over which segmentation is performed. Γ is the set of features on the target object which we are attempting to match in the image. In our current implementation we choose SIFT features [18] but any feature with good invariance to lighting and pose changes could be chosen. To build a library of detectable points for a given instrument, we collect target SIFT features from a sample image of the object in which the instrument pose has been manually aligned, backprojecting them to their intersection with the target object to find their object space coordinates.

The cost function is optimized using gradient descent as this only requires first derivatives yielding faster iterations than other optimization techniques. We additionally use the quaternion representation of angular pose which, although requiring normalization at each step, avoids the singularity problems of the Euler angle representation.

2.4   Initialization and Tracking

To initialize our pose estimate we follow the method of [14]. Frame by frame tracking is provided with a linear Kalman filter for both position and orientation. Our state vector for the kth estimate is defined as

$$\mathbf{x}_k = (x, y, z, \dot{x}, \dot{y}, \dot{z}, \theta, \psi, \phi) \quad (3)$$

where the terms have their usual meanings. We transform the quaternion rotation representation to Euler angles to allow linearization of the Kalman filter. We update pose using the standard Kalman Filter equations

$$\mathbf{x}_k = \mathbf{F}\mathbf{x}_{k-1} + N(0, \mathbf{Q}) \quad (4)$$

$$\mathbf{z}_k = \mathbf{M}\mathbf{x}_k + N(0, \mathbf{R}) \quad (5)$$

where $\mathbf{z}_k$ is the measurement vector, $\mathbf{F}$ is the position-velocity state transition matrix and $\mathbf{M}$ is the identity observation model. Both are corrupted by normally distributed noise of zero mean and variance $\mathbf{Q}, \mathbf{R}$. For more details on the linear Kalman filter, the reader is directed to [19].

3   Results

To evaluate the performance of the proposed method we conducted experiments within a controlled laboratory environment where we were able to obtain ground truth data. For comparison to prior work we compared our results to a recent state-of-the-art method [14]. Qualitative evaluation is also reported for *in vivo* surgical videos.

The implementation of the method used in these results is written in C++ and a single iteration of the gradient descent takes approximately 1 second on a 3.0 GHz dual core CPU. As each pixel of the level set optimization is evaluated independently, the method is highly parallelizable and real time performance has been demonstrated for similar techniques on a GPU [15].

3.1   Laboratory Experiments

A mock-up surgical site was constructed with a lamb's liver and an Endopath monopolar dissector (Ethicon Endo-Surgery Inc.) as the working instrument. The scene was visualized with a 3DHD laparoscope (Viking Systems). We attached optical tracking markers to the proximal end of the laparoscope and to the proximal end of the instrument and tracked their locations using an Optotrak Certus system (Northern Digital). Hand eye calibration was performed using OpenCV[1] and Tsai's handeye method [20] implemented within the NifTK

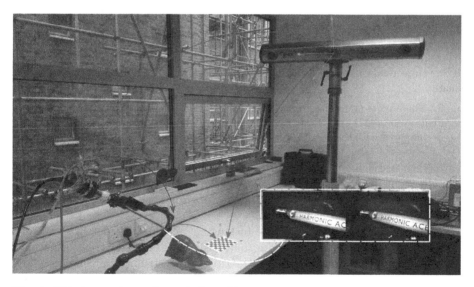

Fig. 1. This image shows the optical tracking system we constructed to capture video with synchronized ground truth data. Inset shows an example frame from our captured video.

---

[1] http://docs.opencv.org/

toolbox[2] to determine the transformations between the optical tracker and the camera coordinate systems (See Figure 1). The location of the instrument tip relative to the tracking markers was found using an invariant point method, also implemented in NifTK. Laparoscope tracking error was experimentally determined to be 1.7mm RMS and instrument tracking error estimated to be 0.7mm RMS, assuming independence this gives a tracking error of 1.8 mm RMS for the instrument tip relative to the laparoscope lens.

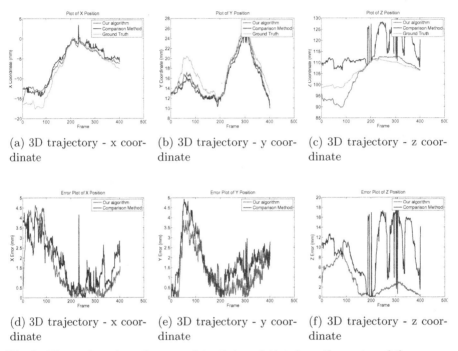

(a) 3D trajectory - x coordinate

(b) 3D trajectory - y coordinate

(c) 3D trajectory - z coordinate

(d) 3D trajectory - x coordinate

(e) 3D trajectory - y coordinate

(f) 3D trajectory - z coordinate

Fig. 2. These plots show the ground truth translation from the center of the camera coordinate system to the tip of the tracked instrument obtained with the Optical tracking system compared with the results obtained from our algorithm and the algorithm of [14]

We learn instrument color models from a single image of the target object manually segmented from a homogeneous background and the background model is learned from a single image of the target environment captured before the instrument is introduced to the scene.

We recorded a single video of the instrument moving in front of the liver synchronising the video and tracking data using NifTK. The transformation from the camera coordinate system to the tip of the instrument is computed for each frame by our algorithm and by the optically tracked markers. Due to the calibration inaccuracy we are forced to manually remove the offset by choosing a frame where the tracking alignment appears most accurate and setting the fixed offset as the difference between the estimates at this point.

---

[2] http://cmic.cs.ucl.ac.uk/home/software/

Table 1. The numerical results showing the mean and std. dev. of error in each axis

	Mean Error (mm)	Std. Dev. Error (mm)
X axis - Our Method	1.51	1.48
X axis - Comparison	1.73	1.21
Y axis - Our Method	1.25	1.04
Y axis - Comparison	1.89	1.17
Z axis - Our Method	3.05	2.68
Z axis - Comparison	9.86	4.89

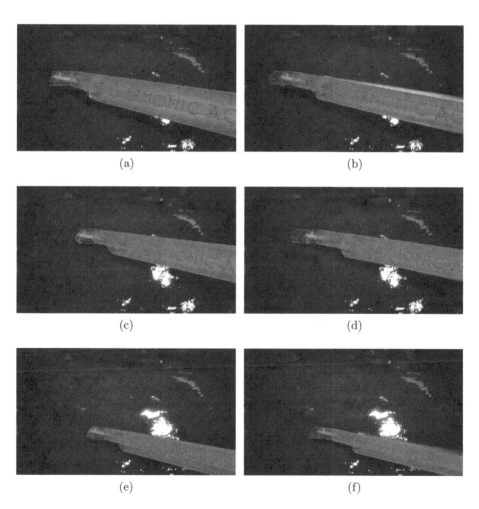

(a)   (b)

(c)   (d)

(e)   (f)

Fig. 3. The images show estimates of the instrument pose overlaid on the video. The left hand column of images show our technique which incorporates stereo, points and a Kalman filter compared with the right hand column showing the method of [14] which does not use these features.

We show quantitative results from the tracking in Figure 2. Selected frames from the tracking procedure compared with the equivalent estimate from our comparison method are shown in Figure 3.

3.2   Qualitative Results

We also demonstrate the qualitative results of our method by performing tracking on several sequences from surgical environments where 3D tracking data is not available. This dataset was not captured with a stereo camera which prevents us from incorporating these constraints in our pose estimation. Selected frames from this validation are shown in Figure 4.

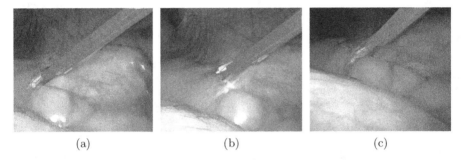

(a)   (b)   (c)

Fig. 4. The frames show select examples from an *in vivo* dataset with the instrument model overlaid at the current pose estimate.

3.3   Failure Modes

The most significant point of failure in our algorithm is dealing with a poor initialization, which is typically due to difficulties in correctly labelling the image pixels using the random forest. When this occurs, the model is placed too far from the ideal location for convergence to occur.

A secondary failure mode occurs due to our treatment of the instrument color model with a bag-of-pixels approach. This means that when the (often different colored) tip of the instrument is occluded behind tissue (e.g. due to cutting) the model can still fit to the image with a high degree of confidence as it doesn't care if the pixels it matches to the tip region of the contour actually match the true surface color at that point, only that they match the appearance model of the whole instrument surface. Potentially the appearance of the instrument model can be broken up into multiple classes [21] but as of yet this is not an area we have investigated.

4   Conclusion and Discussion

In this work, we have presented a novel framework for tracking rigid 3D objects using stereo 2D images. We combine a region based segmentation technique with point based pose estimation simultaneously addressing the weaknesses of both methods. Quantitative validation is performed on optically tracked endoscopic images in a mock surgical environment. Figure 2 shows the estimated (x, y, z) position of the instrument tip compared with the method of [14]. Both methods provide good accuracy in x and y, although ours appears slightly more accurate and there is a significant accuracy improvement in the z direction, which is to be expected given the stereo constraints our method includes. The decrease in error over the duration of the sequence can be explained by the method gradually recovering from inaccuracies in the pose initialization. Table 1 shows the numerical performance improvements of our method. Visual comparison can be seen in sample frames in Figure 3 where both methods converge to an accurate solution but our method more accurately converges around the instrument tip and does not have the same errors in estimating the shaft rotation. The full video can be found online at `https://youtu.be/5VyRmvGBT8k`. Qualitative validation on *in vivo* data demonstrates that our method is feasible in real surgical environments. Sample frames showing the alignment accuracy are shown in Figure 4 which demonstrates the method's robustness to lighting and fast motion as well as the significant articulation in some frames.

Our method presents several areas where improvement is necessary. The most significant of which is the modelling of instrument articulation. Methods of disjoint optimization appear the most simple, where each articulated component is optimized separated however [21] and [22] have both presented methods of 3D pose tracking which handle the articulation as part of a single optimization. Additionally, further constraints need to be added to model the trocar insertion point which would help to improve the accuracy of our system.

Acknowledgements. The authors would like to thank CJMedical for supplying the Viking laparoscope used in the experiments. Danail Stoyanov would like to acknowledge the financial support of a Royal Academy of Engineering/EPSRC Fellowship. Max Allan would like to acknowledge the financial support of the Rabin Ezra foundation as well as the EPSRC funding for the DTP in Medical and Biomedical Imaging at UCL. John Kelly would like to acknowledge the UCL Biomedical Research Centre for their financial support.

References

1. Azimian, H., Patel, R., Naish, M.: On constrained manipulation in robotics-assisted minimally invasive surgery. In: 3rd IEEE RAS and EMBS International Conference on Biomedical Robotics and Biomechatronics, pp. 650–655 (2010)
2. van der Putten Westebring, E.P., Goossens, R.H.M., Jakimowicz, J.J., Dankelman, J.: Haptics in minimally invasive surgery a review. Minimally Invasive Therapy & Allied Technologies 17(1), 3–16 (2008)
3. Speidel, S., Sudra, G., Senemaud, J., Drentschew, M., Müller-Stich, B.P., Gutt, C., Dillmann, R.: Recognition of risk situations based on endoscopic instrument tracking and knowledge based situation modeling. In: Medical Imaging 2008: Visualization, Image-Guided Procedures, and Modeling, vol. 6918 (2008)
4. Chmarra, M.K., Grimbergen, C.A., Dankelman, J.: Systems for tracking minimally invasive surgical instruments. Minimally Invasive Therapy & Allied Technologies 16(6), 328–340 (2007)

5. Mirota, D.J., Ishii, M., Hager, G.D.: Vision-based navigation in image-guided interventions. Annual Review of Biomedical Engineering 13, 297–319 (2011)
6. Stoyanov, D.: Surgical vision. Annals of Biomedical Engineering 40(2), 332–345 (2012)
7. Uecker, D.R., Lee, C., Wang, Y.F., Wang, Y.: Automated instrument tracking in robotically assisted laparoscopic surgery. Journal of Image Guided Surgery 1(6), 308–325 (1995) PMID: 9080352
8. Sznitman, R., Ali, K., Richa, R., Taylor, R., Hager, G., Fua, P.: Data-driven visual tracking in retinal microsurgery. In: Ayache, N., Delingette, H., Golland, P., Mori, K. (eds.) MICCAI 2012, Part II. LNCS, vol. 7511, pp. 568–575. Springer, Heidelberg (2012)
9. Richa, R., Balicki, M., Meisner, E., Sznitman, R., Taylor, R., Hager, G.: Visual tracking of surgical tools for proximity detection in retinal surgery. In: Taylor, R.H., Yang, G.-Z. (eds.) IPCAI 2011. LNCS, vol. 6689, pp. 55–66. Springer, Heidelberg (2011)
10. Zhao, T., Zhao, W., Halabe, D.J., Hoffman, B.D., Nowlin, W.C.: Fiducial marker design and detection for locating surgical instrument in images. Patent US 068 395, 07 08 (2010)
11. Voros, S., Long, J., Cinquin, P.: Automatic detection of instruments in laparoscopic images: A first step towards high-level command of robotic endoscopic holders. The International Journal of Robotics Research 26(11-12), 1173–1190 (2007)
12. Reiter, A., Allen, P.K., Zhao, T.: Appearance learning for 3d tracking of robotic surgical tools. The International Journal of Robotics Research (2013)
13. Austin, R., Allen, P.K., Tao, Z.: Articulated surgical tool detection using virtually-rendered templates. Computer Assisted Radiology and Surgery (2012)
14. Allan, M., Ourselin, S., Thompson, S., Hawkes, D.J., Kelly, J., Stoyanov, D.: Toward detection and localization of instruments in minimally invasive surgery. IEEE Transactions on Biomedical Engineering 60(4), 1050–1058 (2013)
15. Prisacariu, V.A., Reid, I.D.: PWP3D: Real-Time segmentation and tracking of 3D objects. Int. J. Computer Vision 98(3), 335–354 (2012)
16. Maier-Hein, L., Mountney, P., Bartoli, A., Elhawary, H., Elson, D., Groch, A., Kolb, A., Rodrigues, M., Sorger, J., Speidel, S., Stoyanov, D.: Optical techniques for 3d surface reconstruction in computer-assisted laparoscopic surgery. Medical Image Analysis 17(8), 974–996 (2013)
17. Cremers, D., Rousson, M., Deriche, R.: A review of statistical approaches to level set segmentation: Integrating color, texture, motion and shape. Int. J. Comput. Vision 72(2), 195–215 (2007)
18. Lowe, D.G.: Distinctive image features from scale-invariant keypoints. Int. J. Comput. Vision 60(2), 91–110 (2004)
19. Prince, S.: Computer Vision: Models Learning and Inference. Cambridge University Press (2012)
20. Tsai, R., Lenz, R.: A new technique for fully autonomous and efficient 3d robotics hand/eye calibration. IEEE Transactions on Robotics and Automation 5(3), 345–358 (1989)
21. Pezzementi, Z., Voros, S., Hager, G.D.: Articulated object tracking by rendering consistent appearance parts. In: IEEE International Conference on Robotics and Automation, ICRA 2009, pp. 3940–3947 (May 2009)
22. Prisacariu, V.A., Reid, I.: Nonlinear shape manifolds as shape priors in level set segmentation and tracking. In: Proceedings of the 2011 IEEE Conference on Computer Vision and Pattern Recognition, CVPR 2011, pp. 2185–2192. IEEE Computer Society, Washington, DC (2011)

Robust Real-Time Visual Odometry for Stereo Endoscopy Using Dense Quadrifocal Tracking

Ping-Lin Chang[1], Ankur Handa[1], Andrew J. Davison[1],
Danail Stoyanov[3], and Philip "Eddie" Edwards[1,2]

[1] Department of Computing
[2] Department of Surgery and Cancer
Imperial College London, United Kingdom
{p.chang10,a.handa,a.davison,eddie.edwards}@imperial.ac.uk
[3] Centre for Medical Image Computing and Department of Computer Science
University College London, United Kingdom
danail.stoyanov@ucl.ac.uk

Abstract. Visual tracking in endoscopic scenes is known to be a difficult task due to the lack of textures, tissue deformation and specular reflection. In this paper, we devise a real-time visual odometry framework to robustly track the 6-DoF stereo laparoscope pose using the quadrifocal relationship. The instant motion of a stereo camera creates four views which can be constrained by the quadrifocal geometry. Using the previous stereo pair as a reference frame, the current pair can be warped back by minimising a photometric error function with respect to a camera pose constrained by the quadrifocal geometry. Using a robust estimator can further remove the outliers caused by occlusion, deformation and specular highlights during the optimisation. Since the optimisation uses all pixel data in the images, it results in a very robust pose estimation even for a textureless scene. The quadrifocal geometry is initialised by using real-time stereo reconstruction algorithm which can be efficiently parallelised and run on the GPU together with the proposed tracking framework. Our system is evaluated using a ground truth synthetic sequence with a known model and we also demonstrate the accuracy and robustness of the approach using phantom and real examples of endoscopic augmented reality.

1 Introduction

Visual odometry is the process of determining the position and orientation of a camera moving in 3D space using only the associated image data. In minimally invasive surgery (MIS), visual odometry is an element of surgical vision that enables endoscope/laparoscope tracking without additional hardware such as optical or electromagnetic trackers [16]. Such tracking is crucial for image-guided surgery because the accuracy of camera tracking dominates the stability of applications such as registering a preoperative model to the surgical site [3] or building a mosaic for dynamic view expansion [17]. By using a visual odometry approach it is possible to overcome the hand-eye calibration and to reduce error propagation while simplifying clinical translation.

D. Stoyanov et al. (Eds.): IPCAI 2014, LNCS 8498, pp. 11–20, 2014.
© Springer International Publishing Switzerland 2014

Camera tracking based on photometrics in endoscopic scenes is difficult because of the homogeneous appearance of certain tissues, tissue deformation and severe specularities caused by the strong illumination intensity. Previous works have adopted a sparse feature based simultaneous localisation and mapping (SLAM) approach to stereo laparoscope tracking [6,11]. In such systems, salient features build a long-term map in order to globally correct for camera drift, but however they are severely affected by large highlights and lack of scene rigidity. Recent dense approaches have shown promising results where the camera tracking benefits from using the entire image data resulting in a very robust motion estimation even without bundle adjustment in a texture-poor or occluded scene [5,12].

In this paper, we propose a dense approach for real-time stereo laparoscope tracking. Our method uses a combination of stereo reconstruction, which is effective at recovering snapshots of the surgical site geometry [9], and quadrifocal tracking. Benefiting from recent GPU technology and parallelisable optimisation algorithms, the proposed dense visual odometry can reach real-time performance. We validate the proposed approach by a ground truth study using a photo realistic surgical scene rendition. We also demonstrate the robustness of the tracking on a real phantom video as well as *in vivo* clinical MIS sequences.

2 Method

The proposed system for dense stereo visual odometry has two main components: 1) stereo reconstruction and 2) quadrifocal tracking. The first reconstruction step is crucial because it initialises point correspondences for the later quadrifocal warping. Importantly both components rely purely on photometric information.

2.1 Preliminaries

Consider an image function $\mathbf{I}(\mathbf{p}) : \Omega_I \to \mathbb{R}$ where the $\mathbf{p} = (u, v)$ is the pixel location in the domain $\Omega_I \subseteq \mathbb{R}^2$. In the rectified stereo geometry, point $\mathbf{p}_l$ in the left image has its correspondence $\mathbf{p}_r = (u - \mathbf{d}(\mathbf{p}_l), v)$ in the right image found by the disparity function $\mathbf{d} : \Omega_I \to \mathbb{R}_\mathbf{d}$, where $\mathbb{R}_\mathbf{d}$ is the range of the disparity in subpixel accuracy.

To represent variables in the two-view stereo, it is convenient to consider the set of image measurements in a vector form such that $\mathcal{I} = (\mathbf{I}_l, \mathbf{I}_r)^\top$ is a vector of stacked intensity values. The stereo disparity can be represented in a similar way, i.e., $\mathcal{D} = (\mathbf{d}_l, \mathbf{d}_r)^\top$ which also implicitly defines the correspondence set $\mathcal{P}$.

2.2 Dense Stereo Reconstruction

The task of stereo reconstruction is to optimise the disparity function $\mathbf{d}$ in order to establish point correspondence $\mathcal{P}$ across the stereo pair. We exploit the recent real-time stereo reconstruction algorithm [4], which optimises a variational energy function with respect to $\mathbf{d}$:

$$\mathring{\mathbf{d}} = \arg\min_{\mathbf{d}} E_r(\mathbf{d}), \quad \text{where}$$

$$E_r(\mathbf{d}) = \sum_{\mathbf{p} \in \Omega_I} \left\{ \|\gamma(\mathbf{p})\nabla\mathbf{d}(\mathbf{p})\|_\varepsilon + \lambda C(\mathbf{p}, \mathbf{d}(\mathbf{p})) \right\}. \tag{1}$$

The data term C is a 3D disparity cost-volume which is built up by zero-mean normalised cross-correlation (ZNCC) to save the photometric similarity between left and right pixels within the determined disparity range $\mathbb{R}_{\mathbf{d}}$.

The variational model is regularised by disparity gradient, which takes the assumption that the disparity shall be smooth in areas of homogeneous appearance. To preserve discontinuities, which usually occur along image edges, we adopt the anisotropic diffusion tensor for the weighting function:

$$\gamma(\mathbf{p}) = \exp(-\alpha|\nabla\mathbf{I}(\mathbf{p})|^\beta)nn^\top + n^\perp n^{\perp^\top},$$

where n is the normalised image gradient $n = \frac{\nabla\mathbf{I}(\mathbf{p})}{|\nabla\mathbf{I}(\mathbf{p})|}$ and $n^\perp$ its perpendicular vector and α and β define the weighting strength [18]. The effects of the data and the regularisation term are controlled by the λ.

The energy function is optimised by a GPU-implemented primal-dual algorithm which provides a linear convergence rate $O(1/N)$ [2]. The optimisation parameters are determined by preconditioning which significantly reduces the number of iterations to converge [13]. Note that the Eq. 1 is a first-order total generalized variation (TGV) model which is only able to reconstruct fronto-parallel structure [14]. However we have observed that instead of applying a rather expensive second-order TGV to reconstruct the affine structure, using the Huber-norm $\|\cdot\|_\varepsilon$ for the regulariser term is a good approximate to avoid the staircasing effect caused by L^1-norm, which is sufficient for reconstructing general endoscopic scenes.

2.3   Dense Stereo Camera Tracking

The camera motion $\mathbf{x}$ is minimally parameterised by $\mathfrak{se}(3)$ Lie algebra. Specifically the 6-vector $\mathbf{x} = (\nu, \omega) \in \mathbb{R}^6$ consists of $\nu \in \mathbb{R}^3$ for the linear velocity and $\omega \in \mathbb{R}^3$ for the angular velocity of the motion. The smooth and invertible rigid-body transformation $\mathbf{T} \in \mathbb{SE}(3)$ based on the 6-vector can be obtained by the exponential map of $g(\mathbf{x})$:

$$\mathbf{T}(\mathbf{x}) = \exp(g(\mathbf{x})) = \begin{pmatrix} \mathbf{R} & \mathbf{t} \\ \mathbf{0} & 1 \end{pmatrix} \in \mathbb{R}^{4\times4},$$

where $\mathbf{R} \in \mathbb{SO}(3)$ and $\mathbf{t} \in \mathbb{R}^3$. Details of the $\mathbb{SE}(3)$ Lie group and its generator function g can be found in [15].

Given a reference frame pair $\mathcal{I}^*$ and the reconstructed disparity $\mathcal{D}$, we can track the camera by continuously registering the current frame pair $\mathcal{I}$ with the reference pair using a generative model called quadrifocal warping $w(\boldsymbol{\mathcal{P}}^*, \mathbf{T}_{rl}, \mathbf{K}_l, \mathbf{K}_r; \mathring{\mathbf{T}})$. The $\mathring{\mathbf{T}} \in \mathbb{SE}(3)$ is the current pose with respect to the reference one in camera coordinate. We assume that the stereo laparoscope is calibrated in advance and the intrinsic matrices $\mathbf{K}_l$, $\mathbf{K}_r$ and the extrinsic matrix $\mathbf{T}_{rl}$ are constant.

The registration warping with respect to the camera motion $\mathbf{x}$ can be obtained by optimising the photometric energy function:

$$\mathring{\mathbf{x}} = \arg\min_{\mathbf{x}} E_t(\mathbf{x}), \quad \text{where}$$

$$E_t(\mathbf{x}) = \sum_{\boldsymbol{\mathcal{P}}^* \in \boldsymbol{\mathcal{R}}^*} \left(\boldsymbol{\mathcal{I}}\big(w(\boldsymbol{\mathcal{P}}^*; \mathbf{T}(\mathbf{x})\hat{\mathbf{T}})\big) - \boldsymbol{\mathcal{I}}^*(\boldsymbol{\mathcal{P}}^*) \right)^2. \tag{2}$$

All the corresponding pixels from the reference frame pair form the set $\boldsymbol{\mathcal{R}}^* = \{\{\mathbf{p}_l^*, \mathbf{p}_r^*\}_1, \{\mathbf{p}_l^*, \mathbf{p}_r^*\}_2, \dots, \{\mathbf{p}_l^*, \mathbf{p}_r^*\}_n\}$ which mutually includes the left and right matching pair with in total n number of correspondences used for tracking. The optimisation incrementally updates the warping motion $\hat{\mathbf{T}} \leftarrow \mathbf{T}(\mathbf{x})\hat{\mathbf{T}}$ toward the minimum. It is assumed that the truth motion parameter $\mathbf{x}$ exists so that $\exists \mathring{\mathbf{x}} : \mathbf{T}(\mathring{\mathbf{x}})\hat{\mathbf{T}} = \mathring{\mathbf{T}}$.

Quadrifocal Geometry. To maximally exploit the stereo image data for tracking, the quadrifocal geometry is a constraint for associating geometric entities across the four views. However, instead of adopting the rather complicated quadrifocal tensor, two trifocal tensors are decoupled from the four-view in order to bring the quadrifocal geometry constraint into the optimisation [5]. Fig. 1 shows an example of the trifocal geometry for the left view. Note that we will elaborate only the left trifocal tensor, and the right one is exactly its inverse.

A trifocal tensor $\mathcal{T} = [\mathcal{T}_1(\mathbf{x}), \mathcal{T}_2(\mathbf{x}), \mathcal{T}_3(\mathbf{x})]$ is a $3 \times 3 \times 3$ matrix. Each slice in the tensor is defined by $\mathcal{T}_j = \mathbf{a}_j \mathbf{b}_4^\top(\mathbf{x}) - \mathbf{a}_4 \mathbf{b}_j^\top(\mathbf{x})$ where $\mathbf{a}_j$ are the columns of $\mathbf{T}_{rl}$ and $\mathbf{b}_j(\mathbf{x})$ are the columns of the motion matrix $\mathbf{T}(\mathbf{x})$. We use the point-line-point configuration in which the correspondent line $\mathbf{l}_r = (-1, -1, u+v)$ with each of the three tensor slices form the columns of a homography matrix:

$$\mathcal{H}(\mathbf{x}) = [\mathcal{H}_1(\mathbf{x}), \mathcal{H}_2(\mathbf{x}), \mathcal{H}_3(\mathbf{x})] \quad \text{and} \quad \mathcal{H}_j(\mathbf{x}) = \mathcal{T}_j^\top(\mathbf{x})\mathbf{K}_r^{-1}\mathbf{l}_r.$$

The corresponding point $\mathbf{p}_l$ in the current image can be simply obtained by the homography transformation of the reference point $\mathbf{p}_l^*$. We can now define the warping function in Eq. 2 for each correspondence as:

$$w(\mathbf{p}_l^*; \mathbf{x}) = \pi\left(\mathbf{K}_l \mathcal{H}(\mathbf{x})\mathbf{K}_l^{-1} \begin{bmatrix} \mathbf{p}_l^* \\ 1 \end{bmatrix} \right), \tag{3}$$

where π is the dehomogenisation function projecting a point to its image coordinate.

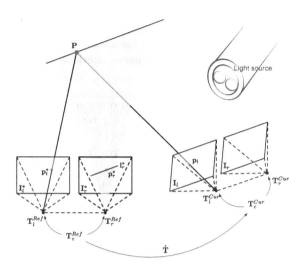

Fig. 1. Point-line-point trifocal geometry: The point $\mathbf{p}_l^*$ in the left reference frame is transformed to the point $\mathbf{p}_l$ in the left current frame using the homography formed by back-projecting the corresponding line $\mathbf{l}_r^*$, which defines an incidence relation $\mathbf{p}_l^* \leftrightarrow \mathbf{l}_r^* \leftrightarrow \mathbf{p}_l$

Note that the incremental update motion $\mathbf{T}(\mathbf{x})$ is applied to the centralised pose $\mathbf{T}_c$ at the middle of the stereo-rig baseline as shown in Fig. 1. This establishes a canonical coordinate for the stereo geometry, in which the left and right camera poses can be obtained via:

$$\mathbf{T}_c = \exp^{\log(\mathbf{T}_{rl})/2}, \quad \mathbf{T}_l = \mathbf{T}_c^{-1} \quad \text{and} \quad \mathbf{T}_r = \mathbf{T}_c \mathbf{T}_{rl}^{-1}. \tag{4}$$

Robust Tracking. The original energy function in Eq. 2 is the standard least-square method which assumes the residuals have a zero-mean Gaussian distribution. However, the residual distribution is usually not Gaussian, especially when there are outliers appearing in the scene. For example, occluding objects which do not belong to the original reconstructed model, lighting changes or specularities will generate a considerable number of outliers.

We can instead reformulate Eq. 2 in terms of using a different norm $\rho(r)$. For a least-square norm, $\rho(r) = \frac{1}{2}r^2$:

$$E_{robust}(\mathbf{x}) = \sum_{\mathcal{P}^* \in \mathcal{R}^*} \rho\Big(\mathcal{I}\big(w(\mathcal{P}^*; \mathbf{T}(\mathbf{x})\hat{\mathbf{T}})\big) - \mathcal{I}^*(\mathcal{P}^*)\Big). \tag{5}$$

We use the non-convex Tukey M-estimator which essentially rejects outliers above the tuning threshold [19]. This results in very robust tracking even with the appearance of instruments occluding the endoscopic scene.

Rapid Motion. Because the Tukey norm is not a convex function, one cannot expect to find the true global minimum. Furthermore the linearization with respect to the parameters $\mathfrak{se}(3)$ only holds for small camera motions. To make the method more robust towards rapid camera motions we adopt a common coarse-to-fine scheme.

Optimisation. We adopt the efficient second-order minimisation (ESM) algorithm for optimising Eq. 5. ESM is mainly the combination of a forward and an inverse compositional algorithm, which can avoid local minima and takes fewer iterations to converge [10]. The optimisation of quadrifocal warping can be easily framed using ESM due to the fact that the warping is simply two homography transformations in which the warped current image pair and the reference image pair have a linear relationship. Dense tracking by warping a 2.5D surface projection image has no such property and can only use the first-order forward compositional algorithm [1, 12].

The ESM optimisation for solving Eq. 5 is performed with an iteratively reweighted least squares (IRLS) scheme, which will require three Jacobians: $\mathbf{J}_{\mathcal{I}^*}$, $\mathbf{J}_{\mathcal{I}}$ and $\mathbf{J}_w$, the Jacobians of the reference image, the current image and the warping function (Eq. 3) respectively. It can be shown that the overall approximate second-order Jacobian can be derived as:

$$\mathcal{J} = \frac{(\mathbf{J}_{\mathcal{I}} + \mathbf{J}_{\mathcal{I}^*})}{2}\mathbf{J}_w. \tag{6}$$

Derivations of these Jacobians can be found in [5]. Using the common normal equation solver with IRLS, the update parameter $\mathbf{x}$ can be obtained by :

$$\mathbf{x} = -(\mathbf{W}\mathcal{J})^+\mathbf{W}(\mathcal{I} - \mathcal{I}^*), \tag{7}$$

where the $\mathbf{W}$ is the diagonal weighting matrix determined by the Tukey M-estimator and $(\cdot)^+$ is the pseudo-inverse operator.

2.4   Reference Frame Selection

The proposed dense stereo visual odometry has the advantage that the reconstruction can be done any time to provide a dense model for the quadrifocal tracking without the need of a bootstrapper. However, reconstructing a model for every frame is unnecessary and in fact frame-to-frame tracking is susceptible to drift. To constrain tracking and prevent drift, we adopt frame-to-model tracking which is essentially the same concept as the keyframe strategy in visual SLAM systems [8, 12].

Whether a subsequent stereo frame pair is selected as the reference frame is based on two criteria: 1) if the overlay between the warping image and the reference image is below a threshold; 2) if the root-mean-square error of Eq. 5 is larger than a threshold. The first criterion occurs when the scope explores a sufficiently large area of the scene, so that there is not enough of the previous reference model in view. The second criterion can also be associated with insufficient overlap one but it is additionally useful that when the scene is invaded by other objects and we have to immediately reconstruct a new reference model for tracking.

3   Empirical Studies

The system is implemented in C/C++ and CUDA running on a Nvidia GeForce GTX 670 with 2GB GPU memory. The real video sequences are acquired from da Vanci robot's stereo endoscopy with size 720×576 and downsampled to 360×288. The stereo reconstruction for two frames takes about 100ms and the tracking for per subsequent stereo pair takes about 40ms.

3.1   Sythetic Ground Truth Study

In order to have a ground truth dataset, we use POV-Ray for realistic rendering for a bladder and a pelvis phantom model. The luminance is intentionally set as using a point light source and materials with strong specularity to simulate the real surgical scene where the only light source is at the middle of the endoscopy cameras as shown in Fig. 1. Fig. 2a shows a realistically rendered stereo frames. Following the same methodology in [7], we use the proposed approach to track a real phantom model using the da Vinci robotic platform as shown in Fig. 3b to generate a realistic camera motion. We then use this camera trajectory to render the ground truth sequence. The ground truth trajectory is shown in Fig. 2c.

The first frame is used as the reference frame for tracking the rest. The methodology for the validation is to add white noise to the reference model with different standard deviation and observe how this will affect the tracking. Fig. 2b shows the tracking errors along the x-axis under different level of white noise. It reveals several important results. Firstly, as the green curve shows, tracking with a perfect model gives almost no drift but in practice a perfect reconstruction is never achievable. The blue curve is closer to the real situation where we have a decent reconstruction but not perfect. Due to using the imperfect model, the camera drifts about 0.5mm after tracking for 100 frames. The cyan curve shows that with a very bad reconstructed model, the tracking can still work but with a significant drift.

3.2   Real Sequences

To validate the proposed approach on real data, we use a phantom and a clinical endoscopy sequence to conduct a qualitative evaluation. The phantom is an anatomical pelvis and prostate model from Educational and Scientific Products Limited with added surrounding tissue features made from coloured silicone and outer areas filled with polyeurathane expanding foam to avoid unrealistic sharp edges as shown in Fig. 3a. Fig. 3c shows the reconstructed disparity map of the

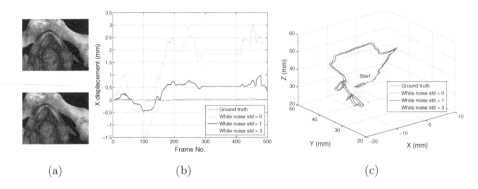

(a)   (b)   (c)

Fig. 2. The ground truth study. (a) The realistically rendered stereo frames with a pelvis and bladder models. (b) The displacement of the tracked x-translation away from the ground truth. (c) The trajectories. The figures are best viewed on screen with colour and zoomed in.

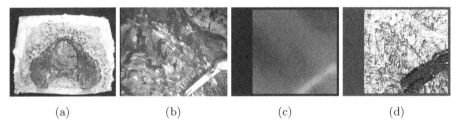

(a)   (b)   (c)   (d)

Fig. 3. (a) The painted plastic phantom. (b) A viewport from the da Vanci robot's endoscopy. (c) The reconstructed disparity map used for quadrifocal tracking. (d) The Tukey M-estimator weighting image where the blue pixels are rejected and gray pixels from black to white corresponds to the weight value from 0.1 to 1.0.

Fig. 3b where the depth discontinuity around the instrument is preserved. With this well-reconstructed model, when the instrument starts to move, the robust estimator assigns low weight for the tracked pixels which do not belong to the model or even completely rejects them, as shown in Fig. 3d.

The proposed dense approach can be applied to a variety of applications. We demonstrate augmented reality (AR) using the reconstructed dense model. As shown in Fig. 4a, we can draw text on the dense model and maintain their position on the surface. Note that this is not possible for sparse feature approach in which there is no a dense geometry to be drawn on. This method could be useful as it allows surgeons to tag AR annotation in the endoscopic scenes. Fig. 4b shows another application where we augment the preoperative models into the endoscopic scene.

Another useful function of the robust tracking using a dense model is to detect occlusions. As shown in Fig. 4c and Fig. 4d, the dense reference model provides a strong prior to reject the occluding instrument which is judged directly by

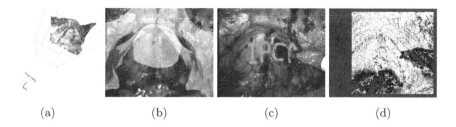

(a)   (b)   (c)   (d)

Fig. 4. (a) Text drawn on the 3D dense reconstructed model. (b) Preoperative models augmented into the *in vivo* endoscopic scene. (c) An example for occlusion detection. (d) The Tukey weights of (c) showing that the pixels from the invading instrument together with the specularities are mostly rejected.

Tukey's weight. When a new reference model is added, the occlusion can be also detected by comparing the depths between the tagged markers and the new model. Note that in Fig. 4d, those specularities are also rejected for the quadrifocal tracking. The tracking quality can be observed in the supplementary video[1].

4   Conclusions

In this paper, we proposed a dense visual odometry method for tracking the motion of the stereo laparoscope in MIS by using quadrifocal constraints. The dense approach has been shown to achieve promising results for synthetic, phantom and clinical data even in sequences with instruments occluding the surgical site. Promising applications of the proposed technique include image-guided surgery with AR overlay onto the laparoscopic images. In our future work we will focus on building a fully dense SLAM system with keyframes refined by pose graph optimisation to accurately maintain a global map while efficiently selecting known keyframes for tracking.

References

1. Baker, S., Patil, R., Cheung, K.M., Matthews, I.: Lucas-kanade 20 years on: Part 5. Tech. Rep. CMU-RI-TR-04-64, Robotics Institute (2004) 16
2. Chambolle, A., Pock, T.: A first-order primal-dual algorithm for convex problems with applications to imaging. Journal of Mathematical Imaging and Vision (JMIV) 40(1), 120–145 (2011) 13
3. Chang, P.-L., Chen, D., Cohen, D., Edwards, P.'.: 2D/3D registration of a preoperative model with endoscopic video using colour-consistency. In: Linte, C.A., Moore, J.T., Chen, E.C.S., Holmes III, D.R. (eds.) AE-CAI 2011. LNCS, vol. 7264, pp. 1–12. Springer, Heidelberg (2012) 11

---

[1] http://www.doc.ic.ac.uk/~pc3509

4. Chang, P.L., Stoyanov, D., Davison, A.J., Edwards, P.E.: Real-time dense stereo reconstruction using convex optimisation with a cost-volume for image-guided robotic surgery. In: Mori, K., Sakuma, I., Sato, Y., Barillot, C., Navab, N. (eds.) MICCAI 2013, Part I. LNCS, vol. 8149, pp. 42–49. Springer, Heidelberg (2013) 12

5. Comport, A., Malis, E., Rives, P.: Real-time quadrifocal visual odometry. The International Journal of Robotics 29(2-3), 245–266 (2010) 12, 14, 16

6. Grasa, O., Civera, J., Montiel, J.M.M.: EKF monocular SLAM with relocalization for laparoscopic sequences. In: IEEE International Conference on Robotics and Automation (ICRA), pp. 4816–4821 (2011) 12

7. Handa, A., Newcombe, R.A., Angeli, A., Davison, A.J.: Real-time camera tracking: When is high frame-rate best? In: Fitzgibbon, A., Lazebnik, S., Perona, P., Sato, Y., Schmid, C. (eds.) ECCV 2012, Part VII. LNCS, vol. 7578, pp. 222–235. Springer, Heidelberg (2012) 17

8. Klein, G., Murray, D.: Parallel tracking and mapping for small AR workspaces. In: IEEE International Symposium on Mixed and Augmented Reality (ISMAR), pp. 225–234 (2007) 16

9. Maier-Hein, L., Mountney, P., Bartoli, A., Elhawary, H., Elson, D., Groch, A., Kolb, A., Rodrigues, M., Sorger, J., Speidel, S., Stoyanov, D.: Optical techniques for 3D surface reconstruction in computer-assisted laparoscopic surgery. Medical Image Analysis (MedIA) 17(8), 974–996 (2013) 12

10. Malis, E.: Improving vision-based control using efficient second-order minimization techniques. IEEE International Conference on Robotics and Automation (ICRA) 2, 1843–1848 (2004) 16

11. Mountney, P., Stoyanov, D., Davison, A.J., Yang, G.Z.: Simultaneous stereoscope localization and soft-tissue mapping for minimal invasive surgery. In: Larsen, R., Nielsen, M., Sporring, J. (eds.) MICCAI 2006. LNCS, vol. 4190, pp. 347–354. Springer, Heidelberg (2006) 12

12. Newcombe, R.A., Lovegrove, S.J., Davison, A.J.: DTAM: Dense tracking and mapping in real-time. In: IEEE International Conference on Computer Vision (ICCV), vol. 1, pp. 2320–2327 (2011) 12, 16

13. Pock, T., Chambolle, A.: Diagonal preconditioning for first order primal-dual algorithms in convex optimization. In: IEEE International Conference on Computer Vision (ICCV), pp. 1762–1769 (2011) 13

14. Ranftl, R., Pock, T., Bischof, H.: Minimizing TGV-based variational models with non-convex data terms. In: Pack, T. (ed.) SSVM 2013. LNCS, vol. 7893, pp. 282–293. Springer, Heidelberg (2013) 13

15. Stillwell, J.: Naive Lie Theory. Springer (2008) 13

16. Stoyanov, D.: Stereoscopic scene flow for robotic assisted minimally invasive surgery. In: Ayache, N., Delingette, H., Golland, P., Mori, K. (eds.) MICCAI 2012, Part I. LNCS, vol. 7510, pp. 479–486. Springer, Heidelberg (2012) 11

17. Totz, J., Mountney, P., Stoyanov, D., Yang, G.-Z.: Dense surface reconstruction for enhanced navigation in MIS. In: Fichtinger, G., Martel, A., Peters, T. (eds.) MICCAI 2011, Part I. LNCS, vol. 6891, pp. 89–96. Springer, Heidelberg (2011) 11

18. Werlberger, M., Trobin, W., Pock, T., Wedel, A., Cremers, D., Bischof, H.: Anisotropic Huber-L1 Optical Flow. In: British Machine Vision Conference (BMVC), pp. 108.1–108.11 (2009) 13

19. Zhang, Z.: Parameter estimation techniques: A tutorial with application to conic fitting. Image and Vision Computing 15, 59–76 (1997) 15

Comparative Assessment of a Novel Optical Human-Machine Interface for Laparoscopic Telesurgery

Fabien Despinoy[1,2,3], Alonso Sánchez[1], Nabil Zemiti[1],
Pierre Jannin[2,3], and Philippe Poignet[1]

[1] LIRMM - CNRS, UMR 5506, Université Montpellier 2,
Montpellier, F-34000, France
{despinoy,sanchezsec,zemiti,poignet}@lirmm.fr
[2] LTSI, Université de Rennes 1, Rennes, F-35000, France
[3] INSERM, UMR 1099, Rennes, F-35000, France
pierre.jannin@univ-rennes1.fr

Abstract. This paper introduces a novel type of human-machine interface for laparoscopic telesurgery that employs an optical sensor. A Raven-II laparascopic robot (Applied Dexterity Inc) was teleoperated using two different human-machine interfaces, namely the Sigma 7 electro-mechanical device (Force Dimension Sarl) and the Leap Motion (Leap Motion Inc) infrared stereoscopic camera. Based on this hardware platform, a comparative study of both systems was performed through objective and subjective metrics, which were obtained from a population of 10 subjects. The participants were asked to perform a peg transferring task and to answer a questionnaire. Obtained results allow to confirm that fine tracking of the hand could be performed with the Leap Motion sensor. Such tracking comprises accurate finger motion acquisition to control the robot's laparoscopic instrument jaws. Furthermore, the observed performance of the optical interface proved to be comparable to that of traditional electro-mechanical devices, such as the Sigma 7, during adequate execution of highly-dexterous laparascopic gestures.

Keywords: Infrared stereoscopic camera, human-machine interface, teleoperation, laparoscopic surgery, hand tracking.

1 Introduction

During the last three decades, the field of laparoscopic surgery was constantly subject to technological advances looking to offer better healthcare in terms of safety, patient outcome, medical staff coordination and comfort [1]. Among these advances, the appearance of telesurgical systems represents a major breakthrough. Teleoperated systems enabled surgeons to interact with a distant environment, while providing them with a sense of immersion within the remote environment. To that end, high-resolution endoscopic cameras and intuitive human-machine interfaces (HMIs) for controlling the robotized laparoscopic tools have been developed. Moreover, it is well-known that telesurgical systems allow further performance improvements for surgeons by scaling down the hand motions (i.e. to

D. Stoyanov et al. (Eds.): IPCAI 2014, LNCS 8498, pp. 21–30, 2014.

perform more accurate gestures), filtering involuntary hand tremor and offering, in some cases, force-feedback information [2]. However, the lack of cost-effective, sterilizable, precise and repeatable force sensing solutions represents an open issue, which is clearly reflected in currently available commercial robotic systems such as the *Da Vinci*® surgical system (Intuitive Surgical Inc) or the *Raven-II* platform [3] [4].

The majority of master-slave systems used in telesurgery exchange kinematic information of the operator's hands (e.g. through the system's position and/or velocity channels) in order to define the control reference of the robotic end-effectors [5]. Hence, the HMIs that are used to recover kinematic information from the surgeon do have a direct impact on the overall robotic system performance. For that reason, some recent research focused on the development of novel HMIs to improve dexterity and ergonomy. In [6], for instance, the authors presented an analysis of an electro-mechanical HMI for minimally invasive surgery, which is based on ergonomic principles and on polls carried out within the surgical community. Their results suggested that surgeons' preferences are mainly driven by 2 factors: comfort and precision. Nevertheless, the proposed electro-mechanical HMI is unable of fully exploiting the capabilities of the surgeon's hands. For example, their workspace is limited in order to avoid collisions between the left and right hand devices, whereas a human operator is capable of highly-dexterous and accurate bi-manual surgical manipulations within the frontal region that is unexploited by conventional electro-mechanical HMIs (e.g. the Sigma 7 employed in this work, or the Omega 7 modified in [6]). Therefore, ergonomy and intuitiveness of today's HMIs might be further improved.

In this paper, we address the issue of validating the possibility of performing highly-dexterous and precise telesurgical tasks by means of an infrared stereoscopic camera, the Leap Motion. Furthermore, initial results on the novel possibilities that could be offered by such type of interfaces are also introduced through a comparative study with a high-performance commercial electro-mechanical HMI, the Sigma 7.

Previous works employing optical based sensors in the context of teleoperation can be found in the literature. In [7], the Kinect device (Microsoft Corp) was employed to track the user's upper limbs and to control two industrial robot arms to perform pick and place tasks. Thanks to the anthropomorphic configuration of the robot arms, the user can easily control their motion by using joint angle inputs without major kinematic issues. Similarly, [8] implemented tracking algorithms to segment and detect the hand's thumb and index fingers in order to control the robot end-effector. However, their algorithms were highly sensitive to optical occlusions, and also relied on the detection of the entire forearm. Finally, whether a surgical application is considered, these approaches would fail to accurately distinguish finger motions for fine control of the instrument tips. In consequence, it might be more suitable to state that [7] and [8] employed less accurate hand gesture recognition techniques (e.g. open hand and fist gestures) for control of the robotic end-effectors. Finally, in [9] the authors performed simultaneous tracking of both hands and fingers in a robust manner, accounting for possible optical occlusions by estimating two 26 degrees of freedom (DoFs) hand models and performing optimization to find an unique fitted solution based on Kinect sensor measurements. Nevertheless, one major issue of their work regards its considerable computational complexity due to the solution of a high-order optimization problem using stochastic algorithms. Indeed, time delay and synchronization are two key factors which affect the performance of the entire teleoperation system. Therefore, a simplified and less computationally expensive solution using a 7 DoF hand model is introduced in this paper for tracking of the hand within the context of laparoscopic surgery.

The remaining sections are structured as follows. Section 2 introduces the teleoperation platform with the two different HMIs that were compared. Section 3 describes the methods employed for evaluating the performance of the system and the obtained results are also presented and analyzed. Lastly, in section 4 concluding remarks and future works are discussed.

2   The Teleoperation Setup

In order to effectively compare the relative performance of both HMI technologies, the platform depicted in Figure 1 was employed. Such a scheme was proposed to isolate the influence of the HMIs by keeping constant the other hardware components (i.e master components and the slave robot system). For that reason, an unified HMI application programming interface (API), which allows quick exchange of the interfaces, was implemented by software wrapping of the corresponding device drivers. A footpedal was used in order to activate/deactivate teleoperation when required.

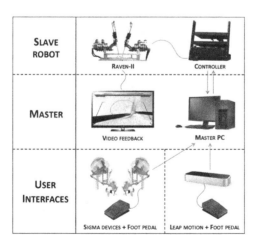

Fig. 1. Overall diagram of the teleoperation setup

In Figure 2, pictures of the actual slave side system components are provided, including the peg board used for laparoscopic task evaluation. The Raven-II robot comprises two robotic arms of 7 DoFs, in which the two distal DoFs are decoupled and allow independent movements of each grasping jaw. During the experiments with both HMIs, the same Cartesian position servoing software routines were employed at a control frequency of 1kHz.

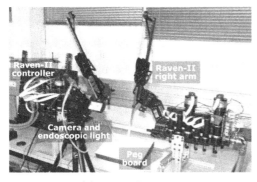 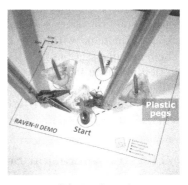

(a) Raven-II system   (b) Peg board

Fig. 2. Slave side hardware

Figure 3 depicts the main master side system components. Each of the Sigma devices has 7 active DoFs. A Cartesian position measurement accuracy of about 0.005 mm (including translation and grasping motions) is reported by the manufacturer. During tests, these devices were polled at a 1 kHz rate. Since the Sigma interfaces were disposed in order to avoid workspace overlapping of the left and right hands, no risk of collision between the HMIs exists.

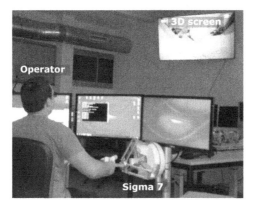

Fig. 3. Sigma 7 based master side hardware

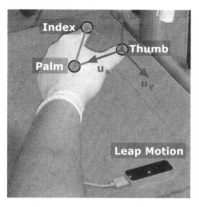 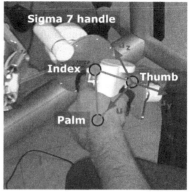

(a) Infrared stereoscopic camera   (b) Electro-mechanical device

Fig. 4. Hand model geometry shown for both HMIs

Regarding the Leap Motion HMI, visible in Figure 4(a), three infrared sensors coupled with an array of two cameras is used to create a depth map of the scene. The Leap Motion's Cartesian position measurement accuracy is about 0.01 mm, and the employed hand tracking refresh rate was ≈110 Hz. The API provided by the manufacturer allows tracking of hand palms and fingers, the latter being classified as pointy objects. Such device could also allow left and right hand workspaces overlapping without the associated risks of HMI collisions. Such possibility might be advantageous during some laparascopic tasks (e.g. intracorporeal knotting and peg or needle transfers from one hand to another), which could otherwise turn to be less comfortable and intuitive. Nonetheless, whether the hand workspaces intersect, particular care should be taken when optical hand occlusions arise. For that reason, a simple model consisting of three points (i.e. index finger, thumb finger and hand palm) was defined in order to allow robust model based tracking using a simple time-consistent Kalman filter. The model geometry is depicted in Figures 4(a) and (b).

Tremor filtering is applied in both HMIs through an autoregressive moving-average (ARMA) low-pass filter, having an attenuation of ≈25 dB at 2 Hz [10]. Finally, whenever hand tracking is lost, special care was taken in order to stop teleoperation (i.e. overriding the footpedal), while avoiding bumps when the tracking is recovered.

3   Performance Assessment of the HMIs

3.1   Methods

A population of ten researchers from the LIRMM Lab were enrolled in the comparative performance evaluation of the HMIs. A video was shown to each candidate in order to introduce the overall system functioning and the demanded peg transferring sequence. The latter sequence consisted in transferring some pegs directly from one pin to another, and takes into account guidelines provided by SAGES and FLS organizations [11]. The sequence is defined as follows:

1. Pick the first peg with the left tool and insert it in target 1 (leftmost pin of Fig. 2(b))
2. Pick the second peg with the right tool and insert it in target 2 (rightmost pin)
3. Pick the latest peg with the left or right tool, then advance towards the center of the peg board to grab it with the other available tool in order to finally insert it in target 3 (uppermost pin)

Each subject began the protocol with a randomly selected HMI and was allowed to freely use the device during 5 minutes, allowing him/her to test-drive the teleoperated system, familiarize with movements and hand coordination. During this test-drive, the participant was taught how the system works, about its possibilities and limitations (i.e. avoiding prolonged-time occlusions when using the Leap Motion or engaging teleoperation at the workspace limits of the Sigma 7). Subsequently, the candidates were asked to repeat the presented peg transferring sequence five times with each device. The last three trials were used for the statistical analysis. Finally, the subjects were asked to grade each HMI through multiple measurements.

3.2   Results

Recorded data were analyzed using the JMP 11 software (SAS Institute Inc). A one-way analysis of variance (ANOVA) was carried out by defining the HMI device as a fixed factor and the duration as the response variable. ANOVA relies on the variance analysis from multiple samples to determine their affiliation and whether a difference between mean durations exists, and thus, to accept or discredit H_0 *hypothesis*, which means that each device allows to perform the same task with the same duration time. Before performing ANOVA calculation, we ensured that data respect a normality function for an homogeneous repartition (i.e. χ^2 normality test).

Figure 5(a) depicts the average value and standard deviation of the total task completion time for all subject trials with each device. It is observed that the candidates were able to execute the task 13% faster in the case of the Sigma 7 device. ANOVA computation results are summarized in Figure 5(b), which shows the mean difference of duration times for each device. With a *p-value* of 0.0172, this analysis highlights that a significant difference between both devices can be confirmed, so that they can constitute two distinct populations. Nevertheless, even though a difference is confirmed, there is only a small gap between both devices (i.e. 14 seconds for a task requiring $\approx$1 min 50 secs).

Figure 6(a) shows the success rate of peg transfers. A fail was attributed to the operator whenever a peg was dropped before reaching the intended target. A higher success rate was observed in the case of the Leap Motion, signifying that,

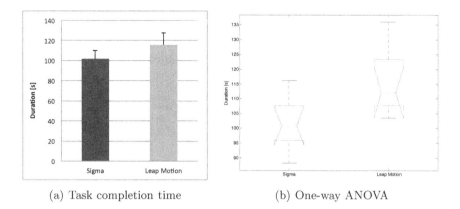

(a) Task completion time   (b) One-way ANOVA

Fig. 5. Duration of the pick and place task for all subjects and repetitions, with standard deviations for each HMI. The one-way ANOVA analysis shows the median, first and third quartiles and highlights the significant mean duration difference of the HMIs based on the variance of each population ($p\text{-}value = 0.0172$).

in spite of the slightly larger task completion times, the operators committed less mistakes with this device.

Similarly, the number of times the users had to clutch the teleoperation system through the footpedal was recorded (see "Clutching" column in Figure 6(b)). Subjects had to do this in order to reposition themselves for being able to carry on with the peg transferring task (e.g. hand tracking loss, reaching the workspace limits). It can be observed that better clutching results could be obtained with the Sigma 7 device, mainly due to the simple occlusions handling strategy that was implemented for the Leap Motion device. Consequently, operators were not able to properly detect the limit of the manipulation workspace, leading to a security lock and forced subjects to clutch in order to recover the hand tracking. Indeed, similar completion times, clutching and success rates can be obtained with both devices (see "Time", "Success" and "Clutching" columns in Figure 6(b)), whereas two additional metrics highlight a significant difference between the HMIs. On the one hand, the cost of each interface is taken into account (see "Cost" column in Figure 6(b)), in favor of the Leap Motion sensor. Even so, the high cost of the Sigma 7 interface is mainly explained by the force-feedback embedded technology which is not employed during the experimentations. Alternative positioning systems such as the *MicroScribe*® (Solution Technologies Inc) or the *Phantom Omni*® haptic device (Sensable, now part of Geomagic) can be taken on board for a more relevant comparison. Nevertheless, the Leap Motion device is still one of the cheaper interactive device present on the market. On the other hand, the sterilization capacity was compared (see "Sterilization" column in Figure 6(b)). This latter measurement refers to the possibility for the surgeon of preserving asepsis (i.e. hygiene without considering the certification requirements) during the whole duration of the procedure, so that he/she can directly operate in the patient, if required, without forced to change surgical gloves.

An upper grade was attributed to the Leap Motion device, since infrared light can easily traverse a thin film of plastic to prevent it from contaminating the sterile environment. In the case of the Sigma 7, a lower grade was attributed to the device, since the presented system is not certified to meet such requirement.

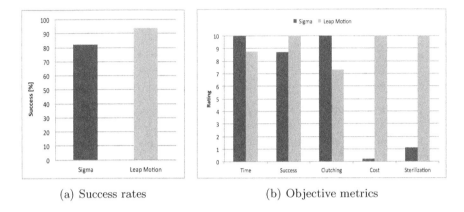

(a) Success rates　　　　　　　　　　(b) Objective metrics

Fig. 6. Success of the pick and place task for all subjects and repetitions. Evaluation of the system through five normalized objective metrics.

Figure 7 summarizes the results that were obtained after questioning each operator. It can be confirmed that the Sigma 7 device outperformed the Leap Motion in terms of perceived reactivity, precision, robustness and comfort. Nevertheless, in terms of intuitiveness, the operators were more satisfied with the contact-less optical device. It is also observed that important ameliorations in terms of robustness are imperative for future experimentations, including an accurate optical occlusion management.

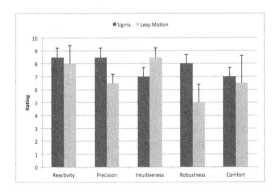

Fig. 7. Attributed grades, for each subjective factor, by all operators

4   Conclusions and Future Works

Considering the advantages and disadvantages of the Sigma 7 and the Leap Motion devices, together with their relative performance during the peg transferring task, our initial results suggest that infrared stereoscopic camera sensors have a promising potential for the development of cost-effective, sterilization compatible, more intuitive and accurate HMIs for laparoscopic telesurgery. Nonetheless, the obtained results also indicate that imperative development are required to improve the robustness of the hand tracking algorithms in the presence of optical occlusions.

Some design recommendations for next-generation HMIs could also be suggested from this first study. Report from experimentation highlights that the enlarged workspace and the freedom of bi-manual interactions between hands was appreciated by subjects. Furthermore, alternative solutions allowing force-reflecting teleoperation might be considered in the future, whether appropriate force sensing solutions for the medical field become available, through the development of wearable antagonistic tendon-like systems, exoskeletons, or through the application of model based electrical stimulation of the upper limbs.

Immediate future works mainly regard the development of a more robust model based hand tracking. Unfortunately, the API of the Leap Motion is closed by the device provider. Therefore, other specific sensors with open APIs, such as the Senz3D (Creative Labs Ltd, time-of-flight sensor), might be employed in the future. Additionally, a complementary study relying on trajectory analysis, from both master and slave sides, should be considered in order to enhance the interpretation of the results obtained during these experimentations.

Finally, other surgical tasks requiring higher accuracy, such as dissection of small targets, suturing and clip application should be studied, including expert and novice surgeon operators, in order to improve the statistical significance of our first results.

Acknowledgements. This work was partially supported by French state funds managed by the ANR within the Investissements d'Avenir programme (Labex CAMI) under reference ANR-11-LABX-0004.

References

1. Sanchez, A., Poignet, P., Dombre, E., Menciassi, A., Dario, P.: A design framework for surgical robots: example of the ARAKNES robot controller. Journal of Robotics and Autonomous Systems, Special issue on Intelligent Autonomous Systems; Lee, S., Lee, J.M., Menegatti, E. (eds.). Elseiver (2013) (in press)
2. Rosen, J., Hannaford, B., MacFarlane, M.P., Sinanan, M.N.: Force Controlled and Teleoperated Endoscopic Grasper for Minimally Invasive Surgery-Experimental Performance Evaluation. IEEE Transactions on Biomedical Engineering 46(10), 1212–1221 (1999)

3. Lum, M.J.H., Friedman, D.C.W., Sankaranarayanan, G., King, H., Fodero, K., Leuschke, R., Hannaford, B., Rosen, J., Sinanan, M.N.: The RAVEN: Design and Validation of a Telesurgery System. The International Journal of Robotics Research 28(9), 1183–1197 (2009)

4. Hannaford, B., Rosen, J., Friedman, D.W., King, H., Roan, P., Cheng, L., Glozman, D., Ma, J., Kosari, S.N., White, L.: Raven-II: An Open Platform for Surgical Robotics Research. IEEE Transactions on Biomedical Engineering 60(4), 954–959 (2013)

5. Lawrence, D.A.: Stability and transparency in bilateral teleoperation. IEEE Transactions on Robotics and Automation 9(5), 624–637 (1993)

6. Santos-Carreras, L., Hagen, M., Gassert, R., Bleuler, H.: Survey on Surgical Instrument Handle Design: Ergonomics and Acceptance. Journal of Surgical Innovation 19(1), 50–59 (2012)

7. Dragan, A.D., Srinivasa, S.S., Lee, K.C.T.: Teleoperation with Intelligent and Customizable Interfaces. Journal of Human-Robot Interaction 2(2), 33–57 (2013)

8. Du, G., Zhang, P., Mai, J., Li, Z.: Markerless Kinect-Based Hand Tracking for Robot Teleoperation. International Journal of Advanced Robotic Systems 9(1), 36–46 (2012)

9. Oikonomidis, I., Kyriazis, N., Argyros, A.A.: Tracking the Articulated Motion of Two Strongly Interacting Hands. In: IEEE Conference of Computer Vision and Pattern Recognition, pp. 1862–1869 (2012)

10. Bo, A.P.L., Poignet, P., Geny, C.: Pathological Tremor and Voluntary Motion Modeling and Online Estimation for Active Compensation. IEEE Transactions on Neural Systems and Rehabilitation Engineering 19(2), 177–185 (2011)

11. Derossis, A.M., Fried, G.M., Abrahamowicz, M., Sigman, H.H., Barkun, J.S., Meakins, J.L.: Development of a Model for Training and Evaluation of Laparoscopic Skills. The American Journal of Surgery 175(6), 482–487 (1998)

Modelling and Control of an ERF-Based Needle Insertion Training Platform

Adrián Graña, Alonso Sánchez, Nabil Zemiti, and Philippe Poignet

LIRMM - Lab., Montpellier, France
adri.gs@gmail.com, {sanchezsec,zemiti,poignet}@lirmm.fr

Abstract. In the medical field, there exists some surgical simulators and training platforms that have been developed for training novice surgeons in order to improve their surgical skills and for performing preoperative planning. In this paper we present a haptic platform for surgical needle insertion training gestures. It uses passive brakes based on Electro-Rheological (ER) fluids to provide a safe and realistic physical feedback to the physician. To achieve this objective, a prototype has been built, its kinematic model has been obtained and experimentally validated. The modelling, the bandwidth analysis and the force control scheme of the platform are also presented.

Keywords: Needle insertion, ERF, Force control, Haptic Feedback.

1 Introduction

Known the risks of letting inexperienced practitioners perform operations on actual patients, it was necessary to develop artificial training methods, which could emulate the conditions of a real operation as faithful as possible.

In the context of medical applications, many industries have created training platforms that would recreate certain parts of the human body, depending on the goal of the training, like the TraumaMan System [1] and the Arthrocentesis model [2], both by Simulab Corporation. Another type of training platforms are virtual platforms, which emulate the conditions of the operation as it were to be remotely performed, like the DV trainer by Mimic Technologies [3]. A major characteristic in training platforms is the feedback illusion given to the user, which has to be the closest possible to the reality.

The most common way of creating a feedback illusion is by using actuators such as electrical motors, working against the user's movements such as the Phantom from Geomagic [4] and the Omega Haptic device from Force Dimension [5].

Another way of giving a force feedback sensation is by using passive devices such as brakes, which impede the movement not by moving actively against it, but creating a passive physical resistance. Such devices do not create energy, so they do not have the stability problems which active devices suffer from, as discussed in [6] and in [7]. This decreases the stability, thus the safety issues related to the operator. These passive devices can be implemented using Magneto-Rheological and Electro-Rheological fluids.

D. Stoyanov et al. (Eds.): IPCAI 2014, LNCS 8498, pp. 31–40, 2014.

Magneto-Rheological Fluids (MRF) increase their apparent viscosity when subjected to a magnetic field, to the point of becoming a viscoelastic solid [8]. Their damping properties can be used to create a haptic illusion, like the proposal of a "Smart Mouse" by K. H. Kim *et al* [9], where a haptic hand master intended to display force feedback at the fingertip of the human user is proposed. The authors in [10] showed also the possibility of directly using a MRF to simulate the behavior of soft tissues in cutting operations, by developing a haptic interface which combines the MRF properties with a moving table.

Electro-Rheological Fluids (ERF), on the other hand, increase their apparent viscosity in the presence of an electrical field [11]. The capacity of ER fluids in increasing or diminishing their shear rate in very short periods of time (under 1 ms) allowed to use them in applications which require a quick response and high dynamics, such as joint damping and, in general, mechatronic devices [12]. In the medical context, ERF-based devices should be thus the suitable candidate to replicate the dynamics of the needle insertion interaction force through soft tissue.

An example of using ERF in the medical context is the Robotic Hand Rehabilitation System presented in [13], which facilitates repetitive performance of low dynamics task specific exercises for patients recovering from neurological motor deficits. Another example is the work presented in [14] where a 4DoF ERF-based haptic interface for teleoperating a slave robot in the context of minimally invasive surgery (MIS) have been developed. The proposed solution can generate a repulsive force/torque with the 4DoF motion.

In the context of surgical training platforms regarding haptic feedback, a needle insertion simulator is proposed in this paper. It features ERF brakes capable of changing its physical resistance in a one DoF motion, to simulate the different tissue behaviors against the movement of a surgical needle without feeling the mechanical impedance of the haptic interface.

In the medical field, there exist some surgical simulators and training platforms that have been developed. However, at this moment and to our knowledge, there exists neither haptic device dedicated to surgical simulations nor needle insertion training platform based on ERF solution. Indeed, all what have been described in the literature regarding needle insertion simulators concerns only the modeling of the needle tissues interaction and all the proposed needle insertion simulators use conventional and commercially available motor based haptic devices [15], [16], [7].

In this work, the ERF based solution has been preferred to homemade or commercially available motor based haptic device since, compared to motor based solutions, ERF based solutions are passive thus stable and safe, reversible, low cost, compact and lightweight, and they can offer a negligible mechanical impedance compared to motor based solutions (even more if geared motors are used).

The proposed study includes a built of a prototype, its mathematical model, parameter estimation, and a PI force control test. These are preliminary tests on this platform to validate the concept and viability of such a device.

2 Design of a Force Simulator Using ERF

The purpose of the platform is to simulate the physical resistance of several tissues against the movement of a surgical needle. The ERF would, thus, change its viscosity as the user moves the knob of the manipulator, giving the mentioned force-feedback. When performing a needle insertion, there are significant experience differences depending on the part of the body where it is performed. Moreover, the tissues' characteristics are different from one patient to another, adding a problem of patient dependance. So, instead of building a physical polymer-based platform for training in each case, it can be easier to have a cheaper, programmable device which can emulate several scenarios, such as inserting a needle through different stiffness tissue layers, which can be easily programmed.

2.1 Prototype Description

This project's object of study is a prototype-state platform which has been developed to study the phenomena and validate the concept of a haptic-feedback simulator for needle insertion. It is based on the Couette flow problem in fluids mechanics. In this problem, a plate is moving above a static surface, with a fluid between them. The shear stress is maximal at the moving plate, and zero at the stationary plate, and depends on the viscosity of the fluid. The main idea is to dynamically modify the fluid's viscosity, so the shear stress is, as well, modified. Thus, the necessary force to move the plate can be dynamically changed using a smart fluid.

The moving plate is a 53x53x1.5 millimeter copper plate, with a soldered electrode and four holes for its attachment to a same-size plastic plate. This plastic plate is mounted to a rounded-bearing profile rail guide to ensure minimum friction. The static plate is a 243x196x1.5 millimeter copper plate, also with a soldered electrode, but mounted inside an open plastic box, to store the fluid and

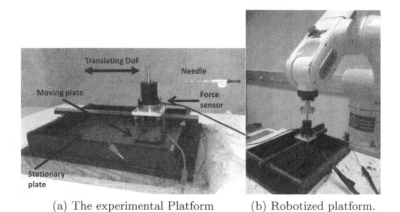

(a) The experimental Platform   (b) Robotized platform.

Fig. 1. Experimental platform

ensure electrical isolation. This box is 30 mm high. The montage allows to select different gap values, by loosening and tightening the threadless screws which connect the small plates. This gap has been experimentally fixed to $1.6mm$ to avoid the apparition of electrical arc and to optimize the time response of the system. During the experiments, the overall platform is kept horizontally and the moving plate is fully immersed within the fluid (see Fig. 1).

The effect of pushing on the copper plate in addition to the friction between the copper plate and the fluid and to the friction at the level of the bearing transmission are felt by the operator. However, the mechanical impedance of the device remains almost transparent to the user and offers 0.2N measured force while no actuation is performed.

2.2   Mathematical Model

The procedure which will be used here to evaluate the parameters and equations of the platform is inspired by the one used in [11] where a rotary knob that dynamically changes its physical resistance using an ERF actuator was studied.

As it was discussed before, the platform works according to the Couette Flow problem, using an ER fluid which behaves under a non-Newtonian model known as Bingham model. Although there are other models which can predict the behavior of these kind of fluids, the Bingham is the most used in these kind of applications, given its linearity and simplicity, according to the literature ([11],[17],[12]). In order to perform a further control of the platform, it is necessary to obtain the relation between the force output F and the voltage input V, starting with the equation which states the relation between the force and the shear stress τ of the Couette flow problem. Force equals to the double integral of the shear stress on a rectangular plate whose sides are a and b. In this particular case, a square plate of area A:

$$F = \iint \tau \cdot db \cdot da = \int_A \tau \cdot dA \qquad (1)$$

The shear stress, τ, in eq.1 can be replaced with the corresponding equation of the Bingham Model,

$$\tau = \mu \cdot \dot{\gamma} + \tau_{y,d} \qquad (2)$$

where the shear rate $\dot{\gamma}$ is a function of the speed of the sliding plate, $\frac{dx}{dt}$, and the gap, h, between both plates.

$$\dot{\gamma} = \frac{dx}{dt} \cdot \frac{1}{h} \qquad (3)$$

Also, the documentation of the commercial fluid used in this project states that both terms $\tau_{y,d}$ (dynamic yield stress) and μ (plastic viscosity) are functions of the squared value of the electrical field applied, E, and two constants, Cd and Cv, [18].

$$\tau_{y,d} = Cd \cdot E^2 \qquad (4)$$

$$\mu = \mu_0 - Cv \cdot E^2 \tag{5}$$

where μ_0 is the zero field viscosity.

The combination of equations 1 to 5 leads to the relationship between force and electrical field applied:

$$F = \int_A [(\mu_0 - Cv \cdot E^2) \cdot \frac{dx}{dt} \cdot \frac{1}{h} + Cd \cdot E^2] \cdot dA \tag{6}$$

As the relationship between the applied field, E, the voltage output of a high voltage source, and the gap between the two plates is $E = \frac{V}{h}$, the final equation of the platform is, after replacing and integrating:

$$F = [(\mu_0 - Cv \cdot \frac{V^2}{h^2}) \cdot \frac{dx}{dt} \cdot \frac{1}{h} + Cd \cdot \frac{V^2}{h^2}] \cdot A \tag{7}$$

To evaluate those parameters more easily, the equation will be modified to be expressed as a combination of three scalar constants, so the final model can be written as:

$$F = (a_0 - a_1 \cdot \frac{dx}{dt}) \cdot V^2 + a_2 \cdot \frac{dx}{dt} \tag{8}$$

where $a_i, i\epsilon \{1, 2, 3\}$ are constant positive scalars given by:

$$\begin{cases} i = 0 & a_0 = \frac{A \cdot Cd}{h^2} \\ i = 1 & a_1 = \frac{A \cdot Cv}{h^3} \\ i = 2 & a_2 = \frac{A \cdot \mu_0}{h} \end{cases} \tag{9}$$

Also, the inverse model of the system, needed for control, is obtained writing the value of the voltage as a function of the rest of the parameters:

$$V = h \cdot \sqrt{\frac{\frac{F}{A} - \frac{\mu_0}{h} \cdot \frac{dx}{dt}}{Cd - \frac{Cv}{h} \cdot \frac{dx}{dt}}} \tag{10}$$

It is necessary, then, to obtain the parameters which lead to the direct and inverse model of the platform to perform a control, with desired force as input, to obtain it as output.

2.3   Prototype Testing and Parameter Estimation

In order to evaluate the mathematical model and estimate the values of the parameters, an experimental setup was built. The goal is to measure the force when applying an increasing electrical field to the platform, with the plate moving at a desired speed. To do so, a six-axis Viper s650 articulated robot designed for assembly applications was chosen. An ATI Nano43 force sensor was attached to the upper platform to measure the interaction force, and the robot arm attached to it (see Fig. 1b). Although the final objective is to manually operate the simulator, a robot-controlled experimentation was chosen over manually-controlled in order to guarantee the repeatability of the experiment and the soundness of the results and their analysis. To create the needed electrical field, an EMCO C80R DC/DC High Voltage converter was used. The ERF used was the Smart Technologies LID 3354S, made up of polymer particles in a non density matched silicone based oil [18] (for more information, see www.smarttec.co.uk). The parameters of the liquid, such as dynamic yield stress, plastic viscosity and density are provided by the developer and are ambient temperature dependent. However, to our knowledge, there is no study in the literature that has shown that the ER fluid heated up over time and through continuous use. Consequently, it is necessary to run identification experiments in order to obtain, with the greatest accuracy, the real parameters of the platform and of the fluid, which may differ from the ones given in the literature. The robot and the voltage control was performed by a RTAI Linux PC running at $1kHz$ commanding a National Instruments DAQ Card (NI 6034e) that drives the voltage controller.

The purpose of the experiment will be the estimation of the parameters a_0, a_1 and a_2 of the eq. 8, i.e., the fluid and the platform parameters : Cd, Cv, μ_0, A and the gap h . Assuming a linear behavior, the mathematical procedure will be the following:

As $\frac{dx}{dt} = v$, for a number of samples n, each sample i corresponds to:

$$F(i) = a_0 \cdot V^2(i) - a_1 \cdot v(i) \cdot V^2(i) + a_2 \cdot v(i) \tag{11}$$

which, written as array, leads to:

$$\underbrace{\begin{pmatrix} F(0) \\ \vdots \\ F(i) \\ \vdots \\ F(n) \end{pmatrix}}_{B} = \underbrace{\begin{pmatrix} V^2(0) & -v(0) \cdot V^2(0) & v(0) \\ \vdots & \vdots & \vdots \\ V^2(i) & -v(i) \cdot V^2(i) & v(i) \\ \vdots & \vdots & \vdots \\ V^2(n) & -v(n) \cdot V^2(n) & v(n) \end{pmatrix}}_{A} \cdot \underbrace{\begin{pmatrix} a_0 \\ a_1 \\ a_2 \end{pmatrix}}_{a} \tag{12}$$

Thus, a simple operation leads to the vector of parameters a, being $A^\#$ the pseudo-inverse of A, as it is not invertible :

$$a = \begin{pmatrix} a_0 \\ a_1 \\ a_2 \end{pmatrix} = A^\# \cdot B \tag{13}$$

The identification experiments were carried away with the robot arm performing a continuous sinusoidal movement $(0.2Hz, 1.5cm/s)$, while different voltage steps $(0.5, 1, 1.5, 2KV)$ were applied. A voltage ramp was finally applied while the platform's speed reaches its maximum value. The objective here is to provide an as rich as possible signal excitation to guarantee the good conditioning of the matrix A and thus the parameters identification success. This has been evaluated here using the "COND()" Matlab function which gave the satisfactory value $cond(A) > 10^3$. The data registered is the speed, the force, and the voltage. The obtained data leads to the successful calculation of the parameters and the force output during the estimation procedure reaches values between 2.5 and $3N$, suitable quantities to simulate the resistance of soft tissues, according to [19].

Beside these results, the maximum force that has been obtained with the current version of the prototype is more than $10N$ for a voltage input of $5kV$. If we increase the input voltage, electrical arcs should appear and disturb the measurements. Moreover, beyond $10N$ of input force, the plate started to stick-slip and electrical arcs appear again. If needed, higher force capabilities should be obtained by increasing the contact surface between the electrodes and by increasing the voltage input. Optimizing the gap between the electrodes should reduce the appearing of electrical arcs.

2.4   PI Force Control of the Platform

To assess the quality of the model and the parameter estimation procedure, a PI type force control was developed. According to [11], a PID controller is unstable due to the derivative term, in this type of fluid application, so a PI type controller was chosen. Since the prototype is at an early design state, it was necessary to make an on-line calibration on each control experiment, to avoid issues regarding parameters temperature dependency and the variability of the boundary conditions.

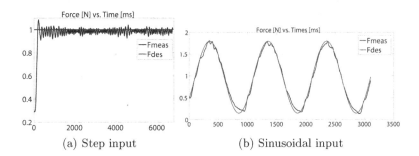

(a) Step input   (b) Sinusoidal input

Fig. 2. PI control results

Fig. 2 shows the PI force control results of the experiment. In a first experiment, the robot arm is moving at a speed of $6mm/s$, and the desired force was a step of $1N$ (see Fig. 2a). In a second experiment, a desired sinusoidal force of $0.8N$, 1Hz of frequency, and a mean value of $1N$ was specified as an input for the system (see Fig. 2b). As seen in Fig. 2, the proposed PI force controller gives very promising results in terms of tracking errors and dynamics. Indeed, the steady state error (step response) and the dynamic error (sinusoidal response) of the system are both less than $0.15N$. On the other hand, the closed loop force feedback bandwidth of the platform is capable of managing a step response and a $1Hz$ sinusoidal force signal. One can conclude that the controller could withstand, with an affordable error rate, the soft tissues needle insertion forces, under non-optimal conditions.

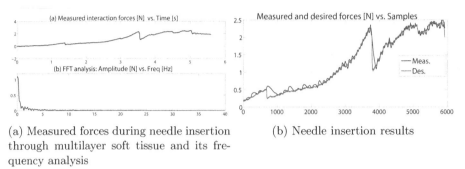

(a) Measured forces during needle insertion through multilayer soft tissue and its frequency analysis

(b) Needle insertion results

Fig. 3. Measured needle interaction forces

2.5   Needle Insertion Interaction Forces Experiments

In order to validate the reliability of the ERF-based platform and its force feedback control scheme, it is fundamental to analyze the measured interaction force during a needle insertion on soft tissue in terms of time and frequency variation. To do so, we have measured the interaction forces during an ex-vivo robotized needle insertion experiment through a multilayer soft tissue (two different bovine slices of approx. the same depth 18mm) [20] (see Fig. 3a-up). In this ex-vivo experiment, the two soft tissue layers were horizontally superposed and attached together and a 18 gauge beveled biopsy needle was vertically inserted into the tissues. As it can be observed on the Fig. 3a-up, it appears three "puncture points". The first one at the needle entry point (at approx. 1.5s), the second one at the boundary between the two layers (at approx. 3.5s) and the last one at approx. 5.2s which corresponds to a tissue inhomogeneity.

The Fig. 3a-down presents the frequency analysis (FFT) of the measured force and shows that the energy of the interaction force is mainly located at the very low frequencies $(0 - 2Hz)$ and the force amplitude can be almost neglected beyond $10Hz$ since it is less than $0.15N$ which corresponds to the previously obtained PI force controller error. One can thus conclude that the bandwidth of the proposed device should be sufficient to realistically feedback this needle interaction forces to the user. Indeed, as shown in the Fig. 3b, we have performed a last validation experiment where the desired controlled force was the one recorded in Fig. 3a during the multi-layer needle insertion procedure on soft tissue.

As one can see on the Fig. 3b, the measured interaction forces correctly reaches the desired value. However, the measured force lags somehow behind the desired force when the latter makes a discrete change which corresponds to the first and the second "points of puncture" (at approx. 750 samples and 3750 samples) but surprisingly not at the last discrete change (at approx. 5200 samples). This lag phenomena should be related either to the overall system bandwidth (including the high voltage converter) or the the presence of the integral term in the controller. This result has to be deeply investigated and fixed in a future work.

Beside this lag phenomena, the obtained results are very promising and showed that ERF-based technology is a good candidate to safely simulate the physical resistance of soft tissues.

3 Conclusions and Future Work

The goal of this research was to test the possibilities of a simple, programmable ERF-based platform, as a linear haptic-feedback device simulating different stiffnesses. A prototype was built, its mathematical model has been obtained, and experimentally validated. The inverse model was used in a PI force controller. The control experiments showed the capabilities of the platform to exhibit a fast and accurate response, given the design limitations of the device. The preliminary experimental results are very promising and showed the great potential of the ERF-based platform to simulate the physical resistance of soft tissues against the movement of a surgical needle. However, many improvements in terms of mechatronic, modeling and control have to be considered before to link the ERF-based needle training platform to a FEM-based virtual needle insertion simulator as the one presented in [21]. User trials experiments have also to be conduced to evaluate the quality of the force feedback rendering and to improve the platform design and control.

References

1. Traumaman system website,
   http://www.simulab.com/product/surgery/open/traumaman-system
2. Arthrocentesis trainer website,
   http://www.simulab.com/product/critical-care/arthrocentesis-mode
3. Dv trainer from mimic simulation,
   http://www.mimicsimulation.com/products/dv-trainer/
4. Phantom haptic device from geomagic,
   http://geomagic.com/en/products-landing-pages/haptic/
5. Omega haptic device from force dimension,
   http://www.forcedimension.com/omega7-overview/
6. An, J., Kwon, D.-S.: Haptic experimentation on a hybrid active/passive force feedback device. In: ICRA, vol. 4, pp. 4217–4222. IEEE (2002)
7. Hamza-Lup, F., Bogdan, C., Popovici, D., Costea, O.: A survey of visuo-haptic simulation in surgical training. In: Proceedings of the 3rd International Conference of Mobile, Hybrid and on-line Learning, pp. 57–62 (2011)
8. Jolly, M.R., Bender, J.W., Carlson, J.D.: Properties and applications of commercial magnetorheological fluids. Journal of Intelligent Material Systems and Structures 10(1), 5–13 (1999)

9. Kim, K.-H., Nam, Y.-J., Yamane, R., Park, M.: Smart mouse: 5-dof haptic hand master using magneto-rheological fluid actuators. Journal of Physics: Conference Series 149(1), 012062 (2009)

10. Tsujita, T., Ohara, M., Sase, K., Konno, A., Nakayama, M., Abe, K., Uchiyama, M.: Development of a haptic interface using mr fluid for displaying cutting forces of soft tissues. In: ICRA, pp. 1044–1049. IEEE (2012)

11. Vitrani, M.A., Nikitczuk, J., Morel, G., Mavroidis, C.: Torque control of electrorheological fluidic actuators for haptic vehicular instrument controls. In: ICRA (2004)

12. Mavroidis, C., Bar-Cohen, Y., Bouzit, M.: Haptic interfaces using electrorheological fluids. In: Electroactive Polymer Actuators as Artificial Muscles: Reality, Potentials, and Challenges, pp. 567–594 (2001)

13. Unluhisarcikli, O., Weinberg, B., Sivak, M., Mirelman, A., Bonato, P., Mavroidis, C.: A robotic hand rehabilitation system with interactive gaming using novel electro-rheological fluid based actuators. In: ICRA, pp. 1846–1851. IEEE (2010)

14. Oh, J.S., Shin, W.K., Uhm, C.H., Lee, S.R., Han, Y.M., Choi, S.B.: Control of haptic master - slave robot system for minimally invasive surgery (mis). In: Journal of Physics 412(1) (2013); 13th Int. Conf. on ERF and MRF Suspensions

15. Chan, S., Conti, F., Salisbury, K., Blevins, N.: Virtual reality simulation in neurosurgery: technologies and evolution. Neurosurgery 72, 154–164 (2013)

16. Coles, T.R., Meglan, D., John, N.: The role of haptics in medical training simulators: A survey of the state of the art. IEEE Trans. on Haptics 4, 51–66 (2011)

17. Cho, H.J., Oh, J.S., Choi, S.B.: Design and performance evaluation of haptic master device using er spherical joint. Advanced Materials Research 317, 577–580 (2011)

18. U. K. Technical Information Sheet, Electro-rheological fluid lid 3354s, ER Fluids Developments Ltd. (2003)

19. Okamura, A.M., Simone, C., O'Leary, M.D.: Force modeling for needle insertion into soft tissue. IEEE Transactions on Biomedical Engineering 51(10), 1707–1716 (2004)

20. da Frota Moreira, P.L.: Model based force control for soft tissue interaction and applications in physiological motion compensation, Ph.D. dissertation, Université de Montpellier (December 2, 2012)

21. Duriez, C., Guébert, C., Marchal, M., Cotin, S., Grisoni, L.: Interactive simulation of flexible needle insertions based on constraint models. In: Yang, G.-Z., Hawkes, D., Rueckert, D., Noble, A., Taylor, C. (eds.) MICCAI 2009, Part II. LNCS, vol. 5762, pp. 291–299. Springer, Heidelberg (2009)

Intraoperative Cone Beam CT Guidance
for Transoral Robotic Surgery

Wen P. Liu[1,*], Jeremy D. Richmon[2], Mahdi Azizian[3],
Jonathan M. Sorger[3], and Russell H. Taylor[1]

[1] Department of Computer Science, Johns Hopkins University
[2] Department of Otolaryngology - Head and Neck Surgery,
Johns Hopkins Hospital
[3] Intuitive Surgical Inc., Sunnyvale, USA
wen.p.liu@jhu.edu

Abstract. We have developed an intraoperative image guidance system that integrates information from cone beam computed tomography with video augmentation for transoral robotic surgery. A proposed workflow to overlay critical structures with relative tool positions on stereoscopic endoscopy for resection of base of tongue neoplasms was evaluated using ex vivo and in vivo animal models. Results included visual confirmations of augmented critical anatomy during controlled arterial dissection and successful mock tumor resection. The proposed image-guided robotic system also achieved improved resection ratios of mock tumor margins (1.00) when compared to control scenarios (0.0) and alternative methods of image guidance (0.58).

Keywords: Transoral robotic surgery, video augmentation, *daVinci*®, cone beam computed tomography, image-guided robotic surgery.

1   Introduction

The rising incidence of oropharyngeal cancer related to the human papilloma virus has become a significant health care concern. Both surgical and non-surgical treatment modalities have been advocated. Recently, transoral robotic surgery (TORS) has become an increasingly utilized minimally invasive surgical intervention for treatment of base of tongue (BOT) oropharyngeal cancer. TORS allows for the en bloc removal of oropharygneal tumors with minimal adjacent tissue injury, thereby optimizing functional results. Surgical strategy and navigational approaches to excise a specific tumor with adequate margins are derived from merging preoperative volumetric data (i.e. computed tomography (CT) and magnetic resonance (MR)), obtained in the supine position with a meticulous evaluation of the patient in clinic. The integration of preoperative planning to the surgical scene is conducted as a mental exercise; thus the accuracy of this practice is highly dependent on the surgeon's experience with this operative technique and subject to inconsistencies. This is further complicated by the

---

* Corresponding author.

D. Stoyanov et al. (Eds.): IPCAI 2014, LNCS 8498, pp. 41–50, 2014.

fact that patient positioning for a TORS procedure requires the patient neck to be extended, mouth open, and tongue pulled anteriorly, presenting a surgical workspace highly deformed from that of preoperative acquisitions.

Research groups have sought to overcome some of the above limitations by integrating information from medical images through augmented reality in orthopedics [1], laparoscopy [2-4], and other head and neck interventions. Approaches differ in visualization from projective and smart displays, to head mounted gear, x-ray and video overlay [5], in addition to direct augmentation of the endoscope [4, 6]. Presenting supplementary navigational information to the surgeon directly within the primary means of visualization (i.e. the endoscopic video) has shown to be advantageous in biliary surgery [4] and skull base studies [7]. Image guidance derived from preoperative data [2-4, 6] benefit from the ability of multiple modalities to target different anatomies, however intraoperative imaging [5, 8] can capture real-time patient positioning and tissue deformation during surgery.

We previously investigated an augmented reality workflow for overlaying graphical information about critical anatomic structures onto stereo endoscopic video during TORS procedures with the *daVinci®* robot (Intuitive Surgical, Inc., Sunnyvale, CA) [9] as a means of assisting the surgeon in accurately resecting tumors. In this approach, graphic models of TORS critical structures (i.e. lingual arteries, tumor) are segmented from standard diagnostic CT or MRI images. Intraoperatively, a CBCT image is acquired after the patient is prepared for surgery and just before the robot is docked next to the operating table. An intensity-based algorithm developed by Reaungamornrat *et al.* [10] is used to deformably register the preoperative image to the intraoperative CBCT, and the deformation field is then used to update the graphical models of the anatomic structures. In this paper, we propose identifying critical structures directly from intraoperative cone beam computed tomographic angiography (CBCTA). A series of experiments resecting BOT mock tumors were conducted on ex vivo and in vivo animal models comparing the proposed workflow for video augmentation to simulated control and fluoroscopy-based image guidance.

2   Materials and Methods

2.1   System Overview and Workflow

In our proposed workflow, the patient is positioned in a standard intraoperative position, contrast material is injected to enable visualization of critical oropharyngeal structures, while an intraoperative CBCTA image is obtained. Critical data as well as registration fiducials are manually segmented from the CBCTA using ITK-Snap and registered to the stereo video camera of the *da Vinci* robot. Segmentation by intensity-based thresholds (manual initialization) from angiographies can be accomplished on order of seconds. Alternatively, detailed preoperative planning based on standard diagnostic CT/MRI can be created prior to the operation, thus does not contribute to the overall intraoperative time. Guidance through video augmentation (refer to [9] for details of system architecture), is implemented by extending the SURGICAL ASSISTANCE WORKSTATION (SAW) open-source toolkit [11], developed at the Engineering Research Center for Computer Integrated Surgery (CISST ERC, Johns Hopkins University). Visual overlay of TORS resection targets (tumor/ margins) and the lingual artery are directly rendered within the endoscopic video to guide the surgeon during BOT tumor resection. The augmentation follows camera kinematics, provided by the *daVinci®* application programming interface (API), and intraoperative tracking of custom fiducials. Orthogonal views of tracked tools relative to the critical data are added to supplement the surgeon's stereo perspective in depth, (i.e. parallel to the camera axis).

2.2   Porcine Models

Ex vivo (EV) Porcine Tongue Phantoms

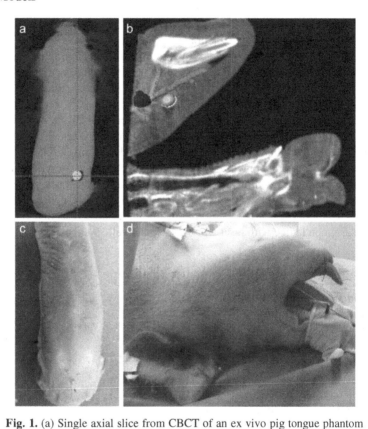

Ex vivo excised porcine tongues (Fig. 1c) were used in simple experimental scenarios. To simulate current standard of practice, as a control scenario, EV models were used in mock tumor resec-tion without integrated image guidance (i.e. CBCT viewed in off-line displays). Custom features and settings (i.e. determining color and opacity values for augmented structures and thresholds for tool tracking) for the user interface (UI)

Fig. 1. (a) Single axial slice from CBCT of an ex vivo pig tongue phantom with embedded tumor (green). (b). Single sagittal slice CBCTA of an in vivo pig phantom with segmented models of the right lingual artery (orange), and two base-of-tongue tumors (right in yellow, left in blue). (c). Photograph of an ex vivo pig tongue phantom affixed with green registration fiducials. (d) Photograph of an in vivo pig phantom supine and readied for tumor placement.

was initially tested using ex vivo models prior to in vivo experiments. Each EV tongue was embedded with a synthetic mock tumor, an 8 mm diameter nitrile sphere (green in Fig. 1a), and five to eight 3.2 mm diameter nylon spheres (green in Fig. 1c) were affixed to the tongue surface, which served as registration and landmark fiducials. A CBCT (109 kVp, 290 mA, 0.48x0.48x0.48 mm^3 voxel size) was then acquired with the tongue secured onto a flat foam template.

In vivo (IV) **Porcine**

For in vivo experiments a live pig was placed supine on an operating table (Fig 1d), anesthetized, catheterized and a tracheostomy tube was inserted. The specimen's jaw was opened with a triangular wooden block, wedged between the molars and the tongue was pulled anteriorly with suture, configuring the BOT in an intraoperative position for TORS. Standard clinical mouth and tongue retractors (ex: Feyh Kastenbauer (FK) Gyrus ACMI/Explorent GmbH, Tuttlingen Germany) were avoided because of metal artifact in CBCT. Radiolucent retractors or advanced reconstruction algorithms [12] with metal artifact reduction could address artifacts from metal but are topics beyond the scope of this paper. An intraoperative angiography was acquired with an injection of 40 ml of iodine (MD-76R®) during a volumetric CBCT scan (90 kVp, 290 mA, 0.48x0.48x0.48 mm^3 voxel size). Two mock tumors (Urethane, medium durometer spherical medical balloons, 10 mm diameter) were placed anterior/ superior to bilateral lingual arteries (using a radiopaque FEP I.V. catheter (Abbocath®-T 14G x140 mm) in the BOT (Fig. 1ab). Balloons were injected with a mixture of 0.5 ml rigid polyurethane foam (FOAM-IT®) and 0.25 ml iodine (MD-76R®) to retain shape and provide tomographic contrast, respectively. Acrylic paint (0.25 ml) was also added to the filling mixture to provide visual feedback. For S1 eight 3.2 mm diameter nylon spheres (Fig. 1c) were placed on the tongue surface as registration fiducials, but for S2 these were replaced by a custom resection fiducial (Fig. 2 triangular green lattice with inset white, black and yellow spheres).

2.3   Image Guidance

Video   Augmentation and Tool Tracking

During mock tumor resection, the stereographic projection viewed through the *daVinci® Si* surgeon side console (SSC) was superimposed with mesh models of critical data segmented from intraoperative CBCTA. Augmentation for EV models included the synthetic tumor and surface fiducials while IV models also included segmented lin-

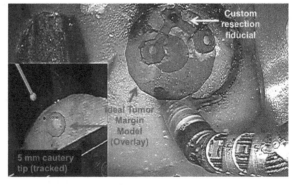

Fig. 2. Screen capture of an ex vivo phantom experiment using video augmentation of margins (green sphere) and tool tracking in novel views (lower left picture-in-picture) for image guidance

gual arteries. IV experiments for S2 added a spherical margin (Fig. 2, green sphere) bounding the mock tumor to provide the surgeon with the overlay of an ideal margin resection (i.e. spherical volume with a 10 mm radius, concentric with the tumor). This was facilitated by the change of sphere's color indicating a breach in the distance between the margin and the tumor. A default blue hue changed to green (large sphere in Fig. 2 is green since tool tip is in proximity) when the tool tip of the primary instrument (5 mm monopolar cautery) was determined to be within +2 mm outside of the margin, then yellow and red when the tip moved within the margin by -2 mm and -4 mm, respectively. In addition to these chromatic cues, a numeric label, on the wrist of the instrument was also displayed, thereby showing a real-time update of the relative distance of tool to the ideal margin boundary.

To provide navigational information in the axis orthogonal to the camera plane, i.e. depth, we implemented supplemental camera views of tracked tools within the virtual scene (model meshes of critical information and CBCT slices and volumes). This auxiliary camera perspective, rendered picture-in-picture (Fig. 2, lower inset left) can be dynamically changed but was observed to be most useful in the lateral, left-to-right sagittal plane, orthogonal to the primary stereo endoscopy view axis. We implemented the picture-in-picture (PIP) display by extending the OpenIGTLink module for Slicer 3D [13] (https://www.slicer.org) with a bidirectional interface to the image guidance program. Registration and tool transformations were streamed to the Slicer module, which rendered the tools, CBCT data, and tumor models in the PIP display.

For S1, superimposed virtual structures were initially, rigidly registered by identifying point-based correspondence with artificial surface spheres (Fig. 1c), visible in stereo video and segmented from CBCTA. In experiments for S2, as a first step toward intraoperative updates, we continuously tracked a custom rigid fiducial attached directly above the resection target (Fig. 2). Assuming a constant spatial relationship within the resected volume (i.e. between the fiducial and targets) we update the overlay of the tumor and margin mesh with the transformation of the tracked custom fiducial. This fiducial was fabricated on a 3D printer and designed as a planar right isosceles triangular lattice with a hypotenuse of 10 mm in length. Each corner of the symmetric triangle was connected by an annulus, a ring with an inner radius of 1.5 mm. The triangular frame, 1 mm in width was painted green, while white, yellow and black 1.6 mm (radius) Teflon spheres were each inserted into corner annuli.

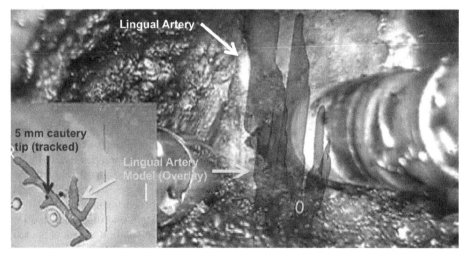

Fig. 3. Screen capture of lingual dissection during an in vivo porcine lab experiment using video augmentation as image guidance

Using color thresholds, the green framework of the fiducial was first located as an initial region of interest. Corner annuli of the green frame created circular negatives that were segmented using contours detection, and matched by their average color to the nylon spheres. Chromatic thresholds, updated on successful fiducial segmentations, were designed to be dynamically adaptive in order to be robust to fiducial color changes due to pollution from cautery. A rigid transformation from point-based tracking of the spheres on the customized fiducial updated the locally rigid transformation of the attached resected volume.

Forward kinematics from instrument joint encoders, as provided by the API, has been measured with error ≤ 25 mm [15]. To correct for this offset, necessary for tool tracking, we tested two methods: 1). Establish the euclidean transformation corresponding tool tip locations in stereo video and the API in several tool poses. 2). Derive setup joint corrections through vision-based processing of markers attached to the shaft of the instrument (a proprietary function developed by Intuitive Surgical Inc.)

Fluoroscopy Augmentation

For comparison with video-based augmentation we also tested scenarios with fluorscopy-based image guidance using the Siemen's Syngo workstation. For the IV experiments, after docking the robotic arms to the operating table, the C-Arm was placed laterally to capture sagittal x-rays of IV experiments. For intraoperative fluoroscopic-guided experiments the surgeon side console was setup in radiation-shielded workspace with access to manually activated x-ray on request. The live fluoroscopic images and its overlay onto the CBCTA of the head of the porcine specimens was rendered in 2D in the bottom left and right corners of the SSC through TilePro®.

3   Experiments

During two sets of experiments (S1 and S2), a head and neck surgeon (second author) resected embedded mock tumors, commensurate with standard surgical practice (i.e attempting to achieve a 10 mm margin around the tumor while avoiding and/or controlling the lingual artery), from EV and IV phantoms using a research *da Vinci®* Si console with variations of the proposed image guidance. Each set of experiments (variable scenarios summarized in Table 1) included: (a). control with EV phantom, (b) video augmentation with EV phantom, (c) Fluoroscopy augmentation with IV on left BOT and (d). video augmentation with IV on right BOT.

Two EV specimens, S1a and S2a, were used as control (i.e. preoperative images were available offline but not integrated to the robotic system) in order to simulate current standards of practice. The clinician was given access to view preoperative CBCTs, with visible tumors and surface landmark fiducials on offline monitors displaying the reconstructed volumes in MPR (Multi-Planar Reconstruction) views. Scenarios S1b and S2b served to gauge user experience and feedback on proposed features of the video augmentation software on simple EV specimens prior to testing on comprehensive IV models. Experiments comparing video to fluoroscopic augmentation were conducted on IV specimens, which provided a realistic, oropharyngeal workspace. While both S1c and S2c used fluoroscopic augmentation, the S2c setup included the capability to enlarge (4x) regions of interest.

Table 1. Experimental Scenarios

Experiment	Model	Image Data	Guidance	Margin	Image Guidance
S1a	EV	Intraop CBCT	None	No	The control for the first set, simulated current practice with preoperative CBCT shown in offline 2D display, i.e. separate from surgeon's console
S1b	EV	Intraop CBCT	Video	No	Represented the basic proposed image guidance workflow where stereo video endoscopy was superimposed segmented tumor and fiducials from CBCT along with tracked tools in novel virtual views, picture-in-picture.
S1c	IV	Intraop CBCTA	Fluoro	No	Superimposed fluoroscopy on CBCTA used for guidance in tumor resection and lingual dissection.
S1d	IV	Intraop CBCTA	Video	No	Used video augmentation guidance similar to S1b, however with in vivo porcine lab requiring lingual dissection
S2a	EV	Intraop CBCT	None	No	The control for the second lab, with the same guidance given as S1a
S2b	EV	Intraop CBCT	Video	Yes	Included all features implemented for S1b, but extended image guidance for margins with resected specimen tracking using a custom fiducial
S2c	IV	Intraop CBCTA	Fluoro	No	Fluroscopic guidance, as given in S1c, with extended capabilities to zoom up to 4x on region of interest
S2d	IV	Intraop CBCTA	Video	Yes	The same guidance and scenario as S1d, but extended image guidance for margins with resected specimen tracking using a custom fiducial

(Rows S1a–S1d are labelled "Set 1"; rows S2a–S2d are labelled "Set 2".)

Video augmentation for S1 differed from S2 as follows. For tool tracking, to calibrate for the inherent offset at the remote center of motion S1 (S1b, S1d) used an initial point-based calibration for corrections while a vision-based technique to track artificial markers was employed for S2 (S2b, S2d). In addition, S2 also tested initial implementation to guide margin resection. Augmented overlays of critical data included an ideal margin, updated during intraoperative tracking of a custom resection fiducial.

4   Results

For both control scenarios (S1a, S2a, i.e. tumor resection without integrated image guidance on an EV tongue), the resected specimen failed to contain the target mock tumor.

All experiments with integrated image guidance successfully resected the whole tumor. In the live animal lab cases accuracy of the lingual artery overlays were visually confirmed (Fig. 3, video augmented

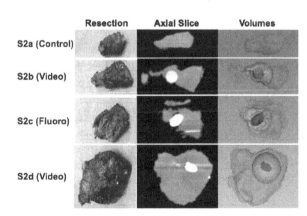

Fig. 4. Resected tumor and margins with corresponding slices (tumor in high intensity, white) and segmented volumes (tumor in blue, intersection with ideal margin in yellow) from postoperative CBCT

overlay of exposed lingual dissection) along with successful arterial dissection and control in both video and fluoroscopic augmentation.

Measurements of the specimen resected from all eight robotic experiments are summarized in Table 2 and Fig. 4 show photographs and corresponding postoperative slices/volumes of the resected tumors (blue in 'Volumes' column) and their intersection with an ideal margin (yellow in 'Volumes' column). Resection ratios (volume of margin resection/volume of ideal spherical margin) in order from high to low was achieved with S2d (1.00), S2b (0.87), S1d (0.81), S1b (0.71), S2c (0.58) and S1c (0.44), respectively. The challenging environment of a featureless ex vivo model, compared to a realistic in vivo model is substantiated with the superior results obtained comparing in vivo to ex vivo experiments which used the same video-based augmentation for image guidance. Improvements achieved by S2d, in reference to S1d (similarly from S2b to S1b) can be attributed to the addition of margin overlay and intraoperative tracking of the resected volume. S1c and S2c, scenarios that utilized fluoroscopic overlays had the advantage of precise tool to tumor distances, but were restricted to a single x-ray (2D) plane.

The margin/specimen ratio on S1c and S2d was large secondary to posterior placement of the IV mock tumor and the custom resection fiducial mandated inclusion with the resection specimen. Most IV specimens in general required longer dissections, resulting in smaller ratios as compared to EV, due to volumes removed for arterial control and workspace limitations of the transoral access.

In addition to resection ratios, two forms of accuracy are of interest here: 1). Projection Distance Error (PDE) – the 2D pixel distance between projected overlay and the true image location of the object 2). Tool Tracking Error (TTE) – the 3D position [mm] of the tool tip compared. Mean PDE, from point-based manual registration, has been previously established at 2 mm using an anthropomorphic skull phantom [9]. During video-based image guidance for S2 visual estimates of tool tracking error (distance of virtual to true tool tip in video) for S2d, was observed to be 5 mm (mean), 10 mm (max).

Table 2. Experimental results

Experiment		Specimen [mm^3]	Margin [mm^3]	Tumor [mm^3]	Margin/ Specimen	Margin/ Ideal Margin	Ideal Tumor/ Margin	Tumor/ Ideal Tumor
Set 1	S1a	N/A	N/A	N/A	N/A	N/A	N/A	N/A
	S1b	8059.67	2960.45	257.99	0.37	0.71	0.09	0.49
	S1c	19602.55	1832.28	280.17	0.09	0.44	0.15	0.54
	S1d	13450.55	3410.59	583.45	0.25	0.81	0.17	1.11
Set 2	S2a	N/A	N/A	N/A	N/A	N/A	N/A	N/A
	S2b	5485.52	3646.92	307.47	0.66	0.87	0.08	0.59
	S2c	6656.81	2429.50	323.08	0.36	0.58	0.13	0.62
	S2d	22287.22	4199.81	220.32	0.19	1.00	0.05	0.42

Ideal Margin: A sphere of radius = 10 mm   Ideal Tumor: A sphere of radius = 5 mm

5   Discussion

This is a proof-of-concept study that assessed the value of augmenting the surgeon's endoscopic view with CBCTA data with the goal of improving surgical accuracy and optimizing margins. Though limited by a single, experienced TORS surgeon performing the resections, results demonstrate the value of augmented endoscopy by improved margin status.

In these experiments, video-based augmentation (S1b, S2b, S1d, S2d) achieved superior tumor resection compared to fluoroscopy-based guidance (S1c, S2c). The improvements by S2d compared to S2c can be attributed to the supplementary guidance with margin delineation. However, superior results achieved by S1 scenarios, where overlays did not include margins, emphasize a disadvantage for 2D fluoroscopy, compared to 3D video augmentation, and the significance of the method of integration between supplemental navigational information and the primary visual field. Rendered through TilePro® (i.e. visible in the SCC), unlike the proposed video augmentation system, the fluoroscopic overlays were shown below the native stereo endoscopy. Informal surveys and similar work for monocular video augmentation in skull base surgery [7] have suggested advantages of guidance through augmentation [14] of the primary, "natural" window. Improvements from S1c to S2c support a necessity to be able to enlarge regions of interest in order to take further advantage of the sub-millimeter resolution of 2D X-rays. The EV phantoms presented an abnormally challenging environment consisting of a featureless tongue volume. As the IV resection proceeded dental, oropharyngeal and neurovascular anatomies serve as landmarks, while our simulated control EV models only provided superficial features (surface fiducials).

Despite encouraging results achieved by the proposed video augmentation system, issues of robustness and accuracy remain. Video augmentation registered initially is reliable on approach, however during intraoperative resection, overlaid models should be updated to reflect surgical deformations. Intraoperative resected volume updates based on custom fiducials was susceptible to failure when the fiducial was not positioned orthogonally to the endoscope. For improvements on robustness we are looking to incorporate Kalman filters and prior state information from tool tracking. In addition a 5 mm (mean) TTE, not acceptable for TORS applications, can be improved through intraoperative fluoroscopy, using 2D3D registration to correct for kinematic inaccuracies, tissue deformation and external forces. Comprehensive phantom studies quantifying TTE and techniques for improvement is currently underway.

6   Conclusions and Future Work

Experimental results show the feasibility and advantages of guidance through video augmentation of the primary stereo endoscopy as compared to control and alternative navigation methods. The small number of experiments conducted is a recognized limitation of the work presented, however future work will not only investigate methods to update navigational information after tissue deformation but will optimize the workflow such that more TORS surgeons can be included, a more realistic tongue/tumor model will be incorporated, and increased iterations will improve the validity of our model.

Acknowledgements. The authors extend sincere thanks to support provided by Intuitive Surgical Inc., Johns Hopkins, NIH-R01-CA-127444, and the Swirnow Family Foundation.

References

1. Van de Kelft, E., Costa, F., Van der Planken, D., Schils, F.: A prospective multicenter registry on the accuracy of pedicle screw placement in the thoracic, lumbar, and sacral levels with the use of the O-arm imaging system and StealthStation Navigation. Spine 37, E1580–E1587 (2012)
2. Su, L.M., Vagvolgyi, B.P., Agarwal, R., Reiley, C.E., Taylor, R.H., Hager, G.D.: Augmented reality during robot-assisted laparoscopic partial nephrectomy: toward real-time 3D-CT to stereoscopic video registration. Urology 73, 896–900 (2009)
3. Hughes-Hallett, A., Mayer, E.K., Marcus, H.J., Cundy, T.P., Pratt, P.J., Darzi, A.W., Vale, J.A.: Augmented Reality Partial Nephrectomy: Examining the Current Status and Future Perspectives. Urology (2013)
4. Volonte, F., Buchs, N.C., Pugin, F., Spaltenstein, J., Jung, M., Ratib, O., Morel, P.: Stereoscopic augmented reality for da Vincii robotic biliary surgery. International Journal of Surgery Case Reports 4, 365–367 (2013)
5. Chen, X., Wang, L., Fallavollita, P., Navab, N.: Precise X-ray and video overlay for augmented reality fluoroscopy. Int. J. Comput. Assist. Radiol. Surg. 8, 29–38 (2013)
6. Volonte, F., Buchs, N.C., Pugin, F., Spaltenstein, J., Schiltz, B., Jung, M., Hagen, M., Ratib, O., Morel, P.: Augmented reality to the rescue of the minimally invasive surgeon. The usefulness of the interposition of stereoscopic images in the Da Vinci robotic console. The International Journal of Medical Robotics + Computer Assisted Surgery: MRCAS 9, e34–e38 (2013)
7. Liu, W.P., Mirota, D.J., Uneri, A., Otake, Y., Hager, G.D., Reh, D.D., Ishii, M.: L., G.G., Siewerdsen, J.H.: A clinical pilot study of a modular video-CT augmentation system for image-guided skull base surgery. In: SPIE Medical Imaging 2012: Image-Guided Procedures, Robotic Interventions, and Modeling, pp. 8316–8112 (Year)
8. Badani, K.K., Shapiro, E.Y., Berg, W.T., Kaufman, S., Bergman, A., Wambi, C., Roychoudhury, A., Patel, T.: A Pilot Study of Laparoscopic Doppler Ultrasound Probe to Map Arterial Vascular Flow within the Neurovascular Bundle during Robot-Assisted Radical Prostatectomy. Prostate Cancer 2013, 810715 (2013)
9. Liu, W.P., Reaungamornrat, S., Deguet, A., Sorger, J.M., Siewerdsen, J.H., Richmon, J.D., Taylor, R.H.: Toward Intraoperative Image-Guided Transoral Robotic Surgery. Robotic Surgery 7, 217–225 (2013)
10. Reaungamornrat, S., Liu, W.P., Wang, A.S., Otake, Y., Nithiananthan, S., Uneri, A., Schafer, S., Tryggestad, E., Richmon, J., Sorger, J.M., Siewerdsen, J.H., Taylor, R.H.: Deformable image registration for cone-beam CT guided transoral robotic base-of-tongue surgery. Phys. Med. Biol. 58, 4951–4979 (2013)
11. Deguet, A., Kumar, R., Taylor, R.H., Kazanzides, P.: The cisst libraries for computer assisted intervention systems. In: MICCAI Workshop (2008), https://trac.lcsr.jhu.edu/cisst/
12. Stayman, J.W., Otake, Y., Prince, J.L., Khanna, A.J., Siewerdsen, J.H.: Model-Based Tomographic Reconstruction of Objects Containing Known Components. IEEE Trans. Med. Imaging (2012)
13. Pieper, S., Lorenson, B., Schroeder, W., Kikinis, R.: The NA-MIC kit: ITK, VTK, pipelines, grids, and 3D Slicer as an open platform for the medical image computing community. In: Proc. IEEE Intl. Symp. Biomed. Imag., pp. 698–701 (2006)
14. Rieger, A., Blum, T., Navab, N., Friess, H., Martignoni, M.E.: Augmented reality: merge of reality and virtuality in medicine. Deutsche Medizinische Wochenschrift 136, 2427–2433 (2011)
15. Reiter, A., Allen, P.K., Zhao, T.: Feature classification for tracking articulated surgical tools. Med. Image Comput. Comput. Assist. Interv. 15, 592–600 (2012)

Robotic Device for Acquisition of Wide and High Resolution MRI Image Using a Small RF Coil

Kohei Miki and Ken Masamune

Graduates School of Information Science and Technology, The University of Tokyo, Japan

Abstract. This paper proposed a prototype of wide and high resolution MRI acquisition system for MRI-guided surgery. Currently, MRI-guided neurosurgical procedures are performed in an operating room with open MRI, and intraoperative MR images are provided with real time rich biological information. However, the low resolution of the MR images is still problem and it is difficult to determine precise boundary of the tumor and normal tissue especially when using a low tesla open-type MRI. To solve this problem, a method to acquire wider and higher resolution MR images using a small RF coil is proposed. The outer diameter of the RF coil is 8 mm and its inductance and resistance of the RF coil were 1.0 μH and 2.0 Ω. To receive MRI signals with high efficiency, 1 DOF bending mechanism, which is mounted on the distal tip of the MRI signal receiver, was developed to control the orientation angle of the RF coil. Bending the distal tip of MRI signal receiver, the transmission efficiency of MRI signals is kept high and SNR of MR images was kept high. The SNR of MR images using MRI signal receiver was 11.3 and the voxel size of MR images is $0.5 \times 0.5 \times 1.0 \text{mm}^3$. We successfully obtained clear MR images of okra and the voxel size of MR images is $0.5 \times 0.5 \times 1.0 \text{mm}^3$. These results show that the MRI signal receiver is useful to acquire wide and high-resolution MR images.

1 Introduction

Magnetic resonance imaging (MRI) can provide high-resolution 3D or 2D images and it is non-invasive medical diagnostic imaging. MRI is able to monitor organ shape, blood flow, and brain function. Currently, MRI-guided procedures are performed in an operating room with open MRI, and intraoperative MR images are provide the real time rich anatomy and function information of the body [1–3]. Intraoperative MRI images can provide brain deformation and residual tumor, and resection rate of the tumor is improved significantly [4]. However, the resolution of the MR images when using a low tesla open type MRI still be low. Resection rate of infiltrative tumor still not be high because it is difficult to identify precise boundary of infiltrative tumor and normal tissue. To solve the problem, it is necessary to improve the resolution of MR images. When acquiring high resolution MR images, signal to noise ratio (SNR) of MR images decrease. SNR of MR images can be enhanced when using a small RF coil. Therefore, to improve the resolution of MR images, a method to improve SNR of MR images is proposed using a small RF coil. Another problem with open MRI is strong gradient non-linearity, which cannot be resolved using the proposed method.

D. Stoyanov et al. (Eds.): IPCAI 2014, LNCS 8498, pp. 51–60, 2014.

Massin and colleagues report magnetic resonance images using high-Q factor microfabricated planar coils [5]. Dave and colleagues report an MR-compatible endoscope with integral coil system [6]. Badilita and colleagues report 3D microcoils for microscale MRI applications [7]. However, the MR imaging area of small RF coil is very narrow and sensitivity of the RF coil depends on the angle of magnetic field and the RF coil.

To acquire wide and high resolution MR images using small RF coil, a manipulator to approach the RF coil to the target area and control orientation angle of the RF coil in MRI operating room is required. Currently, MR-guided surgical manipulator is developed extensively [8, 9]. MR-compatible is required for a manipulator used in the MRI operating room. MR-compatible must meet following requirements: 1) it is safe in the MRI environment, 2) its use in the MR environment does not affect MR imaging quality, and 3) it operates as designed in the MR environment [10].

This paper reports development of a MRI signal receiver and performance evaluation of the MRI acquisition system. To approach RF coil to target area using manipulator which equipped with the receiver, RF coil is attached the distal tip of cylindrically-shaped device. To control orientation angle of the RF coil, bending mechanism is mounted on the distal tip of MRI signal receiver.

2 MRI Signal Receiver

2.1 Design of a Small RF Coil

To design a flat spiral coil for MRI signal receiver, we calculated the electrical characteristics of the coil. Because MRI signal is a high frequency, the characteristics of the high-frequency circuit have to be considered [11]. Frequency of the nuclear magnetic resonance (NMR) signal is given by

$$f_0 = \frac{\omega_0}{2\pi} = \gamma H_0 \tag{1}$$

where γ is gyromagnetic ratio, H_0 is magnetic field intensity, and ω_0 is the angular frequency of the NMR. Frequency of the NMR signal is called larmor frequency. MRI used for the measurement of MR images is 0.2 T vertical magnetic filed open-type MRI (AIRIS Mate; Hitachi medico). Gyromagnetic ratio of hydrogen atoms is $\gamma = 42.58$ MHz/T. From Eq.(1), when hydrogen atom is measured with 0.2 T open-MRI, larmor frequency is 8.5 MHz. In the high frequency circuit, coil can be regarded as equivalent circuit consisting of inductance L and resistance R_L (Fig.1). Impedance of the coil Z_L is shown in the following equation:

$$Z_L = R_L + jX_L \tag{2}$$

where R_L is the real part of the impedance, and $X_L = \omega_0 L$ is the imaginary part of the impedance. Flat spiral coil inductor L and resistance R_L is given by

$$L = \frac{1}{25.4} \frac{N^2 A^2}{80A - 11D_i} \tag{3}$$

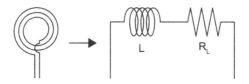

Fig. 1. High-frequency Equivalent Circuit of Coils

Table 1. Designed Value of the RF Coil

Outer Diameter [mm]	8
Inner Diameter [mm]	6
Wire Diameter [mm]	0.05
Number of Turns	9
Inductance [μm]	1.00
Resistance [Ω]	2.04

$$A = \frac{D_o + D_i}{4} \tag{4}$$

$$R_L = \rho \frac{l}{S} = \frac{\rho N(D_o - D_i)}{2d(w - d)} \tag{5}$$

where D_o is outer diameter of the coil, D_i is inner diameter of the coil, w is wire diameter, N is the number of turns of the coil, $l = (\pi N(D_o - D_i))/2$ is wire length, $S = \pi d(w - d)$ is wire section area, and d is the skin depth. High frequency current flows mainly at the skin of the wire. When the frequency is 8.5 MHz, the skin depth of copper conductor is 22.7 μm. Table 1 shows design value of the RF coil. The inductance and the resistance of the RF coil is 1.0 μH and 2.0 Ω.

2.2   Design of MRI Signal Receiver

To transmit MRI signal efficiently, it is necessary to match the impedance of the MRI signal receiving circuit and MRI. The MRI signal receiving circuit consisting variable capacitor is connected to RF coil and the impedance of MRI signal receiving circuit is match to the impedance of MRI Z_c at 8.5 MHz (Fig.2). The tuning capacitor C_1 and the matching capacitor C_2 is shown in the following equation:

$$C_1 = \frac{\Delta B}{2\pi f_0} \tag{6}$$

$$C_2 = \frac{1}{2\pi f_0 \Delta X} \tag{7}$$

$$\Delta B = \frac{X_L}{R_L^2 + X_L^2} - \sqrt{\frac{R_L}{Z_c(R_L^2 + X_L^2)} - \left(\frac{R_L}{R_L^2 + X_L^2}\right)^2} \tag{8}$$

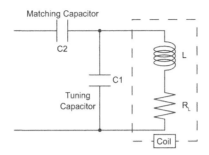

Fig. 2. Impedance Matching Circuit

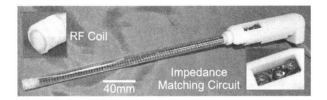

Fig. 3. The MRI Signal Receiver

$$\Delta X = \sqrt{\frac{Z_c(R_L^2 + X_L^2)}{R_L} - Z_c^2} \qquad (9)$$

A MRI signal receiver was developed using a 3D printer and $\phi 10$ mm acrylic pipe was connected to the end of the MRI signal receiver (Fig.3). Impedance matching circuit is mounted within the MRI signal receiver and RF coil is attached the distal tip of acrylic pipe. Sensitivity of the RF coil depends on the angle between the RF coil and magnetic field. MRI signal ξ_0 is given by

$$\xi_0 = \omega_0 B_1 M \left(1 + \frac{\omega_0^2 + r_0^2}{c^2}\right) \exp(j\omega_0 t) \qquad (10)$$

where ω_0 is the angular frequency of the NMR, B_1 is the magnetic field at the center of the RF coil, M is the bulk nuclear magnetic moment, r_0 is the radius of the coil, and c is the speed of light [12]. The vertical component of the magnetic field is $B_1(\phi) = B_1\sin(\phi)$, and MRI signal is $\xi(\phi) = \xi_0\sin(\phi)$. ϕ is the angle of magnetic field and the RF coil. Sensitivity of the RF coil is highest when the angle of magnetic field and the RF coil is $90°$. To control the angle of magnetic field and the RF coil, bending mechanism is mounted on the distal tip of MRI signal receiver (Fig.4). Bending mechanism is a 1-DOF linkage mechanism. The linkage mechanism converses linear slide motion using linear actuator into bending motion of the distal tip. The range of bending motion is $-20° \sim +20°$.

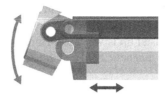

Fig. 4. Bending Mechanism of the MRI Signal Receiver

3 Experiment

3.1 SWR

To evaluate the transmission efficiency, we measured the impedance of the MRI signal receiving circuit using a vector network analyzer and calculated the standing wave ratio (SWR) of the MRI signal receiver. SWR indicates the relationship between the traveling wave and the reflected wave in the AC circuit and means the reception efficiency in the high-frequency circuit. SWR is shown in the following equation:

$$SWR = \frac{1 + \Gamma}{1 - \Gamma} \tag{11}$$

$$\Gamma = \left| \frac{Z - Z_c}{Z + Z_c} \right| \tag{12}$$

where Z is measuring impedance of MRI signal receiving circuit, Z_c is the impedance of MRI, and Γ is reflection coefficient. Fig.5 shows the results of SWR of the MRI signal receiver. Left is SWR of MRI signal receiver when the frequency of signal is 8 - 9 MHz and the angle of distal tip is $0°$. Right is SWR of MRI signal receiver when frequency is angle is $-20° \sim +20°$ and the frequency of signal 8.5 MHz. The minimum value of SWR is 1.04 ± 0.01 when the angle of distal tip is $-10°$ and the maximum value of SWR is 1.02 ± 0.01 when the angle of distal tip is $10°$. When SWR is 1.04,

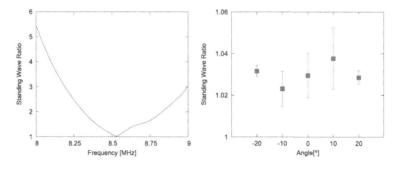

Fig. 5. SWR of MRI Signal Receiver. Left: SWR when frequency is 8 - 9 MHz and angle is $0°$. Right: SWR when frequency is angle is $-20° \sim +20°$ and frequency 8.5 MHz.

transmitting efficiency of MRI signal receiving circuit is 99.97 %. The result shows that transmission efficiency of MRI signals is high and the reduction of transmission efficiency by bending of the distal tip is very few. Transmission efficiency can be kept high regardless of the angle of magnetic field and the RF coil.

3.2   SNR Measuring Experiment

We measured the SNR of MR images of phantom using the MRI signal receiver with 0.2 T open MRI. Fig.6 shows the SNR measuring setup. Aqueous solution of nickel chloride is filled into the phantom. Aqueous solution of nickel chloride is used MRI phantom for performance evaluation of the open type MRI. Table 2 (a) shows imaging parameters of SNR measuring experiment. Measured voxel size of MR images is $0.5 \times 0.5 \times 1.0 \text{mm}^3$ and slice plane is transverse plane. The signal region is 8 mm circle region at the center of MR images and the noise region is 11.7 mm circle at four corners of the MR images (Fig.7). The signal intensity is the average signal intensity of signal region and the noise intensity is the average signal intensity of noise region. SNR of MR images is given by the ratio of signal intensity to noise intensity. The SNR of MR images using the MRI signal receiver were 11.3 with the voxel of $0.5 \times 0.5 \times 1.0 \text{mm}^3$. The SNR of the MR images by the MRI signal receiver and MR images by medical coil, the improvements of SNR are 3 times.

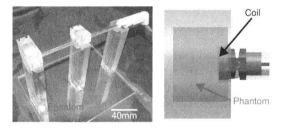

Fig. 6. MR Images of Phantom Acquisition Setup

Table 2. Imaging Parameters of MRI

	(a)	(b)
Imaging Sequence	Spin-Echo Sequence	
TR (Repetition Time) [msec]	250	
TE (Echo Time) [msec]	22	
NSA (Number of Signals Averaged)	16	
Slice Thickness [mm]	1	
Field of View [mm^2]	80×80	
Frequency	160	80
Phase	160	80
Voxel Size [mm^3]	$0.5 \times 0.5 \times 1.0$	$1.0 \times 1.0 \times 1.0$

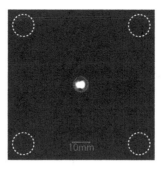

Fig. 7. The MR Image of Phantom

3.3   Sensitivity of the RF Coil Experiment

Sensitivity of the RF coil depends on the angle between the RF coil and magnetic field. We measured the SNR of MR images using MRI signal receiver with 0.2 T open MRI. Fig.8 shows experiment setup. Table 2 (b) shows imaging parameters. Measured voxel size of MR images is $1.0 \times 1.0 \times 1.0 \text{mm}^3$ and slice plane is transverse plane. The angle

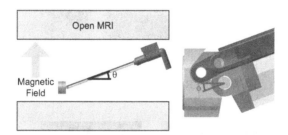

Fig. 8. Sensitivity of the RF Coil Measuring Setup. Left: the angle between the RF coil and magnetic field. Right: the angle of distal tip of MRI signal receiver.

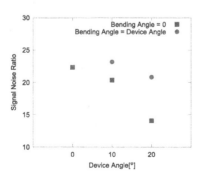

Fig. 9. SNRs of MR Images using MRI Signal Receiver

between MRI signal receiver and magnetic field θ is $0°$, $10°$, and $20°$. When the angle between MRI signal receiver and magnetic field $\theta \neq 0°$, the angle of distal tip of MRI signal receiver ϕ is $0°$, and equal to the angle between MRI signal receiver and magnetic field θ. Fig.9 shows the results. SNR of MR images reduced with the increasing the angle between MRI signal receiver and magnetic field θ. Compared $\theta \neq 0°$ to $\theta = \phi$, SNR of MR images was improved 13.7 % at $\theta = 10°$, and 47.1 % at $\theta = 20°$.

3.4   Image Acquisition Experiment

We measured MR images of okra. Fig.10 shows measuring of Okra images setup. Table 2 (a), (b) shows imaging parameters. Measured voxel size of MR images is $0.5 \times 0.5 \times 1.0\text{mm}^3$ and $1.0 \times 1.0 \times 1.0\text{mm}^3$. Slice plane is transverse plane and sagittal plane. Fig.11 shows MR images of okra. Direction of transverse plane is equal to cross-sectional of okra. Top left is transverse plane at $0.5 \times 0.5 \times 1.0\text{mm}^3$, bottom left is sagittal plane at $0.5 \times 0.5 \times 1.0\text{mm}^3$, top right is transverse plane at $1.0 \times 1.0 \times 1.0\text{mm}^3$, and bottom left is sagittal plane at $1.0 \times 1.0 \times 1.0\text{mm}^3$. We can identify the inner structure of okra at $0.5 \times 0.5 \times 1.0\text{mm}^3$ that it is difficult to identify from MR images by medical.

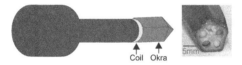

Fig. 10. MR Images Acquisition Setup

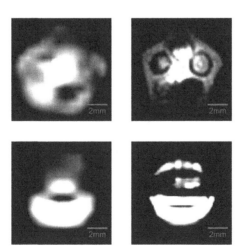

Fig. 11. MR Images of Okra. Top Left: TRS $1.0 \times 1.0 \times 1.0[\text{mm}^3]$, Bottom Left: SAG $1.0 \times 1.0 \times 1.0[\text{mm}^3]$, Top Right: TRS $0.5 \times 0.5 \times 1.0[\text{mm}^3]$, Bottom Right: SAG $0.5 \times 0.5 \times 1.0[\text{mm}^3]$.

4   Discussion and Conclusion

The paper proposed high resolution MR images acquisition system using the flat spiral coil and develop MRI signal receiver mounting the RF coil and the MRI signal receiving circuit. The outer diameter of the RF coil is 8 mm and its inductance and resistance of the RF coil were 1.0 μH and 2.0 Ω. The bending angle of distal tip is $-20° \sim +20°$.

SWR is less than 1.04 when the frequency of signal 8.5 MHz and transmitting efficiency of MRI signal receiving circuit is 99.97 %. Transmission efficiency can be kept high regardless of the angle of magnetic field and the RF coil. The SNR of MR images using the MRI signal receiver was 11.3 with the voxel size of $0.5 \times 0.5 \times 1.0 \text{mm}^3$. Comparing MR images by the MRI signal receiver and MR images by medical coil, the improvements of SNR are 3 times. When SNR of MR images is more than 10, we were able to observe structure of imaged object. So, we were able to observe structure of imaged object using MRI signal receiver with the voxel size of $0.5 \times 0.5 \times 1.0 \text{mm}^3$. However, SNR of the transverse plane away from coil 2mm is 5.8 and we cannot observe structure of imaged object. Precise positioning is required for acquisition high resolution MR images. To keep the angle between the RF coil and magnetic field is 90° using bending of the distal tip, the SNR of MR images is improved when the angle between MRI signal receiver and magnetic field $\theta \neq 0°$. The use of MRI siganal receiver using small RF coil, SNR of MR images can be enhanced and we successfully obtained clearly MR images of okra with the voxel size of $0.5 \times 0.5 \times 1.0 \text{mm}^3$. These results show that the MRI signal receiver is useful to acquire wide and high-resolution MR images.

In future work, we developed 5 DOF coil positioning manipulator to ensure good SNR from the whole imaged volume. Controlling the position and orientation angle of the RF coil using manipulator, high resolution MR images is acquired with MRI signal receiver.

References

1. Iseki, H., Muragaki, Y., Taira, T., Kawamata, T., Maruyama, T., Naemura, K., Nambu, K., Sugiura, M., Hirai, N., Hori, T., Takakura, K.: New Possibilities for Stereotaxis. Stereotactic and Functional Neurosurgery 76(3-4) (2002)
2. Seifert, V., Zimmermann, M., Trantakis, C., Vitzthum, H.-E., Kuhnel, K., Raabe, A., Bootz, F., Schneider, J.-P., Schmidt, F., Dietrich, J.: Open MRI-guided neurosurgery. Acta Neurochir. 141(5), 455–464 (1999)
3. McDannold, N., Clement, G., Black, P., Jolesz, F., Hynynen, K.: Transcranial MRI-guided focused ultrasound surgery of brain tumors: Initial findings in three patients. Neurosurgery 66(2), 323–332 (2010)
4. Iseki, H., Muragaki, Y., Nakamura, R., Hori, T., Takakura, K., Sugiura, M., Taniguchi, H., Ozawa, N., Sirakawa, H.: Intelligent Operating Theater and MR-compatible Operating System. MEDIX 39, 11–17 (2003)
5. Massin, C., Eroglu, S., Vincent, F., Gimi, B.S., Besse, P.-A., Magin, R.L., Popovic, R.S.: Planar microcoil-based magnetic resonance imaging of cells. In: 12th International Conference on TRANSDUCERS, Solid-State Sensors, Actuators and Microsystems, vol. 2, pp. 967–970 (2003)

6. Umakant, R., Dave, M., Andreanna, D., Williams, M., Jason, A., Wilson, M., Zahir Amin, M., David, J., Gilderdale, M., David, J., Larkman, M., Mark, R., Thursz, M., Simon, D., Taylor-Robinson, M., Nandita, M., deSouza, M.D.: Esophageal Cancer Staging with Endoscopic MR Imaging Pilot Study. Radiology 230(1), 281–286 (2004)

7. Badilita, V., Kratt, K., Baxan, N., Mohmmadzadeh, M., Burger, T., Weber, H., Elverfeldt, D.V., Hennig, J., Korvink, J.G., Wallrabe, U.: On-chip three dimensional microcoils for MRI at the microscale. The Royal Society of Chemistry 10, 1387–1390 (2010)

8. Krieger, A., Susil, R.C., Menard, C., Coleman, J.A., Fichtinger, G., Atalar, E., Whitcomb, L.L.: Design of a Novel MRI Compatible Manipulator for Image Guided Prostate Interventions. IEEE Transactions on Biomedical Engineering 52(2) (2005)

9. Fischer, G.S., Iordachita, I., Csoma, C., Tokuda, J., Dimaio, S.P., Hata, N., Fichtinger, G.: MRI-Compatible Pneumatic Robot for Transperineal Prostate Needle Placement. IEEE/ASME Transactions on Mechatronics 13(3) (2008)

10. Chinzei, K., Miller, K.: MRI Guided Surgical Robot. In: Australian Conference on Robotics and Automation, pp. 50–55 (2001)

11. Elster, A.D., Burdette, J.H.: Question & Answer in Magnetic Resonance Imaging, 2nd edn. Mosby, A Harcourt Health Sciences Company (2001)

12. Hoult, D.I., Ginsberg, N.S.: The Quantum Origins of the Free Induction Decay Signal and Spin Noise. Journal of Magnetic Resonance 148(1), 182–199 (2001)

Building Surrogate-Driven Motion Models from Cone-Beam CT via Surrogate-Correlated Optical Flow

James Martin, Jamie McClelland, Benjamin Champion, and David J. Hawkes

Centre for Medical Image Computing,
University College London, London, WC1E 6BT
james.martin.09@ucl.ac.uk

Abstract. An iterative approach to building a surrogate-driven motion model exclusively from cone-beam CT projections is presented. At each iteration the motion model is updated via an analytical expression derived from an optical flow-based approach, with corresponding improvements in the motion compensated reconstruction. The differences between the actual and estimated motion, as seen in the projections, are incorporated into a modified CBCT reconstruction. The correlations between these differences and the surrogate signals used in the motion model are also taken into account in determining the motion model updates. The updates are then composed with the previous estimate of the motion model and set as the new estimate of the motion model. New updates to this new estimate can then be calculated.

The motion model could be used to better understand respiratory motion immediately prior to a fraction of radiotherapy treatment, or to monitor key regions of interest during tracked treatments. This method would also be a promising candidate to adapt an older model built during planning to the day of treatment. The local, voxel-wise updates to the model can account for large inter-fraction changes, specific to the day of treatment.

Results on a simulated case are presented, derived from an actual patient dataset undergoing radiotherapy treatment for lung cancer. With the fitted motion, simulated projections of the animated patient volume were seen to be more similar to the actual projections than projections of the static patient volume. When compared with the actual motion, the mean L2-error over the entire patient was reduced to 0.46 mm.

1 Introduction

State-of-the-art radiotherapy (RT) rely on accurate identification of targets prior to and during treatment [1]. In treatments such as stereotactic ablative RT (SABR), the dose is delivered in fewer fractions (3-5), with a high dose per fraction. It is important to take tumour respiratory motion into consideration during these treatments [2]. A common approach is to use 4DCT planning scans to identify the extent of respiratory motion and add a margin onto the delineated

D. Stoyanov et al. (Eds.): IPCAI 2014, LNCS 8498, pp. 61–67, 2014.

tumour region. Gated and tracked [3,4] RT treatments account for respiratory motion by delivering dose at select parts of the breathing cycle or tracking the tumour throughout the breathing cycle, respectively. By accounting for respiratory motion of the tumour, gated and tracked approaches would allow a reduction in current margins, potentially allowing increased dose on the tumour region whilst further sparing the healthy region around the tumour. These approaches, however, rely on accurate identification of the tumour region throughout treatment. In addition, knowledge of organs at risk (OAR) respiratory motion would allow the impact on the OAR of adjustments to the dose delivery to also be modelled.

In this work, we propose a method to completely build a surrogate-driven motion model from a cone-beam CT (CBCT) scan. For the surrogate (indicator of respiratory state) we measure the skin surface displacement within a predefined region above the treatment couch. Previous work has included fitting a model of tumour motion directly to a CBCT scan [5,6]. This approach was recently extended to a whole patient motion model [7]. In this work, we build the motion model exclusively from the CBCT by extending an optical-flow-based approach. A novel method to determine voxel-wise updates to the motion model is presented. A modified CBCT reconstruction is proposed, which measures the differences between the actual and current estimate of the motion, and how these differences correlate to the surrogate signals of the motion model. From these reconstructions, the current estimate of the motion can be updated via an analytical expression. It is envisaged that this approach be used to assess respiratory motion immediately prior to treatment, particularly in situations where large inter-fraction variations are expected. These could include weight loss, tumour shrinkage or lung region collapse. Results on a simulated case are presented.

2   Methods and Materials

2.1   Motion Model

Presuming a motion-free image of the patient, V_{ref}, is available, it can be deformed to account for respiratory motion:

$$V_n(x) = V_{ref}\left(x + F_n(x)\right).\tag{1}$$

$x \in \Omega_{CBCT}$, where Ω_{CBCT} is the (3D) region imaged during the CBCT scan and n is an index corresponding to the time of each CBCT projection.

F_n is parameterised by a motion model which can take into account hysteresis and variations in length and depth of breathing cycle:

$$F_n(x) = s_n \Psi_1(x) + \dot{s}_n \Psi_2(x),\tag{2}$$

where s_n and $\dot{s}_n$ are the scalar surrogate signal associated with the nth projection, and its rate of change, respectively. Ψ_1 and Ψ_2 are the motion model deformation fields, which determine a spatially-dependent, linear relationship to s_n and $\dot{s}_n$ respectively.

As with previous work [6], the authors opt to use the Align RT camera system (Vision RT, London, UK) to produce the surrogate signal. The optical stereo-camera system is used to produce high-resolution surface images of the patient's chest. A region of the patient chest (enclosing parts of the thorax and abdomen) is chosen and the average height above the treatment couch within this box is used as the raw surrogate signal. After calculating the derivative trace, both traces are then normalised (mean subtracted; divided by standard deviation) giving the final surrogate traces.

2.2   Determining Ψ_1 and Ψ_2

If the motion free image of the patient were known, a Taylor expansion can be used to approximate the first order correction, δF_n^{est}, to an estimated deformation field, F_n^{est}:

$$
\begin{aligned}
V_n(x) &= V_{ref}\left(x + F_n^{est}(x) + \delta F_n^{est}(x)\right) \\
&\approx V_n^{est}(x) + \nabla V_n^{est}(x) \cdot \delta F_n^{est}(x).
\end{aligned}
\tag{3}
$$

In terms of updates to the motion model, the first order correction can be written:

$$
\delta F_n^{est} = s_n \delta \Psi_1 + \dot{s}_n \delta \Psi_2.
\tag{4}
$$

Note that $\delta \Psi_1$ and $\delta \Psi_2$ are defined in the space of V_n. Substituting the motion model updates (4) into (3), and rearranging:

$$
V_n - V_n^{est} \approx \nabla V_n^{est} \cdot \left(s_n \delta \Psi_1 + \dot{s}_n \delta \Psi_2\right).
\tag{5}
$$

A demons optical flow approach [8] can then be used to specify the form of the motion model deformation fields Ψ_1 and Ψ_2:

$$
s_n \delta \Psi_1 + \dot{s}_n \delta \Psi_2 \approx \frac{\nabla V_n^{est}}{(\nabla V_n^{est})^2}\left(V_n - V_n^{est}\right).
\tag{6}
$$

Updates to each motion model deformation field are desired. This is achievable by exploiting the covariance between the surrogate signals. First multiply both sides of (6) by s_n, sum over all n and divide by the number of patient states seen over the CBCT scan (i.e. number of projections), N:

$$
var(s)\delta \Psi_1 + covar(s, \dot{s})\delta \Psi_2 \approx \frac{1}{N} \sum_n \frac{\nabla V_n^{est}}{(\nabla V_n^{est})^2} s_n(V_n - V_n^{est}),
\tag{7}
$$

where $var(s) = \frac{1}{N}\sum_n s^2(n)$, $covar(s, \dot{s}) = \frac{1}{N}\sum_n s(n)\dot{s}(n)$. Because the surrogate signals have been normalised (mean subtracted; standard deviation divided), var and $covar$ are Pearson correlation coefficients and can be simplified: $var(s) = 1$ and $covar(s, \dot{s}) \ll 1$. The latter simplification comes from the approximation of independence between the surrogate signals. The proposed approach could still be used without this approximation, but an additional set of linear equations would need to be solved. Note that satisfying independence could be used as a condition for choosing a suitable set of surrogate signals. The simplified form of (7) is:

$$\delta\Psi_1 \approx \frac{1}{N} \sum_n \frac{\nabla V_n^{est}}{(\nabla V_n^{est})^2} s_n \left(V_n - V_n^{est}\right). \tag{8}$$

By approximating the sum of all patient states seen over the CBCT by a Feldkamp-Davis-Kress (FDK) CBCT reconstruction [9,10], it is possible to approximate the right side of (8) using an FDK reconstruction [11], giving:

$$\delta\Psi_1 \approx \frac{1}{N} \sum_n \frac{\nabla V_n^{est}}{(\nabla V_n^{est})^2} s_n P_n^\dagger \left(p_n - P_n(V_n^{est})\right), \tag{9}$$

where p_n are the CBCT projections, P_n the projection operator and $P^\dagger$ the FDK back-projection operator. A similar equation results for $\delta\Psi_2$ by multiplying (6) by $\dot{s}_n$ instead of s_n:

$$\delta\Psi_2 \approx \frac{1}{N} \sum_n \frac{\nabla V_n^{est}}{(\nabla V_n^{est})^2} \dot{s}_n P_n^\dagger \left(p_n - P_n(V_n^{est})\right). \tag{10}$$

The approximation is essentially using the reconstruction of the differences (in projection space) as an approximation to the average differences in 3D space. The multiplication by the the surrogate is additionally determining which of the differences are correlated with changes in the surrogate signal. As an analogy, if the projections were simply of the animated patient volume, this approximation would correspond to the assumption that the reconstruction is an estimate of the average of all the states seen over the CBCT in 3D space.

2.3   Iterative Approach

In practice, V_{ref} is not accurately known, as this would require knowledge of the exact respiratory motion from which to perform a motion compensated reconstruction (MCR). In this work, an iterative approach is taken, with improving estimates of the motion model deformation fields and MCR with each iteration. Starting with a zero motion assumption (i.e. $\Psi_1 = \Psi_2 = \mathbf{0}$), perform an MCR, V^0, and set it to V_{ref}. The updates to the motion model deformation fields $\delta\Psi_1^0$ and $\delta\Psi_2^0$ are then calculated, and the fields updated via:

$$\Psi_i^1 = \Psi_i^0 + \delta\Psi_i^0 \quad \text{for} \quad i = 1, 2. \tag{11}$$

The updated motion model deformation fields can then be used to determine the updated MCR and the procedure repeated.

For this work, a fixed number of iterations was set. Ten iterations were run with the updated motion model deformation fields having Gaussian smoothing applied prior to composition. To reduce calculation time, $\frac{V_n^{est}}{(V_n^{est})^2}$ was approximated by a Gaussian blurred V_{ref}, as $\frac{V_{ref}}{(V_{ref})^2}$, allowing it to be moved outside the summation in (9,10) and applied in one step. The Gaussian blurring applied was the same as that used to smooth the motion model deformation fields. To ensure that the optical flow equation is not unstable at small values of ∇V_n^{est}, updates to $\delta\Psi_1$ and $\delta\Psi_2$ were set to zero if $(\nabla V_{ref})^2 + \left(\frac{1}{N}\sum_n \dot{s}_n P_n^\dagger \left(p_n - P_n(V_n^{est})\right)\right)^2 < \varepsilon$, where ε was empically set to 5×10^{-5}.

2.4   Simulated Data

The method was tested on a simulated case, built from the 4DCT of an actual patient undergoing radiotherapy treatment. End exhale was registered to each of the seven other phases of the 4DCT and used to determine a transformation to average 4DCT space. Registrations were used to determine transformations from end-inhale to end-exhale, and from mid-exhale to mid-inhale. These transformations were used to determine Ψ_1 and Ψ_2. The end-exhale phase, moved to

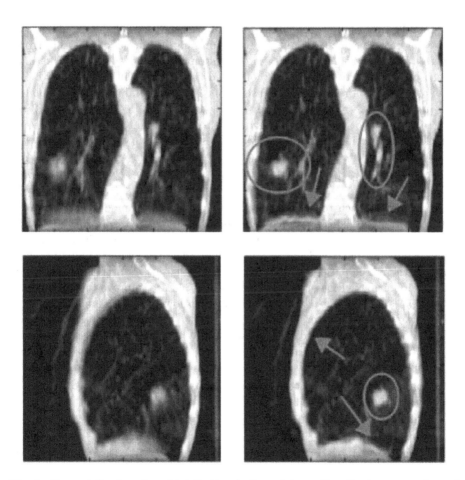

Fig. 1. Coronal (top) and sagittal (bottom) slices, intersecting the tumour region, of MCRs before (left) and after (right) fitting the motion model

average 4DCT space was then animated using Ψ_1, Ψ_2 and an actual patient surrogate trace. The accompanying CBCT geometry information for the respiratory trace was used to simulate a CBCT of the animated volume.

3   Results

After motion correction, improvements in the quality of the MCR were seen. Figure 1 shows coronal slices through the tumour region of the patient volume before and after motion correction. The regions of greatest improvement were in the diaphragm and tumour region. The ribs were also seen to have fewer streak artefacts, especially in the SI direction.

CBCT projections of the animated MCR with the fitted motion were seen to be more similar to the actual projections, than projections of the unanimated no motion reconstruction. Over all the projections, the sum of squared differences (SSD) error was reduced by 12%, from 1.6×10^9 to 1.4×10^9. This also corresponds with an improvement in similarity between actual and fitted motion model deformation fields, compared to assumming no motion. L2-norm errors were calculated for each voxel, between the estimated displacements (at the time of each projection) from the fitted model and the ground truth. Over the whole patient, mean L2-norm errors decreased from 1.4 to 0.46 mm. In the (manually segmented) tumour region, the mean L2-norm error was decreased from 4.2 to 2.6 mm. A movie of the original (left) and simulated (right) CBCT projections with the fitted motion have been included as supplementary material.

4   Conclusions and Future Work

An iterative approach to build a surrogate-driven motion model entirely from CBCT is presented. This approach could be used to reduce respiratory artefacts in CBCT reconstructions, and as an intensity-driven way to estimate patient motion when only the CBCT scan is available. Although an error reduction was seen over the whole patient and within the tumour region, further strategies to improve upon this will be explored. The authors plan to improve this method in multiple areas, including better defined termination conditions and improving the accuracy of the update. The latter improvement would be via the incorporation of a motion corrected reconstruction into the update. The authors are also planning to investigate a more physically justified basis for the direction-vector updates (i.e. alternatives to $\frac{\nabla V_{ref}}{(\nabla V_{ref})^2}$). In its current form, the algorithm takes approximately 10 minutes per iteration. With targeted use of GPU-based acceleration, the authors hope to more than half this figure.

Acknowledgments. James Martin gratefully acknowledges the support of the EPSRC funded UCL VEIV EngD programme and Vision RT. David Hawkes and Jamie McClelland acknowledge the support of EPSRC project EP/H046410/1, and the joint CR-UK & EPSRC funded KCL and UCL Comprehensive Cancer Imaging Centre, in association with the MRC and DoH (England).

References

1. Verellen, D., De Riddeer, M., Linthout, N., Tournel, K., Soete, G., Storme, G.: Innovations in image-guided radiotherapy. Nature Review (2007)
2. Benedict, S.H., Yenice, K.M., Followill, D., Galvin, J.M., Hinson, W., Kavanagh, B., Keall, P., Lovelock, M., Meeks, S., Papiez, L., Purdie, T., Sadagopan, R., Schell, M.C., Salter, B., Schlesinger, D.J., Shiu, A.S., Solberg, T., Song, D.Y., Stieber, V., Timmerman, R., Tomé, W.A., Verellen, D., Wang, L., Yin, F.F.: Stereotactic body radiation therapy: The report of aapm task group 101. Medical Physics 37(8), 4078–4101 (2010)
3. Kubo, H.D., Hill, B.C.: Respiration gated radiotherapy treatment: a technical study. Physics in Medicine and Biology **41**(1) 41(1), 83 (1996)
4. Schweikard, A., Shiomi, H., Adler, J.: Respiration tracking in radiosurgery. Medical Physics 31(10), 2738–2741 (2004)
5. Martin, J., McClelland, J., Thomas, C., Wildermuth, K., Landau, D., Ourselin, S., Hawkes, D.: Motion modelling and motion compensated reconstruction of tumours in cone-beam computed tomography. In: 2012 IEEE Workshop on Mathematical Methods in Biomedical Image Analysis (MMBIA), pp. 281–286 (January 2012)
6. Martin, J., McClelland, J., Yip, C., Thomas, C., Hartill, C., Ahmad, S., O'Brien, R., Meir, I., Landau, D., Hawkes, D.: Building motion models of lung tumours from cone-beam ct for radiotherapy applications. Physics in Medicine and Biology 58(6), 1809 (2013)
7. Martin, J., McClelland, J., Yip, C., Thomas, C., Hartill, C., Ahmad, S., Meir, I., Landau, D., Hawkes, D.: Fully-deformable patient motion models from cone-beam ct for radiotherapy applications. In: Proceedings of the 17th International Conference on the Use of Computers in Radiation Therapy (ICCR 2013). 2013 Journal of Physics: Conference Series (2013)
8. Thirion, J.P.: Image matching as a diffusion process: an analogy with maxwell's demons. Medical Image Analysis 2(3), 243–260 (1998)
9. Feldkamp, L., Davis, L., Kress, J.: Practical cone-beam algorithm. JOSA A 1(6), 612–619 (1984)
10. Lewis, J.H., Li, R., Jia, X., Watkins, W.T., Lou, Y., Song, W.Y., Jiang, S.B.: Mitigation of motion artifacts in cbct of lung tumors based on tracked tumor motion during cbct acquisition. Physics in Medicine and Biology 56(17), 5485 (2011)
11. Rit, S., Wolthaus, J.W.H., van Herk, M., Sonke, J.J.: On-the-fly motion-compensated cone-beam ct using an a priori model of the respiratory motion. Medical Physics 36(6), 2283–2296 (2009)

Vascular 3D+T Freehand Ultrasound Using Correlation of Doppler and Pulse-Oximetry Data

Christoph Hennersperger, Athanasios Karamalis, and Nassir Navab

Chair for Computer Aided Medical Procedures (CAMP), TU Munich, Germany
christoph.hennersperger@tum.de

Abstract. We present a new system to acquire and reconstruct 3D freehand ultrasound volumes from arbitrary 2D image acquisitions over time. Motion artifacts are significantly reduced with a novel gating approach which correlates pulse oximetry data with Doppler ultrasound. The reconstruction problem is split into a ray-based sample selection on a per-scanline basis and a backward algorithm which is based on the concept of normalized convolution. We introduce an adaptive derivation of time-domain interpolation from the correlated pulse-oximetry and Doppler signals as well as an ellipsoid kernel size for spatial interpolation based on the physical resolution of the ultrasound data. We compare pulse-oximetry to classical ECG gating and further show the suitability of our normalized pulse signal for 3D+T reconstructions. The ease of use of the setup without the need of uncomfortable triggering via ECG provides the ability to use 3D+T ultrasound in every day clinical practice.

Keywords: freehand ultrasound, vascular, 4D, cardiac pulse phase, doppler, correlation, adaptive, reconstruction.

1 Introduction

Ultrasound imaging is an essential part of clinical imaging and plays a crucial role in diagnosis of cardiovascular diseases. Three dimensional (3D) ultrasound imaging is already used in obstetrics for diagnosis of facial abnormalities and has high potential for vascular imaging [4]. While 2D matrix array probes are providing 3D and 4D (3D+T) ultrasound information in realtime [10], they are - as conventional 1D array probes - limited in their field of view with respect to transducer design. Freehand ultrasound as an alternative or add-on technique allows the acquisition of high quality 3D ultrasound of steady anatomy; providing an extended field-of-view [11] and thus enables a better overview for physicians. For vascular applications though, the data is acquired over a certain period of time, in which the anatomy changes due to pulsating blood flow.

One major area where avoiding these artifacts is of crucial importance is 3D and 4D volume reconstruction (compounding). The goal here is to interpolate the acquired, irregularly sampled data onto a regular spatial 3D grid to enable an extraction of diagnostic indices (e.g. vessel volume from a segmentation) and visualization of the data in 3D. We propose the use of a fingertip pulse oximetry device,

D. Stoyanov et al. (Eds.): IPCAI 2014, LNCS 8498, pp. 68–77, 2014.

in addition to a 3D freehand ultrasound setup, recording B-Mode and Doppler ultrasound data, to reconstruct 3D volumes for desired cardiac pulse phases. This offers the possibility to accurately reconstruct pulse phase information while avoiding the cumbersome placement of electrodes for ECG gating, which is not applicable in many every-day screening applications with short investigation periods. Pulse oximeters are used as a standard tool in hospitals and allow the monitoring of the patient's oxygen saturation and heart frequency by analyzing the light absorption due to oxygenated red blood cells through thin tissue (i.e. finger or earlobe). However, as the sensors are measuring the local pulsation, which is not synchronous to cardiac excitation due to different patient anatomy, the signals cannot be used for interpolation without a reference to the ultrasound data.

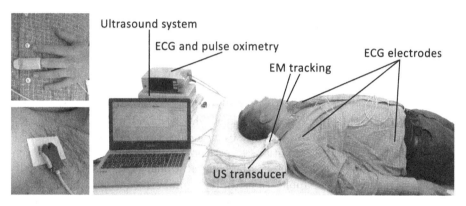

Fig. 1. The experimental setup consists of a combined pulse oximetry / ECG device, an open-access ultrasound system and two electomagnetic trackers mounted on the ultrasound probe. For ECG gating, three electrodes (left bottom) have to be mounted on three torso positions to retrieve a ECG curve, while for pulse-oximetry (left top), only a fingertip is required.

To provide high-quality reconstructions and make full use of the discussed system setup we propose a novel approach to correlate pulse oximetry with Doppler ultrasound information. This allows an automatic and accurate calibration of the pulse oximetry sensor individually for every acquisition. Thus, the pulse oximetry data can be used as a reference for constructing normalized pulse phase signals. The reconstruction of 3D+T volume data from single ultrasound scanlines is computed using a concept similar to normalized convolution [8] for $0-th$ order interpolation. We propose the selection of samples for the reconstruction of every voxel based on an ellipsoid region defined by the US properties around every sample in a backward transformation step. Therefore, we are able to split the sample-selection from the voxel interpolation to reconstruct smooth volumes with respect to the local spatial resolution of the original ultrasound sample data. We compare pulse-oximetry to ECG gating and further demonstrate the advantages of using adaptive time-domain interpolation for the application of carotid artery freehand ultrasound.

2 Related Work

Although ECG can be used to accurately detect cardiac phases for freehand ultrasound [2], the equipment needed is relatively cumbersome and consequently several alternative methods were developed relying on the ultrasound data only. First approaches based on filtering of intermediate signals containing cardiac information calculated from intensity values [13] or via the centroid algorithm [6] demonstrated good performances but needed either user input or were limited to certain areas. Further approaches based on phase correlation [12] and manifold learning with Laplacian eigenmaps [14] were successfully applied to US data for detection of both cardiac and respiratory motion. However, most of the proposed image-based methods rely on a constant pulse frequency for detection [13, 6, 12] and provide rough estimates of cardiac pulse phases [13, 6, 12, 14] which could introduce artifacts in 4D reconstruction with time-domain interpolation.

3D volume reconstruction methods can be grouped into pixel-based methods, voxel-based methods and function-based methods [11]. Pixel-based methods transform pixel values with a forward transformation into corresponding voxels. Voxel-based methods traverse every voxel and map back corresponding pixel values. Function-based methods estimate an interpolation function from the input data and evaluate the function at a regular grid. Recent advances in reconstruction methods also led to improvements by modeling US statistics in a physical way by using Nakagami distributions [7]. Although these methods provide volumetric data of exceptional quality, the computational demands prevent their application in time-critical applications. In [1] a similar reconstruction approach is used to carry out interpolation in the spatio-temporal (4D) domain. However they apply interpolation only in forward direction and do not consider adaptive interpolation in both spatial and temporal domain.

3 Methods

Our goal is to obtain an instensity value $I(v_i, \phi)$ for every voxel $v_i \in V$ in the Cartesian equidistant volume $V \in \mathbb{R}^3$ for a given timepoint ϕ in the cardiac pulse phase. We separate the ultrasound sample selection in spatial and temporal domain from the actual voxel reconstruction, as a sample selection in voxel coordinates (i.e. searching for the k nearest neighbours in the 4D volume) would ignore the physical and temporal information of our acquisition. Instead, we supply temporal and spatial weights for every sample-voxel relation to the reconstruction step. These weights are defined based on either the (temporal) pulse phase information, or the (spatial) ultrasound beam information. Therefore, the reconstruction approach is split into three parts: i) the retrieval of a normalized pulse phase signal for every acquisition; ii) a physics-based selection of ultrasound samples contributing to each voxel; and iii) the reconstruction of the final voxel intensity value from the selected samples.

3.1 Retrieval of Normalized Pulse Signal

We aim to reconstruct 4D data for different points within the cardiac pulse phase and thus introduce a fingertip pulse oximetry device as a reference sensor in the setup, which provides a measure of the oxygen saturation throughout the cardiac pulse phase. As pulse oximetry values are influenced by the percentage of blood that is loaded with oxygen [3], the measured signal changes during cardiac pulse phases and is related to changes in vessel diameter caused by volume-deviations. This is exactly what we are aiming for as changes in vessel diameter are the cause of "pulsatile" artifacts in ultrasound acquisitions. Consequently, the pulse-oximetry signal can not only be used for gating, as it is currently also done with ECG, but also to reconstruct a normalized pulse shape signal. This shape signal can then be used directly within the reconstruction.

In order to be able to utilize the pulse oximetry signal, we first have to carry out a calibration to the ultrasound data, as due to different anatomy and pulse-wave-velocities, the temporal offset between fingertip and target ultrasound location will vary among different acquisitions. For vascular applications, a second signal containing pulse phase information can be retrieved from the Doppler ultrasound components belonging to non-stationary, moving scatterers within the volume of interest. These components can be identified as the sum of all non-zero Doppler data components after clutter filtering of the ultrasound ensemble, where stationary and slowly moving components are removed from the signal. By having two signals containing pulse information, we can automatically map US data to cardiac pulse phases for individual acquisitions without any preconditions of a constant pulse frequency or the absence of arrhythmia. To enable a direct correlation, we extract an arterial flow velocity signal - corresponding to Doppler signals - from the pulse oximetry data by taking the gradient of the signal [3] (see Fig. 2a). Consequently, the time offset $o_{d \to p}$ between the corresponding data can be retrieved by finding the maximum cross-correlation of both real signals as:

$$o_{d \to p} = \arg\max_{l} \sum_{k=0}^{K-l-1} d_{k+l} * p'_k \quad w.r.t. \quad p'_k = \frac{\partial p_k}{\partial k}, \tag{1}$$

with p'_k and d_{k+l} representing the pulse derivative and shifted Doppler data with offset l respectively. Based on the calibration, we can use the pulse-oximetry signal to reconstruct a normalized pulse shape signal $\bar{p}$. Therefore, we first automatically detect the set of M pulse periods $[m_1, \ldots, m_M]$ in the pulse oximetry signal corresponding to the sets of pulse samples $p_{i \to j}^m = [p_i; p_j]$ as follows. As the distance $j - i$ between the peaks varies even within one acquisition, we use the average peak-to-peak distance $D = mean(j - i) \quad \forall i,j$ with $0 \le i < j \le K$ to map all pulse periods $p_{i \to j}$ to the same interval

$$\overline{p_{i \to j}^m} = p_i \ldots p_j \to p_1 \ldots p_D. \tag{2}$$

To preserve the shape of every pulse signal in an optimal way, we use cubic spline interpolation to conduct this mapping to the normalized pulse shapes.

To reconstruct a normalized pulse shape $\hat{p}$ from $m = 1 \ldots M - 1$ pulse periods $\overline{p_{i \to j}}$, we use a weighted average of all normalized pulse shapes, where the weight is defined by the deviation of the original shape period length to the average peak-to-peak distance

$$\hat{p} = \frac{1}{\Omega} \sum_{\forall m \in M} w_m \cdot \overline{p_{i \to j}^m} \qquad (3)$$

$$w_m = 1 - \frac{|D - (j - i)|}{D}, \qquad \Omega = \sum_{\forall m \in M} w_m. \qquad (4)$$

The normalized pulse phase signal $\bar{p}$ can then be retrieved by mapping $\hat{p}$ to every peak-to-peak interval of M accordingly by spline-interpolation. Figure 2b shows an example for resulting normalized pulse phases from given input data.

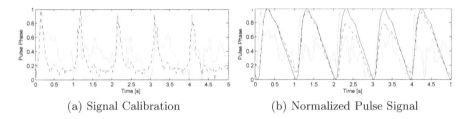

(a) Signal Calibration   (b) Normalized Pulse Signal

Fig. 2. Left: arterial flow signal extracted from pulse oximetry (blue, dashed) used for time calibration with the Doppler signal (green, solid). Right: normalized pulse phase $\bar{p}$ (blue, solid) retrieved from Doppler data (green solid) and pulse oximetry (blue, dashed) for a freehand scan of the carotid artery.

3.2   Ultrasound Sample Selection

Before reconstructing a final intensity value, we have to select and weight contributing samples for every voxel based on spatial and temporal constraints. Every sample has a position s_j, normalized pulse value $\bar{p}_j$ and an intensity value $I(s_j)$. We first select samples for every voxel based on the voxel position in the sample coordinates. To do so, we set an ellipsoid around every sample, representing its corresponding influence region

$$G_s(v_i, s_j) = \begin{cases} K(v_i, s_j) & \text{if } \frac{\left(v_{i,x}^{s_j} - s_{j,x}\right)^2}{d_{mx}^2} + \frac{\left(v_{i,y}^{s_j} - s_{j,y}\right)^2}{d_{my}^2} + \frac{\left(v_{i,z}^{s_j} - s_{j,z}\right)^2}{d_{mz}^2} \leq 1 \\ 0 & \text{otherwise,} \end{cases} \qquad (5)$$

where s_j is the position of sample j in volume coordinates and $v_i^{s_j}$ the i-th voxel position in coordinates of sample j. The maximum spatial distances d_{mx}, d_{my}, d_{mz} to the sample location are set according to the axial, lateral and elevational resolution of the ultrasound data, defined by the transducer and acquisition properties [9] given by our US system (see Sec 3.4). We define the spatial weight of every US sample with respect to a target voxel based on the voxel position in relation to a three-dimensional exponential decay centered at the sample position $s_{j,x}, s_{j,y}, s_{j,z}$ of the current scanline ray sample j

$$K(v_i, s_j) = \frac{1}{(2\pi)^{\frac{3}{2}} |B|^{\frac{1}{2}}} e^{-\frac{1}{2}(v_i^{s_j} - s_j)^T B^{-1}(v_i^{s_j} - s_j)}, \quad B = diag(\sigma_x^2, \sigma_y^2, \sigma_z^2). \quad (6)$$

The spatial variances are set to $\sigma_x = \frac{1}{2}d_{mx}, \sigma_y = \frac{1}{2}d_{my}, \sigma_z = \frac{1}{2}d_{mz}$ to assure the ellipsoid cut-off at 2σ (95.4%). By specifying these distances based on the physical properties, only samples fullfilling these prior information are contributing to the final voxel intensity.

For the temporal selection of samples, weights are retrieved from a linear decay, according to the distance of the normalized pulse phase sample point $0 \leq \phi \leq 1$ to the desired reconstruction point ϕ with

$$G_t(\overline{p_j}, \phi) = \begin{cases} 1 - \frac{|\overline{p_j} - \phi|}{d_{mt}} & \text{if } |\overline{p_j} - \phi| \leq d_{mt} \\ 0 & \text{otherwise} \end{cases}, \quad (7)$$

which enables a reconstruction for any pulse point ϕ throughout the cardiac pulse phase.

3.3   Normalized Backward Reconstruction

In order to obtain the final intensity value $I(v_i, \phi)$ from our (sparse) set of samples, we make use of the concept of normalized convolution. Therefore, we modifiy the orginal concept [8] and apply it as a backward-transformation. By doing so, we can incorporate our spatial and temporal weights directly, while for a forward normalized convoluation, the weights would be retrieved from the convolution of the sample space with a fixed kernel, which would be unrelated to the ultrasound physics. We calculate the cumulative intensities $I_{cum}(v_i, \phi)$ and certainties $C_{cum}(v_i, \phi)$ by traversing all input samples $S = \{s_1, \ldots, s_j, \ldots, s_N\}, s_j \in \mathbb{R}^3$ for every voxel as

$$C_{cum}(v_i, \phi) = \sum_{\forall j \in S} G_s(v_i, s_j) \cdot G_t(\overline{p_j}, \phi) \cdot C(s_j) \quad (8)$$

$$I_{cum}(v_i, \phi) = \sum_{\forall j \in S} G_s(v_i, s_j) \cdot G_t(\overline{p_j}, \phi) \cdot I(s_j) \cdot C(s_j). \quad (9)$$

Here, $C(s_j) \in [0 \ldots 1]$ is a given certainty value for every input sample s_j, representing the reliability of the underlying data sample and G_s and G_t are the spatial and temporal weighting functions. Once all voxels have been traversed, $C_{cum}(v_i, \phi)$ states the total certainty of the individual voxels. It is noteworthy that $|G_s(v_i, s_j)| \leq \frac{1}{(2\pi)^{3/2} \sigma_x \sigma_y \sigma_z}$ for a single sample contributing to the surrounding voxels, thus $C_{cum}(v_i, \phi)$ is not limited to a specific value range. Consequently, the final volume intensity values can be reconstructed as:

$$I(v_i, \phi) = \frac{I_{cum}(v_i, \phi)}{C_{cum}(v_i, \phi)}. \tag{10}$$

3.4   Experimental Setup Protocol

All experiments in this work were carried out with an open access ultrasound system (Aurotech ultrasound AS, model MANUS) with a linear array probe (128 elements - single element width $0.27mm$, height $4mm$, focal depth $30mm$, 45 aperture elements) operating at 8MHz. For every dataset, pulse-oximetry as well as ECG data was acquired synchroneously with a combined POX-ECG system (Medlab GmbH, model P-OX100). An overview of the whole system is shown in Fig. 1.

ECG Cross-Validation: As ECG gating still is mostly considered as the only alternative to achieve an accurate pulse gating, we validated our calibrated pulse-oximetry signals versus ECG slopes. For 6 subjects, 2 records each were acquired. As the total blood volume in the fingertip is influenced by the relative position of the finger w.r.t. the heart, signals could change for varying positions. In our experimental setup the overall patient position (lying on table, similar to conventional ultrasound examinations) was kept constant throughout the experiments, but the position of the fingertip changed for the two recordings to analyze POX signal changes. For the first records, the fingertip was placed at a relaxed position at the table, while for the second recordings the patients had to lift their fingers as high as possible. Scans of about $10s$ were acquired for each position. Subsequently, automatic pulse-oximetry to ultrasound calibration was carried out and additionally, a vessel-tracking method based on [5] employed to the ultrasound data to extract a vessel lumen diameter signal from the recorded 2D frames as an index of vessel expansion and compression. For validation, the pulse peaks were extracted manually from the ECG, the lumen diameter and our normalized pulse signals to compare the distances between the diameter signal and the ECG and POX signals respectively.

Evaluation of Resolution-Preserving Reconstruction: Without time-domain interpolation, cardiac pulsation will either cause the appearance of a "pulsating" vessel in the 3D volume for low frame density or a loss of contour sharpness in regions where deformation is visible throughout the cardiac cycle. The consequence is that a potential diagnostic value would be falsified and the robustness and accuracy of image processing methods affected in general. Thus we evaluate the suitability of our novel normalized pulse phase signal for both cases and compare it to i) a constant volume without time-domain consideration; ii) a linear monotonic increasing pulse phase signal between subsequent pulse peaks, and iii) a linear pulse signal from mininmum to maximum peaks and vice versa. As before, scans of 6 volunteers were conducted, where for every subject both a slow (mean length $58.48s$) and a fast scan (mean length $22.32s$) of the carotid artery was acquired. For all datasets, volumes were reconstructed with a spacing of $0.25mm$ for the four compared methods. The maximum temporal distance d_{mt} was decreased stepwise to $d_{mt} = [\frac{1}{2}, \ldots, \frac{1}{20}] = \frac{1}{2n_s}, n_s = 1 \ldots 10$, which is equivalent to a subdivision of each cardiac pulse phase in n_s steps. We compare how well the original US data is preserved in the reconstructed 3D volumes by evaluating the Mean Squared Error (MSE) of the reconstructed volumes $\in [0, 1]$ with respect to the input samples at their corresponding locations.

4 Results and Discussion

The results for the POX-ECG validation of all compared distances are shown in Table 1. It can be seen that i) the peak to peak distance of the normalized pulse signal is almost identical to the ECG data (mean distance of 1.2ms), and ii) the calibrated pulse signals have a mean deviation to the extracted diameter signal of $-34ms$. As the temporal resolution of the diameter signal extracted from the ultrasound data is low compared to the other signals (12Hz compared to 100Hz for POX and ECG signals), a standard deviation approximately equal to the ultrasound sampling period (83.3ms) is considered as optimal, which is facilitated by the standard deviation of the peak-to-peak distances in the vessel diameter signal (104.9ms). As the deviation of the normalized pulse peaks is perfectly within this range, the extracted ultrasound signal is the limiting factor to the general accuracy. This suggests that the pulse oximetry signal is well-suited for gating of ultrasound acquisitions.

Table 1. Signal pulse period results. Shown are the peak distances between the pulse oximetry and ECG signal, as well as the distance from the pulse oximetry and ECG signals respectively to the vessel diameter signal.

Distance Comparison	Finger Position			
	Relaxed		Lifted	
	$\mu[s]$	$\sigma[s]$	$\mu[s]$	$\sigma[s]$
Δ Area	-	0.1049	-	0.1023
$\Delta \bar{p}$ to ECG	0.0009	0.0187	0.0016	0.0229
$\Delta \bar{p}$ to Area	-0.0341	0.0774	-0.0285	0.0799
Δ ECG to Area	-0.2178	0.0858	-0.1349	0.1348

Results for the evaluation fo the time interpolation scheme are shown in Fig. 3 for all methods. When comparing slow and fast ultrasound scans, it becomes clear that for the fast scans, the input ultrasound information is preserved best without time domain consideration. Disregard of the pulse information is still not recommendable, as this would potentially distort diagnostic values extracted from the volume datasets. For both slow and fast scans it can be observed that our normalized pulse phase provides the lowest errors for the different number of time steps and further preserves the input information better as a static reconstruction for slow scans. This preservation is visualized in Fig. 4, where a reconstruction without considering pulse information is compared to our method considering pulse information. For the former, edges are appearing less sharp and details get lost by using all input samples from different pulse phases for the reconstruction. With our method, details and edges are preserved much better.

Beyond that also a time-domain analysis is enabled by having distinct volume datasets for every point along the cardiac pulse phase.

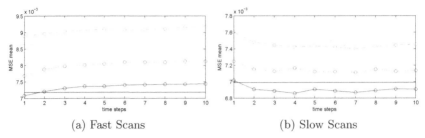

(a) Fast Scans   (b) Slow Scans

Fig. 3. Reconstruction sample preservation. Shown is the mean MSE averaged over all fast/slow scans. The black solid line equals the baseline error without time-domain consideration. Compared is our method (blue, solid) to the linear pulse phase (red, dotted) and the min-to-max linear (green, dash-dotted).

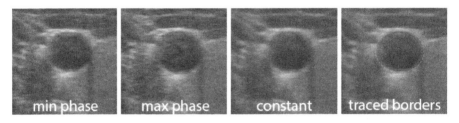

Fig. 4. Reconstruction for different pulse phases. Shown are cross-sectional slices through the vessel for min./max. vessel expansion, a volume without consideration of pulse data (constant) and overlaid contours for min./max. expansion.

Setup Robustness: In respect of the presented experiments, we did not notice significant distortions of the pulse oximetry signals as long as the patients did not move their fingers during acquisition. However, as opposed to pulse oximetry, for placement of the ECG electrodes, full attention was necessary in all experiments to provide useful signals. Thus we suggest that especially for time-critical situations, our technique could be a promising and robust alternative to classical gating. However to confirm these assumptions w.r.t to a direct clinical application, a thorough validation of the presented system is neccessary; especially in regard to different patient conditions (e.g. arrythmia or calloused finger skin) and working environments with possible distortions such as operating lights.

5   Conclusion

We presented a new system to reconstruct 3D+T volume data from freehand ultrasound in combination with a pulse oximetry sensor. We introduced a novel method for correlating pulse oximetry with Doppler ultrasound, enabling an accurate time-calibration on a per-record basis. We further showed how a normalized pulse phase signal can be defined based on the pulse oximetry data to be used directly within time-domain interpolation. The setup can be used to re-construct 3D volume data for cardiac pulse phases superior compared to today's freehand approaches and delievers improved capabilities for vascular ultrasound reconstruction compared to classical ECG gating. Furthermore, the uncomfort-able use of ECG electrodes can be circumvented, which allows a more extensive use of 3D+T in every-day clinical scenarios.

References

[1] Bosch, J., van Stralen, M., Voormolen, M., Krenning, B., Lancee, C., Reiber, J., van der Steen, A., De Jong, N.: Improved spatiotemporal voxel space interpola-tion for 3D echocardiography with irregular sampling and multibeat fusion. In: Ultrasonics Symposium, pp. 1232–1235. IEEE (2005)

[2] Brattain, L.J., Howe, R.D.: Real-time 4D ultrasound mosaicing and visualiza-tion. In: Proc. 14th Intern. Conf. Med. Image Comput. Comput. Assist. Interv., pp. 105–112 (2011)

[3] Cook, L.B.: Extracting arterial flow waveforms from pulse oximeter waveforms. Anaesthesia 56(6), 551–555 (2001)

[4] Forsberg, F.: Ultrasonic biomedical technology; marketing versus clinical reality. Ultrasonics 42, 17–27 (2004)

[5] Guerrero, J., Salcudean, S.E., McEwen, J.A., Masri, B.A., Nicolaou, S.: Real-time vessel segmentation and tracking for ultrasound imaging applications. IEEE Transactions on Medical Imaging 26(8), 1079–1090 (2007)

[6] Karadayi, K., Hayashi, T., Kim, Y.: Automatic image-based gating for 4D ul-trasound. In: 28th Annual International Conference of the IEEE Engineering in Medicine and Biology Society, EMBS 2006, pp. 2388–2391 (2006)

[7] Klein, T., Hansson, M., Navab, N.: Modeling of multi-view 3D freehand radio frequency ultrasound. In: Ayache, N., Delingette, H., Golland, P., Mori, K. (eds.) MICCAI 2012, Part I. LNCS, vol. 7510, pp. 422–429. Springer, Heidelberg (2012)

[8] Knutsson, H., Westin, C.F.: Normalized and differential convolution. In: Proceed-ings of the 1993 IEEE Computer Society Conference on Computer Vision and Pattern Recognition, CVPR 1993, pp. 515–523 (1993)

[9] Ng, A., Swanevelder, J.: Resolution in ultrasound imaging. Continuing Education in Anaesthesia, Critical Care & Pain 11, 186–192 (2011)

[10] Prager, R., Ijaz, U., Gee, A., Treece, G.: Three-dimensional ultrasound imaging. In: Proc. Institution of Mechanical Engineers, Part H: Journal of Engineering in Medicine, vol. 224, pp. 193–223 (2010)

[11] Solberg, O.V., Lindseth, F., Torp, H., Blake, R.E., Nagelhus Hernes, T.A.: Free-hand 3D ultrasound reconstruction algorithms - a review. Ultrasound in Medicine and Biology 33, 991–1009 (2007)

[12] Sundar, H., Khamene, A., Yatziv, L., Xu, C.: Automatic image-based cardiac and respiratory cycle synchronization and gating of image sequences. In: Yang, G.-Z., Hawkes, D., Rueckert, D., Noble, A., Taylor, C. (eds.) MICCAI 2009, Part II. LNCS, vol. 5762, pp. 381–388. Springer, Heidelberg (2009)

[13] Treece, G., Prager, R., Gee, A., Cash, C., Berman, L.: Grey-scale gating for free-hand 3D ultrasound. In: Proceedings of the 2002 IEEE Intern. Symposium on Biomedical Imaging, pp. 993–996 (2002)

[14] Wachinger, C., Yigitsoy, M., Navab, N.: Manifold learning for image-based breathing gating with application to 4D ultrasound. In: Jiang, T., Navab, N., Pluim, J.P.W., Viergever, M.A. (eds.) MICCAI 2010, Part II. LNCS, vol. 6362, pp. 26–33. Springer, Heidelberg (2010)

Semi-automated Quantification of Fibrous Cap Thickness in Intracoronary Optical Coherence Tomography

Guillaume Zahnd[1], Antonios Karanasos[2], Gijs van Soest[3], Evelyn Regar[2], Wiro J. Niessen[1], Frank Gijsen[3], and Theo van Walsum[1]

[1] Biomedical Imaging Group Rotterdam,
Departments of Radiology and Medical Informatics, Erasmus Medical Center,
P.O. Box 2040, 3000 CA Rotterdam, The Netherlands
g.zahnd@erasmusmc.nl
[2] Department of Interventional Cardiology, Thorax Center,
Erasmus MC, Rotterdam, The Netherlands
[3] Department of Biomedical Engineering, Erasmus MC, Rotterdam, The Netherlands

Abstract. Acute coronary syndrome represents a leading cause of death. Events are triggered by rupture of atheromatic plaques, as a result of disruption of the overlying fibrous cap. Pathological studies have shown that cap thickness is a critical component of plaque stability. Therefore, assessment of fibrous cap thickness could be a valuable tool for estimating the risk of future events. To aid preoperative planning and perioperative decision making, intracoronary optical coherence tomography imaging can provide very detailed information about arterial wall structure. However, manual interpretation of the images is laborious, subject to variability, and therefore not always sufficiently reliable for immediate decision of treatment. We present a novel semi-automatic computerized interventional imaging tool to quantify coronary fibrous cap thickness in optical coherence tomography. The most challenging issue when estimating cap thickness is caused by the diffuse nature of the anatomical abluminal interface to be detected. Our method can successfully extract the fibrous cap contours using a robust dynamic programming framework based on a geometrical *a priori*. Validated on a dataset of 90 images from 11 patients, our method provided a good agreement for minimum cap thickness with the reference tracings performed by a medical expert (35.7 ± 33.3 μm, R=.68) and was similar to inter-observer reproducibility (35.2 ± 33.1 μm, R=.66), while being significantly faster and fully reproducible. This tool demonstrated promising performances and could potentially be used for online identification of high risk-plaques.

Keywords: Coronary artery, Optical coherence tomography, Interventional imaging, Thin-cap fibroatheroma, Contour segmentation, Dynamic programming, Preoperative planning.

1 Introduction

Cardiovascular diseases represent the leading cause of mortality in industrialized countries and are responsible of one third of all global deaths worldwide [1].

D. Stoyanov et al. (Eds.): IPCAI 2014, LNCS 8498, pp. 78–89, 2014.

Acute coronary syndrome (ACS) is the most severe manifestation of atherosclerotic disease and is associated with high mortality and morbidity. Pathological studies have shown that the main cause of ACS is acute coronary thrombosis, which is mainly due to plaque rupture [2]. Plaques that bear morphological resemblance to ruptured plaques are called "high-risk" or "vulnerable" plaques and are characterized by a large lipid necrotic core, an overlying thin fibrous cap (FC), and dense macrophage infiltration (Fig. 1a) [3]. These plaques are also called thin cap fibroatheromas (TCFA) and are considered the precursor phenotype of plaque rupture. Among the aforementioned morphological characteristics, FC thickness is considered the most critical component of plaque stability (*i.e.* thinner caps being more vulnerable), and the threshold of 65 μm has been widely adopted to identify high risk lesions [4]. Therefore, identification and quantification of vulnerable plaques *in vivo* prior to the occurrence of events, towards the objective of an appropriate surgical treatment such as percutaneous coronary intervention (*e.g.* balloon angioplasty or stent placement), represents a major clinical challenge.

Intravascular optical coherence tomography (OCT) is a novel biomedical imaging modality that enables detailed visualization of tissues with a near-histology resolution [5]. The main underlying principle of OCT is based on the emission and reception of near-infrared light (center wavelength of $1280 - 1350$ nm). In a similar fashion as intravascular ultrasound, the entire inner circumference of the vessel is investigated by the probe rotating along its axis and acquiring a so-called A-line signal for each angular step. The intensity and echo time of all A-lines are then converted into a gray-scale representation that corresponds to a cross-sectional image of the investigated biological tissues (Fig. 1b). This emerging technology allows minimally invasive acquisition of three-dimensional *in vivo* data (*i.e.* a stack of consecutive cross-sectional images along the length of the assessed artery segment) at very high spatial resolution ($10 - 20$ μm). OCT has been demonstrated to be well suited for accurate characterization of the structure of arterial wall most superficial layers, indicating the degree of subclinical atherosclerotic lesion formation [6]. OCT is the only *in vivo* imaging modality that can accurately assess FC thickness, the most critical component of plaque stability, and thus can be potentially used for *in vivo* identification of high-risk plaques in preoperative planning [7].

Although OCT images are acquired online during intervention, quantification of FC thickness in fibroatheromas is currently performed manually offline [8,9]. This operation is hampered by two major drawbacks, as manual image analysis is generally *i)* cumbersome and time consuming, and *ii)* subject to a certain degree of variability in between different analysts [6,7]. Therefore, the clinical need of immediate and reliable information often remains unsatisfied. Moreover, actual segmentation of the abluminal interface of a fibrous cap remains a challenging task, as the necrotic-core containing fibroatheromas consists in progressively unravelling tissues and are visualized in OCT as a signal-poor region with diffuse contours and high signal attenuation (Fig 1a,b) [9].

In the objective to tackle these issues and permit fast and accurate FC quantification in the intervention room, several teams recently developed various (semi) automated computerized methods to quantify FC thickness. Approaches based on pixel classification using the attenuation coefficient of the backscattered light have been proposed [10–12]. These techniques could successfully identify and locate different types of tissues, among which fibroatheromas, however they are not devised to provide information regarding the actual delineation of anatomical interfaces. Another approach, based on contour segmentation by means of dynamic programming, was proposed to specifically assess FC thickness [13]. This seminal study demonstrated that dynamic programming could accurately and robustly extract the fibroatheromas interfaces and quantify cap thickness, however the proposed scheme relied solely on pixel intensity and did not exploit the information that can be provided by a geometrical *a priori* feature.

The aim of the present study is to propose and evaluate a tool designed to quantify FC thickness of fibroatheromas in intracoronary OCT. The context of our work relates to peri-operative decision making rather than patients screening: the severity of the case is averred and invasive imaging is required. The principal contribution of this work is a robust segmentation method devised to extract the diffuse abluminal interface of FC. The introduced framework is semi-automatic, and based on a contour segmentation approach that previously showed successful results on the common carotid artery wall in B-mode ultrasound [14]. The accuracy of the present method was validated in a set of cross-sectional OCT images acquired *in vivo* from 11 different patients, and demonstrated a similar accuracy compared to the tracings manually performed by two experienced analysts.

2   Material and Methods

We present here in detail our method devised to extract the contours of both luminal and abluminal interfaces to assess FC thickness. Our framework is based on three principal phases, namely *i)* a manual initialization aiming to indicate the presence of the fibrous tissues to be analyzed, *ii)* the automatic delineation of the luminal interface in the objective to localize the wall contour, and *iii)* the automatic extraction of the abluminal interface, which is subsequently exploited to assess the actual cap thickness. An overview of the method is presented in Figure 1.

2.1   Initialization and Lumen Segmentation

Our framework starts with the user manually performing a quick and simple initialization phase. For a given pullback, this operation consists in visually detecting the presence of a necrotic core covered by a FC and indicating its location. More specifically, the user first selects a set of consecutive frames to be analyzed, then, for each frame, a region of interest (ROI) encompassing the FC (Fig. 1a,b). This task is performed in a simple and easy way, thanks to a convenient graphical

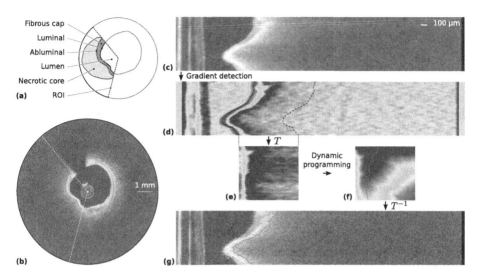

Fig. 1. Segmentation framework. (a) Cartoon depicting the region of interest (ROI, dashed lines) encompassing the fibrous cap. (b) OCT image of an *in vivo* human coronary artery, in Cartesian coordinates, with the resulting luminal (cyan line) and abluminal (magenta line) segmentation contours. (c) Smoothed ROI in polar coordinates, with the luminal contour (cyan line). (d) Cost image C. (e) Transformed sub-image C_T. (f) Cumulated cost $\mathcal{C}$, with the optimal path (magenta line). (g) Resulting abluminal segmentation contour.

interface allowing the user to browse through the pullback. After this operation has been performed, the region shadowed by the guidewire is easily masked out using an approach similar to the one proposed in [13], then the luminal interface is automatically and accurately extracted, using an adapted version of the tool Creaseg [15], based on geodesic active contours [16] minimizing a gradient-based functional.

2.2   Abluminal Interface Segmentation

We now describe the major contribution of our work, namely the contour segmentation of the back-end of the cap. To this purpose, active contours do not provide satisfactory results, as this technique strongly depends on the initial location of the curve, which remains in this case challenging to determine as the location of the back-end of the cap is unknown. Instead, we present a more robust scheme that is independent from initialization and is based on dynamic programming. The contour extraction of the abluminal interface separating FC tissues from the necrotic core is performed in 4 steps, as described below. These operations are realized in the polar domain, within the previously selected ROI, and rely on the *a priori* information provided by the luminal contour segmentation.

Gradient Detection. The first step consists in locally enhancing the regions of the image showing an intensity transition from high (bright fibrous tissues) to low (dark lipid pool) values (Fig. 1c,d). We start by smoothing the image using a Gaussian filter of standard deviation σ to attenuate the degrading noise. Then, the gradient is extracted by means of solving the linear equation that corresponds to the fitting of a degree 1 polynomial onto the intensity profile of the ROI. Each A-line is thus scanned with a sliding window of length L. Finally, a cost function C is built by normalizing the gradient image to the positive interval $[0, 1]$. In this image C, the points most likely to represent the location of the abluminal interface correspond to the points with the lowest cost.

Spatial Transformation T. The aim of the spatial transformation T is to generate a sub-image C_T in which the luminal interface corresponds to a straight vertical line in the polar domain (Fig. 1e). The cost function C is thus shifted line-by-line to match the axial origin with respect to the luminal contour rather than to the probe location. The rationale of our approach is based on the fact that, as the FC thickness does not undergo large variations within adjacent sites, we can exploit a strong geometrical *a priori*. In the transformed sub-image C_T, the abluminal contour that needs to be extracted is henceforth expected to correspond to a nearly-vertical structure.

Dynamic Programming. We now address the issue of determining, among all the potential candidate contours, the one that best describes the actual location of the anatomical interface. Towards this objective, we propose a specific implementation of a dynamic programming framework based on front propagation [17]. Dynamic programming is an efficient method to find the globally optimal solution in combinatory analysis. In our case, we use this strategy to determine the path that runs in the sub-image C_T from top-to-bottom with the minimum cumulated cost. The global cumulated cost $\mathcal{C}$ takes into account both the image feature (*i.e.* strong negative intensity gradient locally corresponding to a low cost in C_T) and a smoothness constraint (*i.e.* the shape *a priori* that describes a nearly vertical structure). Therefore, high cost values as well as non-vertical displacement are penalized when generating the cumulated cost function $\mathcal{C}$, as detailed in Equation 1 (Fig. 1f).

$$\mathcal{C}(r, \theta + 1) = \min_{dr \in \{-N, \dots 0, \dots N\}} \left\{ \mathcal{C}(r + dr, \theta) + C_T(r, \theta + 1)\sqrt{1 + \left(\frac{dr}{N}\right)^2} \right\}, \quad (1)$$

with (r, θ) the horizontal (axial) and vertical (lateral) coordinates, dr the horizontal displacement of the path between two consecutive points, N the number of horizontally reachable neighbors per side, and the uppermost line of $\mathcal{C}$ initialized to zero. The optimal path with the lowest cumulated cost is determined by a classical gradient-descent approach by back-tracking the decreasing values in $\mathcal{C}$ from the bottom border to the top (Fig. 1f). This dynamic programming scheme is performed twice, that is top-to-bottom, then bottom-to-top, the overall optimal path being finally selected.

Inverse Transformation T^{-1}. In the last step of the segmentation process, the actual location of the abluminal interface in the original image is determined by applying the corresponding inverse spatial transformation T^{-1} onto the extracted optimal path (Fig. 1g).

3 Experiments

3.1 Data Collection and Study Population

The OCT imaging database of Thoraxenter, Erasmus MC (Rotterdam, The Netherlands) was screened for native coronary artery OCT pullbacks containing fibroatheromas. Fibroatheromas were defined as necrotic core containing regions with the maximum circumferential extent (arc) exceeding one quadrant of the cross-section. Pullbacks were acquired in the catheterization laboratory of Erasmus MC for clinical indications, using the C7XR frequency-domain system and the Dragonfly intracoronary imaging catheter (Lightlab/St Jude, Minneapolis, MN, USA). Image acquisition was performed with a previously described non-occlusive technique [9]. Briefly, after positioning the OCT catheter distally to the segment of interest, it was pulled back automatically at 20 mm/s with simultaneous contrast infusion through the guiding catheter by a power injector (flush rate $3-4$ ml/s). Images were acquired at the rate of 105 frames/s (corresponding to 54000 A-lines/s), over a total length of 54 mm along the vessel, resulting in a stack of 271 frames. The central bandwidth of the near-infrared light was 1310 nm, and the spatial resolution of the system was 20 μm and 30 μm in the axial and lateral directions, respectively. The depth of the scan range was 4.3 mm, and acquired images were sampled at 504×968 pixels per frame, with a pixel size of 4.5 μm.

3.2 Image Analysis Procedure

For each analyzed pullback, an expert $\mathcal{O}_1$ selected a series of consecutive images where a necrotic core with an overlying FC could be observed visually. Definition of image features identifying a necrotic core was signal-poor regions with diffuse contours and high signal attenuation [9]. Subsequently, $\mathcal{O}_1$ indicated, in each selected frame, the limits of the ROI encompassing the FC (Fig. 1a,b). All that information was stored, and used by our automatic method, the expert $\mathcal{O}_1$, as well as an additional analyst $\mathcal{O}_2$ to perform, blinded from the results of others, the contour extraction of the TCFA. All tracings realized by the human analysts were performed in the Cartesian domain *via* an effective graphical interface that was developed in-house for this purpose. The two experts are specialists in vascular imaging and OCT (5+ years of experience). They received identical instructions, were shown examples of expected segmentation results, and were trained on the new segmentation software during 1 month before the trial.

3.3 Parameters Settings

Our method was applied on all images with the following heuristically-determined (*i.e.* by selecting the optimal configuration out of 12) parameters settings: standard deviation of the Gaussian filter, $\sigma = 18$ μm (in both axial and lateral directions), length of the gradient filter, $L = 185$ μm, number of horizontally reachable neighbors per side, $N = 2$.

3.4 Fibrous Cap Thickness Evaluation

The actual FC thickness was assessed in each analyzed image, for our automatic method as well as the two experts $\mathcal{O}_1$ and $\mathcal{O}_2$. Thickness was defined as the axial distance in between luminal and abluminal interfaces in the polar image. For each image, cap thickness was evaluated using three different measurements, that is *i)* as a vector describing each A-line of the ROI, *ii)* as the average thickness value of the FC per frame, and *iii)* as the thinnest portion within the frame.

4 Results

Eleven patients (mean age 60.8±9.5 y.o., 9 males) suffering from coronary artery disease were identified in the database and included in our study. The average number of analyzed images per individual pullback was 8 ± 2 (range $5 - 10$) consecutive frames, with a total of 90 analyzed images.

For each frame, luminal and abluminal interfaces of the TCFA were automatically extracted within the ROI defined by the expert $\mathcal{O}_1$ (Fig. 1a,b). Representative examples of success and failure in contour extraction are displayed in Figure 2. The two FC anatomical interfaces were successfully localized by our method for all frames in 8 pullbacks among 11. In the remaining 3 pullbacks, our method sometimes failed to localize the abluminal contour for a subset of frames. The results of our segmentation method, compared to the tracings of both observers $\mathcal{O}_1$ and $\mathcal{O}_2$, are presented alongside to the corresponding inter-observer variability in Table 1.

Quantification of FC thickness was derived from the segmented contours of both luminal and abluminal interfaces. Including all the 90 images, the mean cap thickness was 219.6 ± 85.3 μm for all A-lines, and 152.9 ± 63.5 μm for the thinnest point of each frame, as measured by $\mathcal{O}_1$. Results provided by our

Table 1. Segmentation errors (mean ± SD) for extraction of the fibrous cap luminal and abluminal interfaces

Errors (μm)	Luminal		Abluminal	
	Absolute	Signed	Absolute	Signed
Auto *vs* $\mathcal{O}_1$	12.8 ± 17.2	2.7 ± 21.3	41.4 ± 53.9	-1.1 ± 68.0
Auto *vs* $\mathcal{O}_2$	16.2 ± 18.9	9.1 ± 23.1	38.8 ± 44.6	5.6 ± 58.9
$\mathcal{O}_1$ *vs* $\mathcal{O}_2$	10.8 ± 12.3	6.4 ± 15.1	35.3 ± 45.3	6.7 ± 57.0

Table 2. Evaluation of fibrous cap thickness, with absolute error (mean ± SD), bias, 95% limits of agreement (Lim), and Pearson coefficient (R)

Errors (μm)	Average (for all contours)				Average (per frame)				Minimum (per frame)			
	Absolute	Bias	Lim	R	Absolute	Bias	Lim	R	Absolute	Bias	Lim	R
Auto vs $\mathcal{O}_1$	43.8 ± 54.0	-3.8	136.0	.65	34.6 ± 39.3	-17.2	97.2	.75	35.7 ± 33.3	1.4	95.9	.68
Auto vs $\mathcal{O}_2$	42.1 ± 46.3	-3.5	122.5	.66	34.9 ± 32.6	-13.2	90.2	.73	37.2 ± 38.8	3.2	105.4	.52
$\mathcal{O}_1$ vs $\mathcal{O}_2$	37.8 ± 45.4	0.3	115.8	.76	32.9 ± 32.0	4.0	89.9	.79	35.2 ± 33.1	1.8	94.8	.66

method were compared to those obtained with both experts $\mathcal{O}_1$ and $\mathcal{O}_2$, as well as with the inter-observer variability, and showed an overall good agreement, as presented in Table 2. Quantification of minimal cap thickness for each frame is assessed by our method with a similar accuracy as the two experts $\mathcal{O}_1$ and $\mathcal{O}_2$ (Fig. 3a), and the discrepancy between our method and $\mathcal{O}_1$ is similar to the inter-observer variability (Fig. 3b,c). It is noteworthy that, among the 12 evaluated parameters settings, the worst case led to an average error of 71 ± 88 μm for minimum cap thickness. We considered two groups depending on whether the mean cap thickness was higher or lower than the overall median thickness value

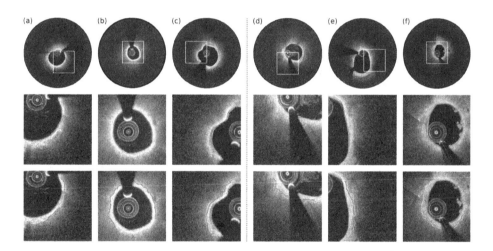

Fig. 2. Results of our segmentation method on 6 frames from different pullbacks, for successful contour extraction (a–c) and failures (d–f). For each example, the top, middle and bottom rows display the full image with the region of interest (ROI, white square), and the luminal and abluminal segmentation results within the ROI, respectively. Tracings realized by our method and observers $\mathcal{O}_1$ and $\mathcal{O}_2$ are represented by magenta, green and yellow lines, respectively. For the 3 unsuccessful pullbacks, probable causes of failure are: (d) The intensity gradient presents several weak fronts. (e) The two analysts disagree when identifying the abluminal interface, while our method estimates a result closer to the contour proposed by $\mathcal{O}_2$. (f) Our method is attracted by a bright spot caused by an image artifact, and fails to detect the abluminal contour.

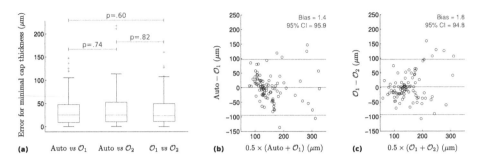

Fig. 3. Evaluation of the minimum cap thickness in all 90 frames with our method (Auto) and the two experts $\mathcal{O}_1$ and $\mathcal{O}_2$. (a) Box plot representing the absolute difference of errors between our method and the experts, with the p-values resulting from the Wilcoxon test. (b) Bland-Altman plot comparing the results of our method with $\mathcal{O}_1$. (c) Bland-Altman plot for the inter-observer variability.

in all frames. In the group of thinner caps our method slightly overestimated the cap thickness (mean error: $11.3 \pm 44.9 \ \mu m$), whereas in the group of thicker caps there was a slight underestimation (mean error: $-18.7 \pm 67.1 \ \mu m$). The present implementation of our computerized method required on average 2 s to perform the contour extraction of both interfaces of the FC and evaluate its thickness for a single image, while the corresponding manual operation required on average 190 s. In both cases and additionally, the average time (per frame) required by the user to define the ROI was 20 s.

5   Discussion and Conclusion

The proposed method was applied *in vivo* on 90 cross-sectional coronary OCT images from 11 patients. In the context of assessing plaque stability and aiming to quantify FC thickness, both luminal and abluminal anatomical interfaces were extracted. The rationale of our study is supported by FC thickness being considered to be the most critical component of plaque stability [4], as well as by a recent longitudinal study demonstrating that lesion morphology was associated with future events [18]. Clinical applicability of our approach is strengthened by an overall good accuracy, provided in a clinically acceptable computation time, *via* an efficient graphical user interface.

Comparing the results of our segmentation method with the reference tracings realized manually by two experts, our framework demonstrated a successful contour extraction of both interfaces in the majority of the pullbacks (8 out of 11). However, matching of the abluminal contour between automated and reference was sub-optimal in 3 cases with a variety of reasons accounting for this discrepancy (*e.g.* presence of several weak gradient fronts, disagreement between the two analysts, or bright spot caused by an image artifact). Nevertheless, the agreement between our segmentation method and reference tracings was in any case similar to the inter-observer agreement, namely $12.8 \pm 17.2 \ \mu m$

vs 10.8 ± 12.3 μm and 41.4 ± 53.9 μm *vs* 35.3 ± 45.3 μm, for luminal and abluminal contours, respectively (Table 1). It is also noteworthy that both manual and automated segmentation errors were roughly three times higher for abluminal compared to luminal interfaces. This lower performance when segmenting the abluminal interface can be explained by the fact that, by definition, a necrotic core has as mild transition, contrary to the luminal interface or a calcific plaque that show a sharp and well perceptible transition [9].

As for the actual FC thickness evaluation (Table 2), we observe that errors introduced by our method remain relatively reduced considering the spatial resolution (*i.e.* 20 μm). Moreover, the accuracy of our method was systematically similar to the inter-observer agreement. This finding tends to indicate that our method performs at least as well as an experienced observer when assessing the cap thickness. We also notice that the error generated by our method when estimating the global thickness (*i.e.* in each A-line of the analyzed ROI) is close to the abluminal interface segmentation error (Table 1), namely 43.8 ± 54.0 μm *vs* 41.4 ± 53.9 μm. This confirms that the most challenging issue to quantify FC thickness is to localize with accuracy the abluminal interface. Furthermore, our method demonstrated a better accuracy when quantifying, for each frame, the thinnest portion of the tissues in comparison to the global thickness evaluation of the whole cap, *i.e.* 35.7 ± 33.3 μm *vs* 43.8 ± 54.0 μm. According to our experience, thickest portions of the cap often present more fuzzy contours, while thinnest portions, which also constitute a more valuable clinical information, tend to present sharper and more defined contours. This is probably caused by two principal reasons, namely *i)* the signal corresponding to deeper tissues is subject to a greater attenuation, and *ii)* the lateral spatial definition decreases along the distance from the probe in the Cartesian domain.

The error introduced by our method when assessing minimal cap thickness was 35.7 ± 33.3 μm, which is relatively large compared to the empirical threshold of 65 μm used to identify rupture-prone sites [2]. Nevertheless, the inter-observer variability also yielded a similar accuracy (35.2 ± 33.1 μm). Moreover, it is noteworthy that the 65 μm threshold may be under-evaluated, as *ex vivo* tissues can undergo a 20% shrinkage during histological preparation [9]. Indeed, recent *in vivo* studies have shown that ruptured plaques in ACS are often associated with a FC thickness of up to 100 μm [19], and that the best cut-off to predict rupture was 151 μm for most representative FCs [20].

It is insightful to compare the results of our approach with the study presented by Wang *et al.* [13], which is, to the best of our knowledge, the only one to report a semi-automatic segmentation scheme dedicated to quantify FC thickness in coronary OCT. That method demonstrated higher accuracy, with errors of 15.7 ± 23.4 μm, 25.3 ± 31.4 μm, and 27.3 ± 26.7 μm for luminal and abluminal contour segmentation and FC thickness evaluation, respectively. Nevertheless, the pertinence of such comparison is limited by the fact that our method was applied onto a different dataset, using a different OCT scanner, and that the protocol followed by the expert $\mathcal{O}_1$ to determine the FCs to be analyzed may also have differed. Moreover, the finding of a higher inter-observer variability as well in our study could imply the presence of challenging cases in our dataset.

Our study presents several limitations that have to be considered. First, our segmentation method is based on 2D cross-sectional images and does not exploit the third dimension along the length of the artery. However, due to the low spatial resolution along the z-axis (200 μm), we would not expect 3D segmentation to greatly improve accuracy. Second, in this pilot study, training and testing datasets are identical. We plan to address this in future work by gathering additional pullbacks to build a testing dataset. Third, the selection of the actual frames to be analyzed, as well as the delimitation of the ROI encompassing the FC, were determined by the single analyst $\mathcal{O}_1$. We could expect that a different expert would occasionally have selected different frames and/or ROI. However, this would probably not have caused a large impact, as previous studies demonstrated a good agreement in between analysts when selecting such lesions [13,20]. Finally, as the present work is focused on the proof of concept that FC thickness can be assessed accurately for a given lesion, we did not investigate here the influence of frame selection. This matter, as well as assessing human inter- and intra-variability with a third analyst, will be assessed in future work. Furthermore, a study combining OCT and biplane angiography is also being conducted by our team, aiming to investigate the association of wall shear stress with FC thickness, to provide further information about plaque vulnerability during the catheterization procedure.

In conclusion, we have proposed a semi-automated method to quantify TCFA in intracoronary OCT, in the objective to assess rupture-prone plaques during percutaneous interventions in the cathlab. The principal challenge of such task is to extract with accuracy the abluminal interface of the FC, consisting of progressively unravelling tissues with poorly defined contours. To cope with this issue, we introduced a robust contour segmentation framework based on the integration of a geometrical *a priori* within a dynamic programming scheme. The proposed method was applied *in vivo* on 90 cross-sectional images from 11 patients, and compared to the reference contours realized by two analysts. Our promising method performed as well as two expert analysts, and could constitute a reliable tool for interventional planning and decision making.

References

1. World Health Organisation: Cardiovascular diseases (CVDs). Fact Sheet 317 (March 2013)
2. Virmani, R., Kolodgie, F.D., Burke, A.P., Farb, A., Schwartz, S.M.: Lessons from sudden coronary death: A comprehensive morphological classification scheme for atherosclerotic lesions. Arterioscler. Thromb. Vasc. Biol. 20(5), 1262–1275 (2000)
3. Burke, A.P., Farb, A., Malcom, G.T., Liang, Y.H., Smialek, J., Virmani, R.: Coronary risk factors and plaque morphology in men with coronary disease who died suddenly. N. Engl. J. Med. 336, 1276–1282 (1997)
4. Narula, J., Nakano, M., Virmani, R., et al.: Histopathologic characteristics of atherosclerotic coronary disease and implications of the findings for the invasive and noninvasive detection of vulnerable plaques. J. Am. Coll. Card. 61(10), 1041–1051 (2013)

5. Brezinski, M.E.: Optical coherence tomography for identifying unstable coronary plaque. Int. J. Cardiol. 107(2), 154–165 (2006)
6. Kume, T., Akasaka, T., Kawamoto, T., et al.: Measurement of the thickness of the fibrous cap by optical coherence tomography. Am. Heart. J. 152(4), 755e1–755e4 (2006)
7. Kubo, T., Imanishi, T., Takarada, S., et al.: Assessment of culprit lesion morphology in acute myocardial infarction: Ability of optical coherence tomography compared with intravascular ultrasound and coronary angioscopy. J. Am. Coll. Card. 50(10), 933–939 (2007)
8. Bezerra, H.G., Costa, M.A., Guagliumi, G., Rollins, A.M., Simon, D.I.: Intracoronary optical coherence tomography: a comprehensive review. J. Am. Coll. Cardiol. Intv. 2(11), 1035–1046 (2009)
9. Tearney, G.J., Regar, E., Akasaka, T., et al.: Consensus standards for acquisition, measurement, and reporting of intravascular optical coherence tomography studies. J. Am. Coll. Card. 59(12), 1058–1072 (2012)
10. Xu, C., Schmitt, J.M., Carlier, S.G., Virmani, R.: Characterization of atherosclerosis plaques by measuring both backscattering and attenuation coefficients in optical coherence tomography. J. Biomed. Opt. 3, 34003 (2008)
11. van Soest, G., Goderie, T., Regar, E., et al.: Atherosclerotic tissue characterization in vivo by optical coherence tomography attenuation imaging. J. Biomed. Opt. 15(1), 011105-1–011105-9 (2010)
12. Ughi, G.J., Steigerwald, K., Adriaenssens, T., et al.: Automatic characterization of neointimal tissue by intravascular optical coherence tomography. J. Biomed. Opt. 19(2), 021104 (2013)
13. Wang, Z., Chamie, D., Bezerra, H.G., et al.: Volumetric quantification of fibrous caps using intravascular optical coherence tomography. Biomed. Opt. Express 3(6), 1413–1426 (2012)
14. Zahnd, G., Orkisz, M., Sérusclat, A., Moulin, P., Vray, D.: Simultaneous extraction of carotid artery intima-media interfaces in ultrasound images: assessment of wall thickness temporal variation during the cardiac cycle. Int. J. CARS (2013) (in press), doi:10.1007/s11548-013-0945-0
15. Dietenbeck, T., Alessandrini, M., Friboulet, D., Bernard, O.: CREASEG: a free software for the evaluation of image segmentation algorithms based on level-set. In: IEEE ICIP, pp. 665–668 (2010)
16. Caselles, V., Kimmel, R., Sapiro, G.: Geodesic active contours. Int. J. Comput. Vis. 22(1), 61–79 (1997)
17. Cohen, L.: Minimal paths and fast marching methods for image analysis. In: Paragios, N., Chen, Y., Faugeras, O. (eds.) Handbook of Mathematical Models in Computer Vision, pp. 97–111. Springer, US (2006)
18. Stone, G.W., Maehara, A., Lansky, A.J.: A prospective natural-history study of coronary atherosclerosis. N. Engl. J. Med. 364(3), 226–235 (2011)
19. Toutouzas, K., Karanasos, A., Tsiamis, E., et al.: New insights by optical coherence tomography into the differences and similarities of culprit ruptured plaque morphology in non–ST-elevation myocardial infarction and ST-elevation myocardial infarction. Am. Heart J. 161(6), 1192–1199 (2011)
20. Yonetsu, T., Kakuta, T., Lee, T., et al.: In vivo critical fibrous cap thickness for rupture-prone coronary plaques assessed by optical coherence tomography. Eur. Heart J. 32(10), 1251–1259 (2011)

A System for Ultrasound-Guided Spinal Injections: A Feasibility Study

Abtin Rasoulian[1], Jill Osborn[3], Samira Sojoudi[1], Saman Nouranian[1],
Victoria A. Lessoway[4], Robert N. Rohling[1,2], and Purang Abolmaesumi[1]

[1] Department of Electrical and Computer Engineering,
University of British Columbia, Vancouver, B.C., Canada
[2] Department of Mechanical Engineering,
University of British Columbia, Vancouver, B.C., Canada
[3] Department of Anesthesia, St. Pauls Hospital, Vancouver, B.C., Canada
[4] RDMS Department of Ultrasound, Women's Hospital, Vancouver, B.C., Canada

Abstract. Facet joint injections of analgesic agents are widely used to
treat patients with lower back pain, a growing problem in the adult
population. The current standard-of-care for guiding the injection is fluoroscopy, but has significant drawbacks, including the significant dose
of ionizing radiation. As an alternative, several ultrasound-guidance
systems have been recently proposed, but have not become the standard-
of-care mainly because of the difficulty in image interpretation by anesthesiologists unfamiliar with complex spinal sonography. A solution is to
register a statistical spine model, learned from pre-operative images such
as MRI or CT over a range of population, to the ultrasound images and
display as an overlay. In particular, we introduce an ultrasound-based
navigation system where the workflow is divided into two steps. Initially,
prior to the injection, tracked freehand ultrasound images are acquired
from the facet joint and its surrounding vertebrae. The statistical model
is then instantiated and registered to those images. Next, the real-time
ultrasound images are augmented with the registered model to guide the
injection. Feasibility experiments are performed on ultrasound data obtained from nine patients who had prior CT images as the gold-standard
for the statistical model. We present three ultrasound scanning protocols
for ultrasound acquisition and quantify the error of our model.

Keywords: multi-vertebrae model, statistical pose+shape model, 3D
ultrasound, spine, registration.

1 Introduction

Lower back pain is one of the most common medical problems in the adult population. It is estimated that up to 80% of adults experience during a lifetime at
least one episode of back pain that is a major cause of disability [12]. Facet joint
injections of analgesic agents have been used for the patients not responsive to
conservative management. The current standard-of-care for guiding the injection is fluoroscopy, but has significant drawbacks, including the significant dose

D. Stoyanov et al. (Eds.): IPCAI 2014, LNCS 8498, pp. 90–99, 2014.
© Springer International Publishing Switzerland 2014

of ionizing radiation and the need for a specialized pain management clinic with access to fluoroscopy equipment. As an alternative, several ultrasound-guidance systems have been recently proposed [2, 7, 14–16], but have not become the standard-of-care mainly because of the difficulty in image interpretation by anesthesiologists unfamiliar with complex spinal sonography. A possible solution to this problem is to register a spine model to the ultrasound images and display it as an overlay. Moore *et al.* introduced an ultrasound-guided system for facet joint injections where the ultrasound transducer was tracked using an electromagnetic tracker [7]. They showed that integration of a virtual CT-based model of the spine improved the accuracy in needle placement. To perform the integration, predefined landmarks on the model were found on the target using the ultrasound, and a point-based registration was performed afterward. To visualize both the target and the needle, the ultrasound transducer has to be oriented in the same plane as the needle, but the ideal spine injection site are easily obscured by the ultrasound transducer. To address this problem, Ungi *et al.* added pre-operative ultrasound snapshots from the target to allow both the transducer and the needle to be placed at the ideal puncture site, i.e., the skin point with the shortest path to the target [15].

In the above-listed image-guided spine injection systems, models are extracted from pre-operative images such as MRI or CT. However, such pre-operative images are not usually available and expose the patient to ionizing radiation in the case of CT. Hence, the use of statistical models is a reasonable alternative.

In this paper, we introduce an ultrasound-based navigation system where the workflow is divided into two steps. Prior to the injection, tracked freehand ultrasound images are acquired from the facet joint and its surrounding vertebrae. The statistical model is then registered to those images. Next, the real-time ultrasound images, augmented with the model, are displayed for needle-guidance.

Statistical shape models have been previously generated for the vertebrae [1, 5, 10, 11]. Boisvert *et al.* studied the statistical variations of relative pose of each two adjacent vertebrae separately. They performed shape analysis of the entire vertebral column and proposed an algorithm for registration of their pose model to radiograph images. Khallaghi *et al.* built separate shape models for each vertebra and by incorporating a biomechanical model to constrain the relative pose of adjacent vertebrae, registered the shape models to an ultrasound volume [5]. This approach has certain disadvantages. Mainly, separate reconstruction of each vertebra neglects the many common shape characteristics between different vertebrae of a given subject which may decrease the accuracy of the registration and add to the computational time. To address these problems, we developed techniques for construction of a statistical multi-vertebrae model with a separate statistical analysis of shape and pose of the vertebrae [10]. The pose statistical analysis in contrast to Boisvert *et al.* are performed on the entire ensemble. We also proposed an algorithm for registration of the model to 3D ultrasound images with only a partial view of multiple vertebrae.

This paper has the following main contributions: first, we implement above mentioned registration technique [10] in a parallelized scheme and adapt it with

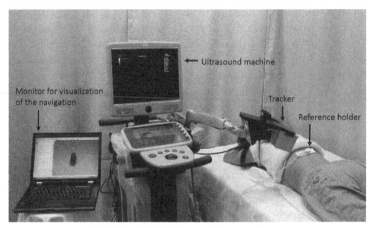

(a) Spinal injection guidance system

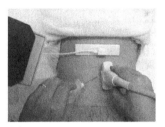

(b) Needle and transducer orientation

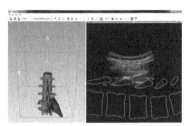

(c) Navigation display

Fig. 1. a) System setup. b) Visualization of the needle and the transducer on the subject's back. c) Guidance system interface. Live ultrasound images are augmented with the registered model, the needle and the transducer.

a navigation system that guides facet joint injections with tracked freehand 2D ultrasound images. As opposed to our earlier work with 3D probes [10], the use of tracked 2D probes is clinically more relevant due to their widespread availability in anesthesiology clinics. Second, experiments are performed on ultrasound data obtained from nine patients who had prior CT images as the gold-standard. This is particularly helpful to determine the accuracy of the registration and the final shape against CT images. Third, current study is performed on patients scheduled for facet joint injections as apposed to our previous study which was on healthy volunteers.

2   Methods

2.1   The Image-Guided System

Figure 1 shows the guidance system. Ultrasound images are tracked by an electromagnetic tracker (Ascension Technology Corporation, Shelburne, VT, USA)

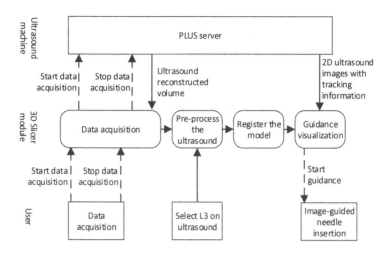

Fig. 2. Overview of the software

and are acquired using an Ultrasonix SonixTouch (Ultrasonix, Richmond, BC) at 30 frames per second. A curvi-linear C5-2 transducer is used which contains a built-in electromagnetic sensor at the tip. The probe is calibrated temporally and spatially at different depths with an average RMS error of 0.94 mm. A reference electromagnetic sensor is attached to the subject skin above the L1 vertebra. The needle tip is also tracked using an electromagnetic sensor. For facet joint injection, no loss-of-resistance is used to guide the placement of the needle, so the EM sensor can be placed directly at the needle tip.

Figure 2 shows an overview of the software design. This software is written on top of the open source library PLUS (Public Library for UltraSound) published by the Perk Lab at Queen's University, Canada [6]. PLUS provides access to ultrasound images, tagged with corresponding transformations of the ultrasound transducer, needle, and the reference sensor in real time. It also provides the reconstruction of the ultrasound volume in real time. 3D Slicer (Harvard Medical School, Boston, MA) is used as the interface for visualization and transmitting the user requests to the plus server [3]. Previously developed application in 3D slicer, called OpenIGTLink Remote, is used for communication with the PLUS server [13].

Conventional 2D ultrasound is used to localize the L1 vertebra by counting-up from the sacrum. The reference sensor is attached to the skin, 3.5 cm above the spinous process of L1. The reference sensor was stabilized in a plastic holder which determines the orientation of the sensor. Therefore, the tracker measurements are mapped into approximately anterior-posterior, lateral, and superior-inferior directions, respectively. Image acquisition for volume reconstruction of the entire lumbar spine is started and terminated by a foot pedal. The ultrasound volume is reconstructed incrementally as the images are acquired. Next, the user is asked to locate the L3 vertebra in the ultrasound volume using a single click in the 3D Slicer interface. The alignment of the model to the volume is performed next, as detailed in the following section. Then, the system automatically switches into real-time guidance by visualizing the live ultrasound images and the needle together with the registered model. The accuracy of needle localization with respect to the ultrasound is mainly determined by the EM-tracker and ultrasound calibration. The EM system used in our research has a static accuracy of 1.4 mm and 0.5 degrees RMS (Ascension Technology Corp, Milton, VT). These should be considered lower limits, since accuracy in vivo will also include some distortion of the EM field.

2.2 Construction of the Multi-vertebrae Model and Its Registration to Ultrasound Volumes

We refer the reader to a detailed description of the model and its registration to ultrasound volumes [10]. Here, we briefly describe the method. The statistical multi-vertebrae shape+pose model is generated from a training set which includes surface points of multiple vertebrae over a range of the population (n=32). Pose statistics are separated from the shape statistics since they are not necessarily correlated and do not belong to the same space [9]. Poses are presented by similarity (rigid+scale) transformations which form a Lie group where linear analysis is not applicable. To address this issue, the transformations are projected into a linear space by logarithmic mapping. Next, Principal Component Analysis (PCA) is performed to extract main modes of variations of poses. A separate PCA analysis is also used to compute the shape statistics. Note that these analyses are performed on the entire ensemble (including all lumbar vertebrae) which results in common statistics of multiple vertebrae. Such analyses result in a mean shape, μ_s, a mean pose, μ_p, and their modes of variations, v_s^k and v_p^k. Linear combination of these modes of variations with the mean shape and mean pose results in a new instance of the ensemble:

$$S = \mathcal{T}(\mu_s, \mu_p, v_s^k, v_p^k, w_s^k, w_p^k), \tag{1}$$

where w_s^k and w_p^k are the weights associated with the corresponding modes of variations. Prior to the registration, ultrasound images are processed to enhance the bone surface. We follow the technique proposed by Foroughi *et al.* where pixels with large intensity and shadow beneath them are considered as bone surface [4]. The registration of the model to enhanced ultrasound images is performed using a GMM-based registration method. In this iterative technique, the previously generated model boundary points are defined as the centroids of the GMM. The target, i.e. the bone surface enhanced in ultrasound images, is considered to be an observation generated by the GMM. The registration is then defined as estimation of proper weights of the modes of variations and a rigid transformation applied to the entire ensemble, to maximize the probability of the GMM centroids generating the target.

The algorithm is parallelized at CPU level, using the Intel Math Kernel Library (Intel, Santa Clara, CA, US). Using this parallelization, the registration, together with the ultrasound pre-processing, takes approximately 10 seconds.

3   Experiments

3.1   Initial Ultrasound Acquisition

Ultrasound images were acquired from a prone subject. To provide maximum similarity to the supine position (subject's posture during CT acquisition) with respect to spine curvature, and also for the subject comfort, a small pillow was placed under the abdomen. Prior to the data collection, brief sonographic study was performed by the sonographer to tune the imaging parameters such as focus and depth. The sonographer also examined the best possible probe trajectory for data collection by marking the spinous processes of L1 and S1. For each experiment, three different scans were performed and corresponding volumes were reconstructed afterward (see Figure 3 for a graphical illustration):

1. Side-sweep scanning was collected from the subject's top-left to bottom-left and back to the top-right ($\sim$ 30 seconds). The transducer angled toward midline and in the transverse plane, 2 cm away from the midline.
2. Transverse midline volume was acquired from top to bottom in the transverse plane ($\sim$ 15 seconds).
3. Sagittal zigzag data collection was performed by moving the transducer laterally in the sagittal plane ($\sim$ 50 seconds).

For the remaining experiments, each of these tracked ultrasound images were reconstructed into a volumetric representation [15].

The standard-of-care for the subjects in this study includes a CT-scan taken several months before the injection session.

The bone surface was also manually segmented from each 2D ultrasound image. The segmentation was then transformed to the subject's coordinate space using the calibration and tracking information. The result is a set of point resembling the surface of the vertebrae in subject's coordinate space. As expected, only some of the posterior aspects of the vertebrae were visible, i.e. laminae, transverse processes, spinous process, and posterior part of the vertebral body.

3.2   Accuracy Validation

For each registration of the model to ultrasound volumes, the following measurements were made:

1. The RMS distance of the manually segmented ultrasound points to the model. Although the manual segmentation does not provide a full representation of the vertebrae, it is used to provide a measure of how well the multi-vertebrae model is registered to the ultrasound features.
2. The RMS distance between the model and the manually segmented CT images. This measure is calculated to estimate how well the patient-specific shape of the vertebrae registered to the ultrasound data matches the patient's anatomy observed in CT images. To this end, each vertebrae of the registered model is separately aligned to the corresponding vertebrae from the segmented vertebrae, using the coherent point drift registration method [8]. Then the RMS surface distance is reported as the shape error.

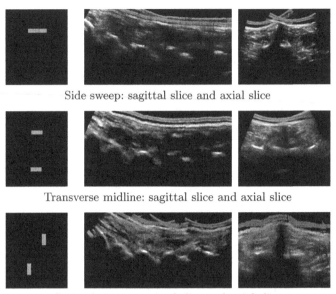

Side sweep: sagittal slice and axial slice

Transverse midline: sagittal slice and axial slice

Sagittal zigzag: sagittal slice and axial slice

Fig. 3. Three different scans were performed on each subject

Experiments were also performed to measure the sensitivity of the algorithm to the initial point selection, i.e. a point around the center of L3, which was marked by the user. To this end, the model is manually well-aligned to the target. The center of mass of the L3 vertebra in the model was extracted. Next, a displacement ranging from 0 to 30 mm, in a random direction, was added to the model, followed by registration. Initial displacements were divided into bins with 5 mm width. For each bin, five experiments were performed for each subject and each ultrasound volume. The mean distance error between the registered model surface to the manually segmented bone surface points in the ultrasound volumes was reported.

4   Results

4.1   Model Construction

The training set for the statistical model was a set of segmented lumbar vertebrae acquired in our previous studies for a total of 32. Manual CT segmentation was performed interactively using ITK-SNAP (www.itksnap.org). 95% of the shape and pose variations are captured by first 25 and 7 modes, respectively. The model is capable of reconstructing an unseen observation with distance error below 2 mm with using the first 20 modes of the variation.

4.2 Registration of the Multi-vertebrae Model to Ultrasound Images

Examples of the registration of the multi-vertebrae model to ultrasound volumes are shown in Figure 4. Distance errors are given in Tables 1. The results for side sweep are significantly better than the other two scans ($p < 0.05$), makes it a preferred scanning protocol. An RMS error of 2.3 mm (maximum 8.4 mm) is adequate for helping to correctly identify the key features in the ultrasound

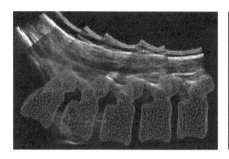
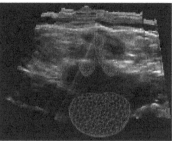

Fig. 4. Example of the registered model to an ultrasound volume

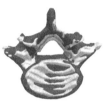

Fig. 5. A comparison of registered model to ultrasound images and the model from CT images. The registered model is highlighted in red and the white surface shows the CT manual segmentation.

Table 1. RMS distance (in mm) between the segmented ultrasound and the registered model. Results for side sweep are significantly better ($p < 0.05$).

	side sweep transverse	midline sagittal	zigzag
RMS distance error	2.3±0.4*	3.2±0.9	3.0±0.5
Maximum distance error	8.9±4.2*	10.6±4.4	13.4±4.9

Table 2. RMS distance (in mm) between the shape of the manual segmentation of the CT and the shape of the registered model to the ultrasound images

	side sweep transverse	midline sagittal	zigzag
L2	1.3±0.3	1.3±0.3	1.3±0.3
L3	1.5±0.4	1.4±0.2	1.3±0.3
L4	1.5±0.4	1.5±0.4	1.5±0.4
L5	1.5±0.3	1.5±0.3	1.5±0.3
All	1.5±0.4	1.4±0.3	1.4±0.3

image. The goal is to interpret the ultrasound and rely on the ultrasound features, not solely the model.

The RMS distance errors between the manual segmentation of the CT and the registered model is given in Table 2. Interestingly, there is no significant differences between the ultrasound acquisition techniques. All vertebrae give errors of $\sim$ 1.5 mm, suggesting that all registered models can accurately generate patient specific vertebrae anatomical shapes.

Results on capture range experiment shows that the error remains the same for variations under 10 mm. This covers a reasonable area (20 mm) within the vertebrae, suggesting the method is robust to initialization errors.

5   Discussion and Conclusion

Our image-guided system can be considered as the evolution of the method presented by Moore *et al.* [7] and Ungi *et al.* [15] by providing the augmentation of the ultrasound with a statistical model. Additionally, the alignment of the model to the ultrasound volume requires minimal interaction, i.e. selection of the L3 vertebra in the ultrasound volume. In the two above mentioned studies, registration is performed by selection of multiple fiducials in both CT and ultrasound. The registration technique used in this work is superior to the one presented by Khallaghi *et al.* [5] in terms of computational time (10 seconds vs. 45 minutes). Additionally, we validate our technique on *in vivo* data.

There are some limitations to this study. Mainly, the training data for reconstruction of the model are segmented vertebrae from the CT images, which are all captured in a supine position. Therefore, the model may not be able to capture all possible spine curvature especially the curvature, when ultrasound and needle insertions are performed.

Future work will be focused on evaluation of the needle injection using this image-guided system and its potential improvement over the conventional manual or fluoroscopy-based technique.

Acknowledgment. The authors would like to thank the Natural Sciences and Engineering Research Council (NSERC) and the Canadian Institutes of Health Research (CIHR) for supporting this research.

References

1. Boisvert, J., Cheriet, F., Pennec, X., Labelle, H., Ayache, N.: Articulated spine models for 3-d reconstruction from partial radiographic data. IEEE Transactions on Biomedical Engineering 55(11), 2565–2574 (2008)
2. Chen, E.C.S., Mousavi, P., Gill, S., Fichtinger, G., Abolmaesumi, P.: Ultrasound guided spine needle insertion. In: Proc. SPIE, vol. 7625, pp. 762538-762538-8 (2010)

3. Fedorov, A., Beichel, R., Kalpathy-Cramer, J., Finet, J., Fillion-Robin, J.C., Pujol, S., Bauer, C., Jennings, D., Fennessy, F., Sonka, M., et al.: 3D slicer as an image computing platform for the quantitative imaging network. Magnetic Resonance Imaging 30(9) (2012)
4. Foroughi, P., Boctor, E., Swartz, M., et al.: 2-D ultrasound bone segmentation using dynamic programming. In: IEEE Ultras. Symp., pp. 2523–2526 (2007)
5. Khallaghi, S., Mousavi, P., Gong, R.H., Gill, S., Boisvert, J., Fichtinger, G., Pichora, D., Borschneck, D., Abolmaesumi, P.: Registration of a statistical shape model of the lumbar spine to 3D ultrasound images. In: Jiang, T., Navab, N., Pluim, J.P.W., Viergever, M.A. (eds.) MICCAI 2010, Part II. LNCS, vol. 6362, pp. 68–75. Springer, Heidelberg (2010)
6. Lasso, A., Heffter, T., Pinter, C., Ungi, T., Chen, T.K., Boucharin, A., Fichtinger, G.: Plus: An open-source toolkit for developing ultrasound-guided intervention systems. In: 4th NCIGT and NIH Image Guided Therapy Workshop, vol. 4, p. 103 (2011)
7. Moore, J., Clarke, C., Bainbridge, D., Wedlake, C., Wiles, A., Pace, D., Peters, T.: Image guidance for spinal facet injections using tracked ultrasound. In: Yang, G.-Z., Hawkes, D., Rueckert, D., Noble, A., Taylor, C. (eds.) MICCAI 2009, Part I. LNCS, vol. 5761, pp. 516–523. Springer, Heidelberg (2009)
8. Myronenko, A., Song, X., Carreira-Perpinan, M.: Non-rigid point set registration: Coherent point drift. In: Advances in Neural Information Processing Systems - NIPS, pp. 1009–1016 (2007)
9. Pennec, X.: Intrinsic statistics on riemannian manifolds: Basic tools for geometric measurements. Journal of Mathematical Imaging and Vision 25, 127–154 (2006)
10. Rasoulian, A., Rohling, R.N., Abolmaesumi, P.: Augmentation of paramedian 3D ultrasound images of the spine. In: Barratt, D., Cotin, S., Fichtinger, G., Jannin, P., Navab, N. (eds.) IPCAI 2013. LNCS, vol. 7915, pp. 51–60. Springer, Heidelberg (2013)
11. Roberts, M.G., Cootes, T.F., Pacheco, E., Oh, T., Adams, J.E.: Segmentation of lumbar vertebrae using part-based graphs and active appearance models. In: Yang, G.-Z., Hawkes, D., Rueckert, D., Noble, A., Taylor, C. (eds.) MICCAI 2009, Part II. LNCS, vol. 5762, pp. 1017–1024. Springer, Heidelberg (2009)
12. Rubin, D.I.: Epidemiology and risk factors for spine pain. Neurologic Clinics 25(2), 353–371 (2007)
13. Tokuda, J., Fischer, G.S., Papademetris, X., Yaniv, Z., Ibanez, L., Cheng, P., Liu, H., Blevins, J., Arata, J., Golby, A.J., et al.: Openigtlink: an open network protocol for image-guided therapy environment. The International Journal of Medical Robotics and Computer Assisted Surgery 5(4), 423–434 (2009)
14. Tran, D., Kamani, A.A., Al-Attas, E., Lessoway, V.A., Massey, S., Rohling, R.N.: Single-operator real-time ultrasound-guidance to aim and insert a lumbar epidural needle. Canadian Journal of Anesthesia/Journal canadien d'anesthésie 57(4), 313–321 (2010), http://dx.doi.org/10.1007/s12630-009-9252-1
15. Ungi, T., Abolmaesumi, P., Jalal, R., Welch, M., Ayukawa, I., Nagpal, S., Lasso, A., Jaeger, M., Borschneck, D., Fichtinger, G., et al.: Spinal needle navigation by tracked ultrasound snapshots. IEEE Transactions on Biomedical Engineering 59(10), 2766–2772 (2012)
16. Yan, C.X., Goulet, B., Pelletier, J., Chen, S.J.S., Tampieri, D., Collins, D.L.: Towards accurate, robust and practical ultrasound-ct registration of vertebrae for image-guided spine surgery. International Journal of Computer Assisted Radiology and Surgery 6(4), 523–537 (2011)

The 'Augmented' Circles: A Video-Guided Solution for the Down-the-Beam Positioning of IM Nail Holes

Roberto Londei[1,*], Marco Esposito[1,*], Benoit Diotte[1], Simon Weidert[2],
Ekkehard Euler[2], Peter Thaller[2], Nassir Navab[1], and Pascal Fallavollita[1]

[1] Chair for Computer Aided Medical Procedures, Technische Univ. Munchen, Germany
[2] Klinik und Poliklinik Innenstadt, Munchen, Germany

Abstract. Intramedullary nailing is the surgical procedure mostly used in fracture reduction of the tibial and femoral shafts. Following successful insertion of the nail into the medullary canal, it must be fixed by inserting screws through its proximal and distal locking holes. Prior to distal locking of the nail, surgeons must position the C-arm device and patient leg in such a way that the nail holes appear as circles in the X-ray image. This is considered a 'trial and error' process, is time consuming and requires many X-ray shots. We propose an augmented reality application that visually depicts to the surgeon two 'augmented' circles, their centers lying on the axis of the nail hole, making it visible in space. After an initial X-ray image acquisition, real-time video guidance allows the surgeon to superimpose the 'augmented' circles by moving the patient leg; the result being nail holes appearing as circles. Our nail pose recovery was evaluated on 1000 random trials and we consistently recovered the nail angulation within 2.76 ± 1.66°. Lastly, in a preclinical experiment involving 7 clinicians, we demonstrated that in over 95% of the trials, the nail hole appeared as a circle using an initial X-ray image.

Keywords: medical augmented reality, interlocking of intramedullary nailing, down-the-beam positioning, freehand distal locking, visualization, orthopedic and trauma surgery.

1   Introduction

Tibial fractures are among the most common lower limb injuries to be treated by an orthopedic & trauma surgeon. Today, the National Center for Health Statistics cites 492,000 tibial fractures per year in the United States [1]. Intramedullary (IM) nailing is the surgical procedure mostly used in fracture reduction of the tibial and femoral shafts. Following successful insertion of the nail into the medullary canal, the nail must be fixed into position in order to prevent rotation or dislocation. This is achieved by inserting screws perpendicular to the nail through the provided proximal and distal locking holes inside the nail shaft. The intramedullary nail is then locked at its two extremities. The insertion of the screws near the entrance point (i.e. proximal) of the nail

---

* Equal contribution.

D. Stoyanov et al. (Eds.): IPCAI 2014, LNCS 8498, pp. 100–107, 2014.

is achieved using an aiming bow attached to the nail. In the distal part of the nail, interlocking is commonly performed freehand with a radiolucent drill attachment (*Synthes Radiolucent Drive Mark II™ 511.300, Synthes GmbH, Switzerland*). Various techniques and devices developed for facilitating interlocking procedures are reviewed in [2]. One of the more challenging tasks for surgeons is achieving the down-beam position of the nail where the distal holes appear as a circles prior to distal locking.

1.1   Review of Literature

Westphal *et al.* first introduced tele-manipulated robot-assisted drill guidance for interlocking of IM nailing which is based on 3D imaging data and automated X-ray image analysis. After final computations of drilling trajectory and planning, the average number of C-arm images required to achieve nail hole circles was four [3]. Two groups have attempted medical augmented reality systems for orthopedic and trauma surgery facilitating the surgical procedure. First, Navab *et al.* augment a regular mobile C-arm by a video camera for X-ray and video image overlay [4]. From a cadaver study, they report 3.7 ± 1.31 X-ray shots versus 4.25 ± 2.16 X-ray shots using conventional fluoroscopy in achieving nail hole circles. Lastly, solutions recovering the pose of the IM nail with a minimum of 2 X-ray shots have been presented— however they rely on external hardware and infrared optical trackers, as proposed by Leloup *et al.* [5] and Zheng *et al.* [6]. These are inspired solutions but are considered expensive and cumbersome by surgeons. The configuration of such systems is not trivial and its accuracy depends on the setup, as described in [7]. Moreover, given the small real-estate left in the operating room for supplemental equipment and lines of sight issues, a more compact and elegant solution is preferable. Commercial technology is also available. Chung *et al.* measure an electromagnetic field to locate the holes. Nevertheless, this requires special custom IM nails with embedded coils to generate the signal [8] and has not found acceptance.

1.2   Contributions

We propose a trivial video-guided process which would allow the intramedullary nail holes to appear as circles. It is an alternative to the intricate and time consuming 'trial and error' process surgeons undertake when repositioning both C-arm and patient leg. After the acquisition of a first X-ray image, our augmented reality solution provides real-time visualization in 3D space of two 'augmented' circles with their center lying on the axis of the hole. The surgeon can then move the patient leg under video guidance until the circles are superimposed in a down-the-beam position w.r.t the X-ray source center. We evaluated our nail pose recovery using computer synthetic data first, and followed the analysis with a preclinical study involving 7 clinicians.

2   Nail Pose Recovery

This section explains the methods used to recover the 6 DOF position of the nail from a single X-Ray image. The portion of the nail that is in the workspace of the surgeon is the distal part with its two holes (labeled as *proximal* and *distal* to discern them). Our aim is to find the position of the nail holes axis, by finding the position of a virtual nail 'tangent' to its distal part. A 3D model of the IM nail is required for the procedure; we replicated one using the Open Source tool Blender. The nail is rendered with Coin3D, using a camera with parameters equal to our calibrated C-arm (details about calibration in [4]). The reference frame for the translation is the standard pinhole camera reference frame, as seen in Fig. 1-left. The origin is in the center of the viewport, with X pointing right, Y pointing down and Z away from the camera. We also assigned names to the Euler angles used to represent the rotation of the nail. The origin of the nail rotation is when the nail is aligned with the x axis (tip pointing to positive X) and with the holes aligned to the Z axis (down-the-beam). The rotation of the nail on the image plane (around the camera axis, Z) is named γ; its rotation along its own axis is named α, and the last angle (on the plane including the camera and the nail) is called β. It should be emphasized that the most important criteria for our application is finding the value of the angles α and β, and that our aim is to minimize them (that is, to align the nail holes with the camera axis).

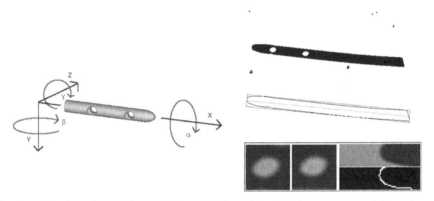

Fig. 1. (Left) The reference frame of the IM nail, and (*Right*) the preprocessed X-ray image with nail and distal holes contouring and tip extraction using OpenCV

2.1   X-ray Image Processing and Segmentation

In the interest of brevity, we omit the details of these steps and direct the reader to the OpenCV toolbox for implementation. All the values were experimentally found and proved to be robust for our hardware and its settings.

X-ray processing: first a thresholding (t = 12) replaces the standard black image frame with a light background uniform to the average X-ray image (~ 150). A median blurring and a morphological closure follows (kernel dimension = 3) accounting against eventual smaller objects and artifacts present inside the X-ray image.

Nail segmentation: a second thresholding (t = 35) leaves just metallic objects in the image; the nail contour is then found among them by geometric constraints on its shape, that is, on its bounding box dimensions. The same process is repeated in finding the contours belonging to the nail holes among the contours included inside the nail contour. The chosen criteria are: absolute dimensions, area, and perimeter/area ratio. If no holes are found a new X-ray must be acquired.

Holes and nail tip: Square patches are extracted around the holes, aligned with the nail axis and positioned about the hole contour centroid. We fit ellipses to each hole and its dimensions and orientation are calculated (Fig. 1-right). Since the proportions of the IM nail are known, we can disambiguate the γ angle (which up to this point is known up to an 180° ambiguity) by searching for the nail tip, at the possible distances from the middle point of the two holes (2 possibilities), or from the only visible one (4 possibilities, since we don't know what hole this is). A patch is extracted at each of these distances, and the Sobel operator is applied. If neighboring maxima are found on each row of the patch, we have found the tip of the nail and we know which hole is what (proximal or distal; relatively, since both are distal holes). Each visible hole is assigned a position given its distance from the nail tip.

Intensity information: The following information is gathered for later use in the nail pose estimation algorithm: the background average color (as visible through the holes of the nail) is computed by averaging it over the central points of the visible holes, while the color of the nail is extracted from the middle point between the two holes, or next to the only visible hole.

2.2   Nail Pose Estimation

Once the nail is successfully identified in the X-ray image, we compute its position with respect to the camera. Our method works, even with a low signal-to-noise ratio, by finding the parameters that make the rendered image of the virtual 3D model of the nail (the DRR) similar to the shape visible in the X-ray image. We developed an incremental heuristic procedure that recovers parameters in the following order (and sets them as rendering parameters for estimation of the successive ones):

- γ, directly measured after segmentation of the nail contour.
- z, found by fitting the diameter of the rendered nail to the actual one from the X-ray; the apparent diameter of the nail on the image is inversely proportional to the distance to the camera.
- (x, y), found by fitting the position of the rendered nail to the actual one. The position is computed as the middle point of the positions of both holes, or of the only visible hole.
- (α, β), found by making the orientation and the minimum axis of the ellipse fitted to the most eccentric hole equal; at greater inclinations, the variation relative to increases of the angle result in greater variations of the image.

The solution for each parameter is then found through a custom coarse gradient descent minimization. Each parameter in the above list is dependent on the preceding one, hence they are found in this order, assuming initial parameter values set to 0 and initial depth position $z_0 = 700$. The assignment $z_0 = 700$ makes the nail visible in our computer simulations and allows the algorithm to initialize. Alternatively, the C-arm device depth can be selected for z_0.

This heuristic procedure works well for the first four parameters (x, y, z, γ) but proved not robust for the last two (α, β). Thus, we fell back to a more conventional algorithm that minimizes the Sum of Squared Differences (SSD) between the patches extracted around the real and virtual nail holes. The nail is rendered in the position composed by the four parameters already found heuristically (x, y, z, γ) and the last two angles α, β, in a range from $\pm40°$ with a step of $0.5°$. This covers the part of the parameter space where the holes are still visible, as we found through inspection of the rendered images. It should be stressed that the first four parameters influence the shape of the holes, and so the first heuristic phase allows this second one to take place.

Algorithm observations: The step size of $0.5°$ was experimentally selected for robustness as larger or smaller values miss the global minimum. This is due to the difficult nature of the problem. Contrary to intuition we were confronted with a non-convex problem with the objective function having thousands of local minima across the search space. This is due to the image discretization: as found by inspection, a small rotation of the hole would change greatly its pixel values, and the ellipse fitted to it. No optimization library succeeded in minimization. This leads to a long execution time (150 s on our setup) which led us to investigate a completely heuristic solution in future work.

Solution uniqueness: The final solution is not unique due to the symmetry of the IM nails. We obtain the magnitude and relative sign of α and β where Pose $= (x, y, z, \alpha, \beta, \gamma)$ gives an identical rendered image to Pose$' = (x, y, z, -\alpha, -\beta, \gamma)$. To rectify this issue in clinical practice, we provide a user interface button that swaps the signs of the two angles instantaneously. A technician can invert manually the angles by clicking on the button and restarting the video guidance of the 'augmented' circles. This leads to a 50% probability of a second X-ray acquisition to verify this case.

3   The 'Augmented' Circles

A trackable object is fixed to the leg of the patient in order to track the movements of the leg (and hence of the nail) after the acquisition of the first X-ray image. As in all orthopedic and trauma clinical applications, the leg is assumed to behave as a rigid object. Hence, the movement of the trackable object is considered rigidly linked to that of the nail. In our scenario, the trackable object consists of two sterile standard AR markers, inclined with respect to each other (see Fig. 2-right). This configuration is crucial in order to maintain a stable detection (i.e. the pose estimation of a marker when it is close to orthogonal to the camera principal axis is very poor). At each time instant during video guidance, the marker that is most inclined with respect to the camera axis is used for the computation of the position of the nail (we reused the tracking software discussed in [4]). The Graphical User Interface (GUI) showcased to the surgeon is composed of two 'augmented' circles, each containing a cross. This configuration was decided alongside the participating surgeons in our study.

The 'augmented' circles are rendered on a line that represents the axis of the hole(s) used to recover the position of the nail. When the circles are superimposed the IM distal holes are in down-beam position to the camera. Visually, the 'augmented circles' are approximately 3 cm apart and provides a clue to the surgeon on how the nail is oriented.

4   Results and Discussion

Computer Simulations: We performed 1000 random tests investigating the robustness of our algorithm for the critical nail angles α and β. The average error for angle α is $1.3 \pm 2.1°$ whereas the error for angle β is $2.0 \pm 4.3°$. We measured the contribution of both angles using the simultaneous orthogonal rotation angle (SORA) metric [10], which is a vector representing angular orientation. The SORA was $2.76 \pm 1.66°$. More than 92.3% of simulations showed β less than 5° compared to 97% of simulations for α. The 5° value represents the tolerance in rotations of the IM nail that surgeons would deem adequate for them to perform distal locking.

Preclinical study: A total of 7 clinicians in the orthopedic and trauma surgery department of the Klinik und Poliklinik Innenstadt, Munich, were involved in the study (2 expert surgeons with vast experience in interlocking of intramedullary nailing procedures, 2 resident surgeons, and 3 last year medical students). An augmented reality fluoroscope [4] was used as the imaging device. A total of 105 C-arm images with various nail inclinations were acquired using bone phantom. Each participant performed the 'augmented' circles technique 15 times. The average time to recover adequate distal holes was 12.7 seconds using an average 2.2 X-ray images total which includes the initial X-ray acquisition. We asked the participants to acquire an additional X-ray to confirm circles if they were not confident on the final orientation of the phantom bone after video guidance. We report a 95.2 % success rate for all trials. The 4.8 % failed cases are due to the nail not being segmented properly because of background clutter present in the X-ray image. Of the 100 successful trials, the UI button was activated in 59 cases to resolve nail ambiguity. Of these cases an additional X-ray image was acquired only twice.

Fig. 2-left provides a visual scenario of the recovered distal holes using our method. The immediate feedback we received by the expert surgeons is that the method stands out for its simplicity, economy, robustness and convenience. In general, the operating room requires complicated workflows and the stressful 'trial and error' task of continuously repositioning the mobile C-arm and/or patient leg is circumvented through our proposed radiation free real-time video guidance. It is worth noting that the students totally relied on our AR visualization while the experts trusted more on their vast clinical experience and thus missed out on important information being depicted to them. The experts failed in their first attempts but then recovered their performance by trusting the 'augmented' circles visualization, realizing that they can use it in their favor.

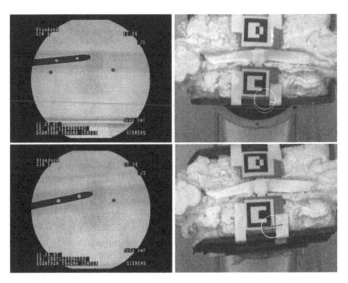

Fig. 2. X-ray images taken prior to and after execution of the 'augmented' circles algorithm

In future, we aim at switching to an RGB-D camera and affixing it to a C-arm device. This would provide depth information and additional clues to help resolve the nail pose uniqueness problem. Also, the estimated distances to the two extrema of the IM nail could be measured and the best fitting solution selected automatically. Regarding the ellipse fitting segmentation, the ideal solution would be developing a new algorithm with sub pixel precision that would smooth the variations of the features detected in X-ray. Our solution tracks the more inclined of the two AR markers in real-time with respect to the camera. Recently, a new type of marker has been developed that allows precise and stable pose estimation at any rotation with respect to a camera (and in particular for small ones). It is called *ArrayMark*, and applies moiré patterns to the surface of a square marker and makes a cross '+' visible inside the marker, at a position dependent from the inclination of the marker (for small angles). Thus a single marker of these would be sufficient for our application. Lastly, the 'augmented' circles can be coupled to that of distal locking presented in [9]. In that work, only a single X-ray image showing adequate circles was required for successful distal locking. As such, we can potentially investigate a full proof augmented reality solution, quasi radiation-free, to complete the entire interlocking procedure.

5   Conclusion

Prior to distal locking of the intramedullary nail, surgeons must position C-arm and/or patient leg in such a way that the nail holes appear in a down-beam position in the X-ray image. We proposed an AR application that visually depicts to the surgeon two 'augmented' circles – the nail and patient leg pose. Using solely video guidance, the surgeon superimposes the circles together to achieve adequate circles. We evaluated our technique using computer simulations and synthetic bones and demonstrated the robustness of the technique by recovering in over 95% of cases and using at most 2 X-ray images.

References

1. Online at,
   http://emedicine.medscape.com/article/1248857-overview#a0199
2. Windolf, M., Schroeder, J., Fliri, L., Dicht, B., Liebergall, M., Richards, R.G.: Reinforcing the role of the conventional C-arm - a novel method for simplified distal interlocking. BMC Musculoskeletal Disorders 13(1), 8 (2012)
3. Westphal, R., Winkelbach, S., Wahl, F., Gösling, T., Oszwald, M., Hüfner, T., Krettek, C.: Robot-assisted Long Bone Fracture Reduction. The International Journal of Robotics Research 28(10), 1259–1278 (2009)
4. Navab, N., Heining, S.M., Traub, J.: Camera Augmented Mobile C-arm (CAMC): Calibration, Accuracy Study and Clinical Applications. IEEE Trans. Med. Imag. 29(7) (2009)
5. Leloup, T., El Kazzi, W., Schuind, F., Warzée, N.: Novel Technique for Distal Locking of Intramedullary Nail Based on Two Non-constrained Fluoroscopic Images and Navigation. IEEE Trans. Med. Imaging 27(9), 1202–1212 (2008)
6. Zheng, G., Zhang, X., Haschtmann, D., Gédet, P., Langlotz, F., Nolte, L.: Accurate and reliable pose recovery of distal locking holes in computer-assisted intra-medullary nailing of femoral shaft fractures: A preliminary study. Computer Aided Surgery 12(3), 138–151 (2007)
7. Liodakis, E., Chu, K., Westphal, R., Krettek, C., Citak, M., Gosling, T., Kenawey, M.: Assessment of the accuracy of infrared and electromagnetic navigation using an industrial robot: Which factors are influencing the accuracy of navigation? Journal of Orthopaedic Research 29(10), 1476–1483 (2011)
8. Chung, T.-K., Chu, H.-J., Wong, T.-H., Hsu, W., Lee, M.-S., Lo, W.-T., Tseng, C.-Y.: An electromagnetic-induction approach for screw-hole targeting in interlocking-nail surgery. In: 2012 IEEE Sensors, pp. 1–4 (2012)
9. Diotte, B., Fallavollita, P., Wang, L., Weidert, S., Thaller, P.-H., Euler, E., Navab, N.: Radiation-Free Drill Guidance in Interlocking of Intramedullary Nails. In: Ayache, N., Delingette, H., Golland, P., Mori, K. (eds.) MICCAI 2012, Part I. LNCS, vol. 7510, pp. 18–25. Springer, Heidelberg (2012)
10. Stančin, S.: Angle Estimation of Simultaneous Orthogonal Rotations from 3D Gyroscope Measurements. Sensors (2011), doi:10.3390/s110908536

CT to US Registration of the Lumbar Spine: A Clinical Feasibility Study

Simrin Nagpal[1], Purang Abolmaesumi[2], Abtin Rasoulian[2], Tamas Ungi[1],
Ilker Hacihaliloglu[2], Jill Osborn[3], Dan P. Borschneck[4], Victoria A. Lessoway[5],
Robert N. Rohling[2], and Parvin Mousavi[1]

[1] Queen's University, Kingston, ON, Canada
[2] The University of British Columbia, Vancouver, B.C., Canada
[3] St. Paul's Hospital, Vancouver, B.C., Canada
[4] Kingston General Hospital, Kingston, ON, Canada
[5] RDMS Department of Ultrasound, Women's Hospital, Vancouver, B.C., Canada

Abstract. Spine needle injections are widely applied to alleviate pain
and to remove nerve sensation through analgesia and anesthesia. Currently, spinal injections are performed using either no image guidance
or modalities that expose the patient to ionizing radiation such as fluoroscopy or computed tomography (CT). Ultrasound (US) is being investigated as an alternative as it is a non-ionizing and more accessible
image modality. An inherent challenge to US imaging of the spine is the
acoustic shadows created by the bony structures of the vertebrae limiting visibility. It is possible to enhance the anatomical information in
US through its fusion with a pre-operative CT. In this manuscript we
propose a clinical feasibility study involving a novel registration pipeline
to align CT and US images of the spine. This pipeline involves automatic global and multi-vertebrae registration. We evaluate the proposed
methodology on five clinical data sets. The proposed method is able to
register the data sets from initial misalignments of up to 25 mm, with a
mean TRE of 1.17 mm, sufficient for many spine needle interventions.

Keywords: Registration, ultrasound, lumbar spine, multi-vertebrae.

1 Introduction

Spine needle injections are commonly used to deliver anesthesia and analgesia.
Facet joint injections are an example of a common spinal intervention to treat
chronic lower back pain [1]. Injections into this region are particularly challenging
due to the deep location and the narrow space of the joint, and proximity to
nerve tissue. These challenges make it difficult to provide accurate treatment to
the target area when the procedure is performed without guidance. The current
gold standard to guide the injection is fluoroscopy or intra-operative computed
tomography (CT), exposing the patient and the clinician to ionizing radiation.

Intra-operative ultrasound (US) guidance for spine needle procedures is an
attractive alternative as US is a non-ionizing and more accessible image modality compared to fluoroscopy or CT [2]. Using US guidance eliminates radiation

D. Stoyanov et al. (Eds.): IPCAI 2014, LNCS 8498, pp. 108–117, 2014.

associated with intra-operative CT or fluoroscopy. Additionally, US images can be taken in any location, as opposed to specialized facilities required for CT or fluoroscopy, improving the accessibility of spine needle interventions. US, however, has not become the standard-of-care for spine needle injections due to the difficulty associated with its interpretation of anatomy. Specifically, acoustic shadows from the bony structures of vertebrae limit the visibility of anatomical targets, such as facet joints in US images. To enhance the interpretation of US images and provide improved guidance, three dimensional (3D) anatomical information (e.g. from a pre-operative CT or a statistical shape model) can be integrated with the intra-operative US images through image registration.

Over the past decade, several point-based methods for registration of CT and US images of boney structures other than the spine have been presented in the literature [3, 4, 6]. A challenge of those techniques has been to reliably extract the bone surface from US images. Recently, local phase-based image processing of US has shown great promise in the automatic enhancement of the US bone surface [7]. To avoid US bone segmentation, intensity-based approaches to registration are also used [8–10]. Our group has also proposed several techniques for the registration of CT and US images [11, 12] based on a biomechanical model of the spine to constrain the possible space of solutions for registration.

Despite this surge of interest, to date, reliable registration of CT and US images of the spine for multiple vertebrae has not been effectively demonstrated, *in vivo*. The closest work is by Winter *et al.* [9] but only for a single vertebra; this approach does not consider the relative change in the pose of the vertebrae with respect to each other that naturally occurs between CT and US data acquisition. Since facet joints lay in the space between two adjacent vertebrae, a fast and robust registration approach of multiple vertebrae is clinically desirable.

In this paper, we present a clinical feasibility study involving a novel registration approach that aligns pre-operative diagnostic CT and intra-operative US images of multiple vertebrae. We validate the approach on data obtained from five patients who were scheduled for a spine injection. The registration approach involves both intensity and point based methods; it starts with global registration of the spine followed by a multi-vertebrae point-based registration.

2   Materials and Methods

2.1   Data Acquisition

Human data sets of the lumbar spine are used to validate the proposed registration method. Following Institutional Research Ethics Board approval, subjects provide informed consent to participate. Data is collected at St. Paul's Hospital in Vancouver, B.C., Canada. Only subjects with previous CT scans are recruited. The population of subjects include female and male patients with ages between 28 and 49 years, and weights between 135 and 202 lbs. The anonymized CT images of patients in supine position, the standard–of–care positioning for spinal CT, are provided as DICOM files by the hospital.

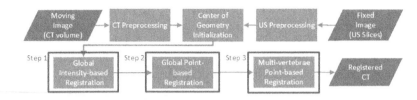

Fig. 1. General overview of the CT to US registration workflow

An imaging protocol is created for freehand US data acquisition that minimizes variability between subjects, and operators, and ensures setup time adheres to clinical practice. A SonixTouch US scanner (Ultrasonix, Richmond, B.C.) equipped with a magnetic tracker (Ascension DriveBay EM tracker, Burlington, VT) and a C5-2 curvilinear transducer are used for US data acquisition. An Ascension 800 EM tracking sensor, affixed to the patient's skin above the T12 vertebra is used as the patient coordinate reference. PLUS, an open-source toolkit [13] is used for US and tracking data recording; US calibration is performed using the N-wire method available in this toolkit as well. Subjects are set in the prone position, with a pillow under their stomach. An experienced sonographer scans the subjects and makes minor adjustments to preset US imaging parameters including depth; the parameters are preset earlier using a population of volunteers. The sonographer places marks on the skin surface corresponding to the T12-L1 and L5-S1 intervertebral spaces to delineate the US scanning region. Data is acquired by moving the US transducer slowly and smoothly in a downward zigzag pattern while holding the imaging plane sagittal, and maintaining contact with the subject's skin. Scanning starts at the left L1 transverse process, moving across to the right L1 transverse process. It then moves down to display the right L2 transverse process and across in the opposite direction, and continues in this zigzag manner to acquire US images of the entire lumbar spine. An US volume is reconstructed using the PLUS toolkit, where the pixel size in each dimension is taken into account. Only the portion of the lumbar spine visible in pre-operative CT, is included in the final US volume.

2.2 Registration

Our proposed method involves intensity- and point-based registration of the bone surfaces to harness the advantages of each method. The general overview of the registration pipeline is illustrated in Fig. 1. In our workflow, pre-operatively, CT volumes are automatically segmented [17]; in addition, points between adjacent vertebrae are manually selected to constrain an intra-operative multi-body registration step. Intra-operatively, registration is performed without any manual intervention. The registration is initialized given the transformation of the center of geometry of the preprocessed CT volume (see below) to the center of geometry of the preprocessed US volume, and assuming that this centre represents similar structures in both image modalities. The method has the following major steps:

Global Intensity-Based Registration: The General Registration (BRAINS) module, within the open source software 3D Slicer (version 4.2), that employs a rigid BRAINSFit algorithm with default parameters, is used to automatically align preprocessed CT and preprocessed US [14] volumes. To enhance the CT bone surface, images are filtered in the frequency domain using local phase image processing [7]. Subsequently, a simple ray-casting is done in the posterior to anterior direction such that the first bone pixel encountered for each column is saved as bone and anything below that pixel is saved as background. The ray-casting helps to remove the bright intensity values that exist in CT, but do not exist in US, since US signals cannot propagate through the bone surface. A sagittal CT slice from one patient overlaid with the enhanced bone surface is seen in Fig. 2, left. The inverse Euclidean distance map is calculated on the enhanced bone surface CT image by computing the distance between each pixel and the nearest non-zero pixel of the image, in physical coordinates (mm). In this map, the intensity values at the bone surface are maximized, and as the distance increases from the CT bone surface, the intensity values decrease.

Local phase filtering of the US volume is performed to automatically enhance the US bone surface relative to the soft tissue. In this approach the US images are filtered with a Gradient Energy Tensor filter. The US local phase filtering differs from the CT phase filtering in that multiple edge features (step edge, line, corner, junction) have to be extracted due to the complex shape of the vertebrae's appearance in US. This method is intensity invariant; a detailed description of its implementation along with robustness studies to noise are available in [7]. The filter parameters are chosen empirically using a small subset of in vivo images to produce a good bone surface localization in the presence of speckle. The parameters are then held fixed all throughout registration. A sagittal US slice of a patient with enhanced bone surface overlaid is shown in Fig. 2, centre.

Global Point-Based Registration: We use the Coherent Point Drift (CPD)[15] to further adjust the result of registration in the previous step. CPD uses probability density estimation to find corresponding points between the CT and US and has a closed-form solution. Myronenko, *et al.* have performed a comparison of the performance of CPD with Iterative Closets Point (ICP) in the presence of outliers and noise, and have demonstrated the robustness of CPD [15]. For each vertebrae in CT data , the vertebrae are automatically labeled pre-operatively using [17]. We automatically extract a single pixel thick bone surface from phase filtered US images by modifying an algorithm originally presented in [16]. In the original algorithm, the US images are smoothed using Gaussian filtering; the bone surface pixels are then enhanced by a combination of two main bone features: high acoustic impedance and acoustic shadowing. Continuity and smoothness of the bone surface are established by minimizing a cost function using dynamic programming [16]. Our modification makes this approach applicable to clinical patient data. Instead of using the intensity values from the smoothed US image, intensity values from a phase filtered US image are used. This results in less noise in the segmented bone surfaces, critical for an accurate point-based registration (Fig. 2, right).

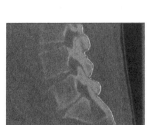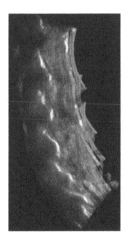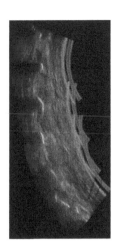

Fig. 2. (left) A sagittal CT slice with the phase filtered and raycasted bone surface overlaid in yellow; (centre) Sagittal US slices with the phase filtered and raycasted bone surface overlaid in yellow (centre) and with the single pixel bone surface (right)

Multi-vertebrae Point-Based Registration: Although vertebrae are rigid bodies, the intervertebral discs are deformable. To account for possible curvature changes of each vertebra along the lumbar spine, we present a novel multi-body rigid CPD registration. At every iteration of the algorithm, each vertebra is transformed individually. As a result, it is possible that they can be transformed into a pose of the lumbar spine that is not physically possible. To overcome this challenge, ten points are chosen pre-operatively on two adjacent vertebra in the CT. Five points on the sagittal slices on the left of the spinous process and five points on the right of the spinous process. Henceforward, these point sets are referred to as springs, since although they are not mechanical springs, they act to constrain the registration similarly to mechanical springs. The points are placed at the midpoint of either the space between the vertebral bodies or the space between the facet joint. Each point is then duplicated to act as a spring, where one point belongs to the superior vertebrae's side and the other point belongs to the inferior vertebrae's side. At each iteration, the springs points are transformed according to the vertebrae they belong to. An example sagittal slice where three points are chosen is shown in Fig. 3. The cost function for CPD, $E(t)$ (where t represents the transformation), has the form of a likelihood function of point correspondences between CT and US data, described as weighted sum of distances [15]. Myronenko *et al.* have provided a closed form solution to $E(t)$; for multi-vertebrae registration, we add a regularization term, $R(t)$ representing springs, to the cost function to achieve the form: $E(t) + \alpha * R(t)$. Here α determines the contribution of the springs. It can be shown that $\alpha * R(t)$ can be combined into $E(t)$, and the closed form solution can be used to minimize the new cost function. As such, in our registration algorithm, springs are integrated into the existing probability density estimations and the cost function is not

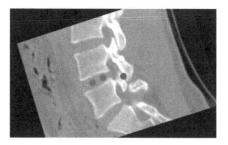

Fig. 3. Sagittal slice of a CT demonstrating three spring points between two vertebrae. Two are at midpoint between vertebral bodies (red) and one is in the facet joint (green).

modified from CPD. Values of α between 2^{-3} to 2^{7} were tested; a value of 2^{5} provided the most accurate registration for all clinical data sets and was chosen.

2.3   Experiments

Since the CT scans are previously acquired, fiducial markers that are visible in both CT and US cannot be used for gold standard evaluation. Instead, anatomical landmarks on the lamina of each vertebra are placed on the US images. Two clinicians with spine anatomy expertise choose these anatomical landmarks and we pool the data. We assume the CT and US to have optimal alignment following registration. To determine the accuracy and precision of the registration method, the CT and the points representing the lamina landmarks are perturbed by a transformation selected randomly from a uniform distribution of $5°$ rotation about each axis and 5 mm translation along each axis. The transformation is applied to the entire lumbar spine that is visible in the CT. The initial misalignment is determined by calculating the target registration error (TRE) between the original position of the lamina landmark points and the position of the landmarks after the initial perturbation. To determine the capture range for the registration pipeline, 20 tests are performed with misalignment errors randomly generated within the range 0 - 25 mm. Registration is then performed and the final TRE is calculated as the root mean square between the transformed lamina landmark points and their original positions. A qualitative clinical validation is also performed. Here, a point is added on the posterior dura between two adjacent vertebra in the US images by both operators. This is where the clinician aims their needle for spinal anaesthesia and thus provides a clinically relevant validation. If the points selected are in the correct region after registering the CT to the US, the registration is potentially suitable for spinal injection.

3   Results and Discussion

For three patient data sets L3, L4 and L5 vertebrae were available in the CT volume for registration, while for the other two patients only L4 and L5 vertebrae were available and used for registration. The mean TRE, maximum point

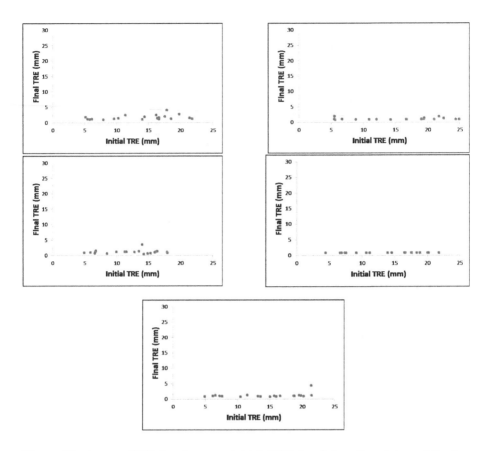

Fig. 4. Final mean TRE (mm) versus initial TRE (mm) for all vertebrae following random misalignment and CT to US registration. The subplots from top left to bottom right correspond to results from patients 1 to 5, respectively.

distance and total success rate for each patient, following the capture range experiments, is depicted in Table 1. The space within a facet joint is reported to be between 2 to 4 mm; previous literature also define 2 to 4 mm as a clinically acceptable accuracy for spinal injections [12]. In our manuscript, we set a more stringent criteria by defining registration success as achieving a mean TRE of 2 mm or less. This provides a conservative estimate for clinical acceptability of our proposed approach. Based on this definition and using Table 1, our average success rate is 97%. The final TRE after each run of the capture range experiment given the initial misalignment TRE for all patients is shown in Fig. 4. All reported values are the average TRE for each individual vertebra. The mean TRE is the average of the TRE values from the 20 runs of the capture experiments. From Table 1, it is evident that the mean TRE is well below 2 mm.

Registration was performed on a Lenovo ThinkCenter, with Intel i5-3570 quad-core CPU and 16 GB of RAM. The runtime for each of the main

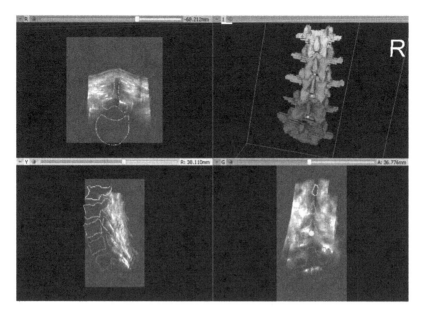

Fig. 5. 3D rendering of CT vertebrae with points on the posterior dura between two vertebrae in yellow (top right); transverse (top left), coronal (bottom right), and sagittal (bottom left) planes showing US slices with CT contours overlaid for one patient

Table 1. Mean TRE (mm), maximum point distance (mm) and total success rate from the CT to US registration for the five patients using the full registration pipeline

dataset	mean TRE ± std (mm)	max point distance (mm)	success rate
Patient 1	1.66 ± 0.77	4.61	16/20
Patient 2	1.09 ± 0.32	3.51	20/20
Patient 3	1.07 ± 0.64	3.76	19/20
Patient 4	0.85 ± 0.01	0.90	20/20
Patient 5	1.18 ± 0.77	4.64	19/20

registration components of the pipeline are as follows: intensity-based (step 1), 5–20 sec, point-based (step 2), 25–45 sec, and Multi-vertebrae (step 3), 20–120 sec.

To provide qualitative validation on successful registration runs, contours of the CT are overlaid on the sagittal, transverse and coronal planes of the US (an example illustrated in Fig. 5). A 3D rendering of the CT with a point on the posterior dura between each two adjacent vertebrae represents the target area for spinal injections. This is placed by our two operators, and provides a clinically relevant result to support quantitative validation. For all patients, the CT contours align in all three planes and the points on the posterior dura are all within the target area for spinal anesthesia (also seen in Fig. 5).

In preliminary analysis we evaluated the significance of the three major registration components. It was observed that both global intensity- and point-based registration steps are necessary for a robust registration especially in cases where there is limited US bone visibility in the data, or one approach does not provide a close initial alignment between the CT and US. We also studied the role of springs to constrain the multi-vertebrae point-based registration. As vertebrae are the rigid bodies transformed individually, registration can result in a pose of the lumbar spine that is not physically possible. This includes having two vertebrae intersect each other (collision). Indeed, our results show that, without the springs, registration of CT and US images resulted in collision in some patients. Capture range experiments when no springs are included to constrain registration, are performed. To determine if there is a significant difference in the TRE using the complete registration pipeline versus one without springs, we use the Wilcoxon Signed-Rank Test, where $p < 0.01$ is considered significant. TRE from all but one patient were statistically significantly worse without using springs.

4   Conclusion and Future Work

We presented a clinical feasibility study involving a novel registration pipeline for the lumbar spine that accurately aligns pre-operative CT to intra-operative US using five clinical data sets. By aligning the CT with the US, anatomical information that is not visible in US is provided to the clinician to guide spine needle interventions. This removes exposure of the physician or patient to radiation intra-operatively. To the best of our knowledge, this is the first work where multiple vertebrae are registered between CT and US using clinical data.

The proposed registration pipeline shows great promise for guiding percutaneous spine procedures, but further improvements are needed for its clinical use. The artificial springs are chosen manually pre-operatively; however, improvements can be made to automate the artificial spring selection for more practical use in the clinic. In addition, the spring parameter α value is set to a constant for all spring points, but could be adaptively adjusted based on the position of the springs on the vertebrae and their anatomical interpretation. Since the CPD registration of individual vertebrae can be parallelized, we can potentially use multi-CPU implementation with the Intel Math Kernel library to gain speed ups of several orders of magnitude. Finally, the registration pipeline includes multiple modules. For clinical applications, it is possible that a simpler pipeline could be selected with only a subsection of these modules, and further steps are only included when registration accuracy does not meet preset thresholds.

Acknowledgments. This work was supported in part by the Natural Sciences and Engineering Research Council of Canada (NSERC), the Canadian Institutes of Health Research (CIHR), and Ontario Early Researcher Award.

References

1. Falco, F., Manchikanti, L., Datta, S., Sehgal, N., Geffert, S., Onyewu, O., Zhu, J., Coubarous, S., Hameed, M., Ward, S., Sharma, M., Hameed, H., Singh, V., Boswell, M.: An update of the effectiveness of therapeutic lumbar facet joint interventions. Pain Physician 15, E909–E953 (2012)

2. Conroy, P., Luyet, C., McCartney, C., McHardy, P.: Real-time ultrasound-guided spinal anaesthesia: a prospective observational study of a new approach. Anesthesiology Research & Practice 2013, 525 818–525 824 (2013)
3. Moghari, M.H., Abolmaesumi, P.: Point-based rigid-body registration using an unscented Kalman filter. IEEE Trans. Med. Imag. 26(12) (2007)
4. Brounstein, A., Hacihaliloglu, I., Guy, P., Hodgson, A., Abugharbieh, R.: Towards real-time 3D US to CT bone image registration using phase and curvature feature based GMM matching. In: Fichtinger, G., Martel, A., Peters, T. (eds.) MICCAI 2011, Part I. LNCS, vol. 6891, pp. 235–242. Springer, Heidelberg (2011)
5. Besl, P., McKay, N.: Method for registration of 3-D shapes. IEEE Trans. Pattern Analysis and Machine Intelligence 14(2), 239–256 (1992)
6. Ma, B., Ellis, R.E.: Robust registration for computer-integrated orthopedic surgery: laboratory validation and clinical experience. Medical Image Analysis 7(3), 237–250 (2003)
7. Hacihaliloglu, I., Rasoulian, A., Rohling, R.N., Abolmaesumi, P.: Statistical Shape Model to 3D Ultrasound Registration for Spine Interventions Using Enhanced Local Phase Features. In: Mori, K., Sakuma, I., Sato, Y., Barillot, C., Navab, N. (eds.) MICCAI 2013, Part II. LNCS, vol. 8150, pp. 361–368. Springer, Heidelberg (2013)
8. Penney, G.P., Barratt, D.C., Chan, C.S., Slomczykowski, M., Carter, T.J., Edwards, P.J., Hawkes, D.J.: Cadaver validation of intensity-based ultrasound to CT registration. Medical Image Analysis 10(3), 385–395 (2006)
9. Winter, S., Brendel, B., Pechlivanis, I., Schmieder, K., Igel, C.: Registration of CT and intra-operative 3-D US images of the spine using evolutionary & gradient-based methods. IEEE Trans. Evol. Comp. 12(3), 284–296 (2008)
10. Yan, C.X.B., Goulet, B., Pelletier, J., Chen, S.J.-S., Tampieri, D., Collins, D.L.: Towards accurate, robust and practical ultrasound-CT registration of vertebrae for image-guided spine surgery. Int. Journal of Computer Assisted Radiology and Surgery 6(4), 523–537 (2011)
11. Gill, S., Abolmaesumi, P., Fichtinger, G., Boisvert, J., Pichora, D., Borshneck, D., Mousavi, P.: Biomechanically constrained groupwise ultrasound to CT registration of the lumbar spine. Medical Image Analysis 16(3), 662–674 (2012)
12. Rasoulian, A., Abolmaesumi, P., Mousavi, P.: Feature-based multibody rigid registration of CT and US images of lumbar spine. Medical Physics 39(6), 3154–3166 (2012)
13. Lasso, A., Heffter, T., Pinter, C., Ungi, T., Fichtinger, G.: Implementation of the plus open-source toolkit for translational research of ultrasound-guided intervention systems. In: Workshop at Medical Image Computing and Computer-Assisted Intervention (MICCAI 2012) - Systems and Architectures for Computer Assisted Interventions, pp. 1–12 (2012)
14. Johnson, H., Harris, G., Williams, K.: Brainsfit: Mutual information registrations of whole-brain 3D images, using the insight toolkit. Insight Journal (2007)
15. Myronenko, A., Song, X.: Point set registration: coherent point drift. IEEE Trans. Pattern Analysis and Machine Intelligence 32(12), 2262–2275 (2010)
16. Foroughi, P., Boctor, E., Swartz, M., Taylor, R., Fichtinger, G.: P6d-2 ultrasound bone segmentation using dynamic programming. In: Ultrasonics Symposium, pp. 2523–2526. IEEE, New York (2007)
17. Rasoulian, A., Rohling, R., Abolmaesumi, P.: Lumbar spine segmentation using a statistical multi-vertebrae anatomical shape+pose model. IEEE Trans. Medical Imaging 32(10) (2013)

A Computer Assisted Planning System for the Placement of sEEG Electrodes in the Treatment of Epilepsy

G. Zombori[1], R. Rodionov[2,3], M. Nowell[2,3], M.A. Zuluaga[1], Matthew J. Clarkson[1],
C. Micallef[2,3], B. Diehl[2,3], T. Wehner[2,3], A. Miserochi[2,3], Andrew W. McEvoy[2,3],
John S. Duncan[2,3], and Sébastien Ourselin[1,4]

[1] Centre for Medical Image Computing, University College London, UK
[2] Dept. of Clinical and Experimental Epilepsy, UCL Institute of Neurology, London, UK
[3] National Hospital for Neurology and Neurosurgery (NHNN), London, UK
[4] Dementia Research Centre, Department of Neurodegenerative Disease,
UCL Institute of Neurology, London, UK

Abstract. Approximately 20–30% of patients with focal epilepsy are medically refractory and may be candidates for curative surgery. Stereo EEG is the placement of multiple depth electrodes into the brain to record seizure activity and precisely identify the area to be resected. The two important criteria for electrode implantation are accurate navigation to the target area, and avoidance of critical structures such as blood vessels. In current practice neurosurgeons have no assistance in the planning of the electrode trajectories.

To provide assistance a real-time solution was developed that first identifies the potential entry points by analysing the entry-angle, then computes the associated risks for trajectories starting from these locations. The entry angle, the total length of the trajectory and distances to critical structures are presented in an interactive way that is integrated with standard electrode placement planning tools and advanced visualisation. We show that this improves the planning of intracranial implantation, with safer trajectories in less time.

1   Introduction

Approximately 20–30% of patients with focal epilepsy are medically refractory to treatment with anti-epileptic drugs. These patients are potential candidates for curative respective surgery [1]. The primary aim of epilepsy surgery is to remove the epileptogenic zone—'the minimum amount of cortex that must be resected (inactivated or completely disconnected) to produce seizure freedom' [2]. The identification of the epileptogenic zone often requires the placement of intracranial electrodes to record where seizures start and rapidly propagate. Stereo-electroencephalography (SEEG) is the practice of recording electroencephalographic signals via depth electrodes that are surgically implanted into the brain tissue. The challenge in epilepsy surgery now is in the treatment of the more difficult patient groups (extratemporal non-lesional) where SEEG is increasingly utilised. This invasive investigation carries the risks of infection, haemorrhage and neurological deficit [3]. In the current work we only consider

D. Stoyanov et al. (Eds.): IPCAI 2014, LNCS 8498, pp. 118–127, 2014.

SEEG electrode implantation where brain shift is anticipated to be negligible due to the borehole surgery approach.

Preoperative planning of SEEG electrode placement is a necessary prerequisite to implantation. Important anatomical and functional landmarks of the brain (such as blood vessels, pial boundaries, nerve tracts, etc.) can be identified with advanced neuro-imaging and image-processing techniques. SEEG electrode trajectories are defined by a target area that has to be reached by the electrode and an entry point where the electrode penetrates the skull. Electrode arrangements are planned to achieve adequate cortical coverage and pass through safe, avascular planes. The large number of electrodes required in SEEG and the cumulative risk associated with this implies that assisted planning (AP) is the most useful in these clinical cases.

Previous publications on pre-operative planning of depth electrode placement describe approaches to find the optimal path either automatically [4-6] or by assisting the decision making process of the neurosurgeon [7-9]. Another state of the art approach [10] proposed a system to assist planning at all stages of the planning from the selection of the target point to the selection of a safe entry point that minimizes the risk of hitting with vital structures. In all of these approaches the operator needs to select the target point precisely and the time required to compute the optimised paths is generally long. A recent article describes a high performance solution to enable quantitative estimation of the risk associated with a particular access path at interactive rates. The authors employ Graphics Processing Units (GPUs) to achieve real-time speed and use risk maps visualisation to aid the planning process [11].

Here we present an advanced set of tools for computer-assisted planning of SEEG electrode placement that come as part of our surgical planning system EpiNav™ (CMIC, UCL, London, UK) that allows neurosurgeons to define safer trajectories in less time. EpiNav™ advances on previous work by offering improved real-time visual feedback to planning; including the addition of several vital structures (such as functional brain regions) into the risk assessment and also factoring the entry angle of the trajectory line with the skull surface.

2   Methods

To enable a faster planning process and ensure safety of the resulting implantation plan the following conditions have to be met with the aid of the planning system:

1. Critical structures have to be clearly identifiable (visualisation).
2. None of the trajectories can intersect any critical tissue to avoid harm to the patient.
3. The trajectory should be further from any critical tissue by a specified safety margin based on the accuracy of the surgical procedure of implanting the electrodes.
4. The trajectory should be as short as possible. It is assumed here that only the tip of the electrode is meant to hit the target. At this stage we are not considering cases of multiple targets sampled by one electrode.
5. The entry angle of the trajectory should be as close to 90 degrees as possible to allow robust implementation of the planned entry angle during the surgical procedure.

To achieve fast processing and real-time interaction EpiNav™ was developed using a cross platform C++ library NifTK (www.niftk.org) that is based on the Medical Imaging and Interaction Toolkit (MITK, www.mitk.org). Furthermore we employ a modern graphics card (GPU) and utilize the OpenCL library to enable parallel programming. EpiNav™ can be installed on any recent PC that runs Mac OS X, Linux or Windows and has a GPU that is OpenCL 1.1 compatible.

2.1   Critical Structures

Identifying critical objects is key to successful estimation of a safe trajectory. The critical structures are imported into an interactive visualisation workstation using the functionality of EpiNav™, then converted into 3D surface mesh objects and coloured using a colour scheme (See Fig. 3/a) as in our previous work [12]. The clinically relevant landmarks are white matter tracts (e.g. cortico-spinal tract, optic radiation tract) derived from DTI data, lesions, eloquent cortex (e.g. language or motor areas) derived from fMRI, areas of ictal hyperperfusion derived from SPECT, areas of hypometabolism derived from PET image, ictal or interictal EEG/MEG sources. Blood vessel images were acquired using CTA, 3D Phase Contrast MR imaging and in some cases ToF MR, then the vasculature was extracted using a custom tool. A surface representation of the skull is used to determine the accurate location of the entry points and to compute the entry angle of the trajectory. The skull surface is usually derived from CT, CTA or pseudo CT synthetized from an MR scan.

2.2   Trajectory Planning

The planning process starts with the selection of the target point. The target point can be placed by clicking on any location within the space of the reference image on one of the 2D or 3D views. If a detailed brain parcellation map is available it can be used to aid the target selection, by highlighting various anatomical regions of the brain. Entry points can only be placed onto the skull surface. In manual mode this is ensured by the entry point selection tool.

2.3   Entry Points Search and Risk Analysis

As soon as the target point is selected the system will analyse the topology of the critical structures and offer a set of entry points that represent minimal risk. The entry point search algorithm is a fully automatic method that is implemented on the GPU. It takes the skull mesh as the input and processes each of its vertices, so the sampling rate is defined by the number of vertices in the skull model. The algorithm takes into account the distance of the target point and the currently evaluated vertex (i.e. the length of the trajectory) and the entry angle of the trajectory starting from this vertex. From a surgical point of view the entry angle has to be as close to perpendicular as possible, otherwise it is not possible to drill the borehole through the skull. As the angle and length analysis is computationally inexpensive it is practical to perform it as the first step and disqualify entry points that are too far, or the entry angle is outside a user-configured range (in our practice ±10 degrees from perpendicular). The remaining entry point candidates are checked for collisions with the critical structures: the ones that do not allow straight access are ruled out. Early exclusion of unsuitable entry points avoids unnecessary evaluations, which enables more detailed risk analysis on the remaining points while maintaining real time performance.

The associated risk to each potential trajectory is evaluated using a GPU based module. Previously published risk metrics would assign risk based on the shortest Euclidean distance from any point on the trajectory, while our new metric provides a full distance profile along it. For each potential trajectory 256 sample locations are considered along the length from entry point to target point. The minimum distance to the critical structures (one at a time) is computed per sample point and the results are aggregated, resulting in an array of values that contains the distance to the nearest critical object per sample point.

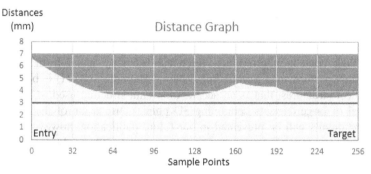

Fig. 1. Distance Graph. The light grey area represents the distance to a critical structure. Green Line - Risk Zone threshold; Red line - Safety margin; Grey/Blue border line - Distance Graph with blue area reflecting risk and grey area reflecting minimal distance to the nearest object.

Once the critical distances have been identified for each potential trajectory the actual risk computation can take place. In this work a new integrative risk metric is introduced that quantifies the level of risk on a 0-1 scale (0 – no risk; 1 – the highest risk which must be avoided). The proposed metric can be extended to include distance, angle of entry and whether the electrode contacts are in grey matter.

A trajectory is considered too risky when the minimum distance to any critical structure is smaller than the "Safety Margin" distance d_{min}. If the trajectory lies further from any structure than a "Risk Zone" margin d_{max} then it represents no potential harm. In EpiNav^{TM} these values can be adjusted by the user when required. The amount of risk that emanates from proximity to critical structures f_{dist} can be quantified within a range of accepted values by computing the area above the curve (See Fig.1 – blue area):

$$S_{risk} = \int_{entry}^{target} (d_{max} - (f_{dist}(x) - d_{min}))dx$$

$$R_{dist} = \frac{S_{risk}}{(d_{max} - d_{min}) * length}$$

This formula yields risk values in the range of 0-1. The quality of the entry angle can be similarly evaluated R_{angle} given the range of accepted values, as well as the length of the trajectory R_{length}. These independent risk components can be combined by applying certain weight factors:

$$R_{total} = w_1 R_{dist} + w_2 R_{angle} + w_3 R_{length},$$

$$where \sum w_i = 1 \ and \ R_i \in [0\sim1]$$

This final metric R_{total} describes the overall quality of the trajectory. After every potential trajectory has been assessed the risk values are visualised in form of a risk-map (Fig. 2.). The planning module will automatically suggest to use the trajectory that has the lowest risk value across the whole map. However, the surgeon can over-ride this by modifying the entry point according to the risk map.

The technical challenges of this work are related to the efficient parallel implementation of collision detection, proximity search and distance evaluations in OpenCL. To allow real-time performance a Bounding Volume Hierarchy (BVH) is built over the cells of critical structures, that is an acceleration data structure used to facilitate the fast traversal of large datasets containing 3D points. Discussion of the specific implementation details will be presented in our future publication, however a good description of the use of BVH for proximity analysis using GPU hardware can be found here [11, 13, 14].

2.4   Visualisation

EpiNav[TM] provides the standard ortho-view (2D planes: axial, coronal, sagittal), combined with 3D visualisation (volume / surface rendering) in a 2x2 layout. The "Probe Eye View" display and a "Distance Graph" widget are placed in a separate window. The Probe Eye View displays an oblique plane (2D) that is always perpendicular to the line of the trajectory (See Fig. 3/b). The distance graph widget (Fig. 3/c) provides the visual representation of the minimal distance information in form of a graph. The length of the graph (horizontal axis) corresponds to the length of the trajectory, while the height of the bars (vertical axis) represent the distance to the nearest critical structure for that particular point of the trajectory. The graph is re-scaled along the vertical axis to focus the representation on the critical sections (Risk Zone).

EpiNav[TM] offers linked visualisation components (similarly to [10]) where the cursor location is synchronised between all visualisation components. For example picking a surface point in the 3D window will update the position of all other views. Similarly, clicking on a point of the distance graph will update the slice positions in the 3 orthogonal plane views and will also update the displayed slice in the probe eye view. This behaviour allows the user to visually identify risky sections of the planned trajectory, by clicking on these sections on the risk display the associated 2D and 3D views will be presented for review.

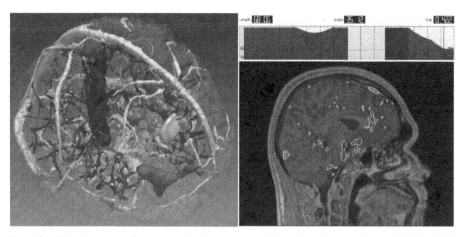

Fig. 3/a. Visualisation of various critical structures. Blue: Cerebrospinal tract (CST), Pink: hypometabolism PET, Deep Pink: SPECT, Cyan-Red: blood vessels, Green arrow: Historical trajectory **3/b**: Probe Eye View displaying a projection that is perpendicular to the trajectory with distance graph showing distances to critical structures along the trajectory. Above the graph the length of the path, angle of entry and the risk are displayed.

The locations of the suitable entry points are marked on the skull surface by colouring their location accordingly (Fig. 4). The risk values are linearly mapped onto a colour lookup table that extends from red to green, red meaning high risk while green symbolising low-risk. All information in the risk map, distance graph, as well as the angle, risk, length and slice position are updated real time as the trajectory being adjusted.

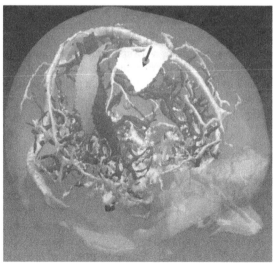

Fig. 4. Risk Map visualisation: The semi-transparent part of the skull represent non-suitable points while the coloured patch shows the potential entry points with associated risk. Green – low risk, red – high risk. In this case the target point was picked at random.

3   Evaluation and Results

3.1   Computational Performance

To evaluate the efficiency each of the proposed methods were tested several times using different input data and the average execution time was recorded for each case. In the evaluation 4 surface meshes were used: skull surface (185k vertices); cerebrospinal tract (33k vertices); veins (91k vertices); arteries (70k vertices). The process times were recorded using OpenCL time events, including both the execution time of the OpenCL kernels, task executions scheduling and the time of data transfer between host and device. The desktop computer that was used in the tests has the following configuration: Intel XEON 16core CPU, 16 GB of RAM and an NVidia Quadro K2000 2 GB GPU.

The first step of the risk analysis is the entry point search algorithm that aims to reduce the number of trajectory candidates. To test this the skull surface model was loaded and 10 historical electrode target points were selected. The average time to complete was measured to be 2.7ms, while the average reduction factor was 97%, resulting between 200-6000 entry point candidates. The next step is the construction of the BVH that only needs to be constructed once at the start. For the reference skull image (the largest mesh used in the test) the construction took 50ms on average.

Table 1. Computation time of risk evaluation for software generated trajectories

Total Num. of Trajectories	Risk Evaluation (ms)
1	1.3
5	7.1
50	13.4
500	96.7
5000	248.1

To evaluate risk computation times various number of trajectories were generated by specifying a target point and assigning a number of random entry points. The computation time was found to be a linear function of the number of trajectory candidates, for the expected maximal number of entry points (~6000) the AP module provides close to real time interactions with 4fps (Table 1).

3.2   Neurosurgical Evaluations

To evaluate the benefits of employing the new risk estimation, the risk map and distance graph, 30 electrode trajectories in 6 patients were evaluated, and their length (Fig. 5), angle of entry (Fig. 6) risk value (Fig. 7) were compared to results of non-assisted planning. The analysis was performed using historical data, where the original electrode trajectories were planned by expert neurosurgeons who relied only on traditional 2D visualisation. The average time to plan one electrode using the non-assisted approach is estimated as 10-15 min based on our previous experience. The new trajectories were planned by a neurosurgeon using the computer assisted planning (AP), keeping the same target points for the purpose of comparison.

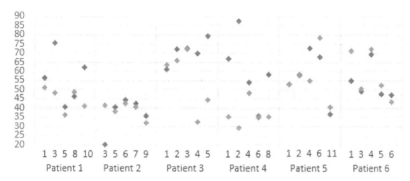

Fig. 5. Comparison of length. Values in blue represent trajectories that were planned without AP, while results in orange were acquired using the AP module.

For each target point, the AP module analysed the topology of the critical structures to find potential entry points and computed the risks for them. Based on these risk values the system automatically offered an optimal entry for the new trajectory.

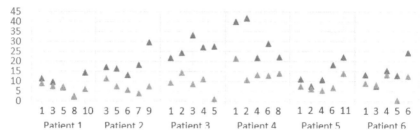

Fig. 6. Comparison of entry angle. Values in blue represent trajectories that were planned without AP, while results in orange were acquired using the AP module.

The new trajectories were inspected by the surgeon to validate the safety profile and feasibility. The entry point has changed in all cases (Fig. 8), while the target point had to be adjusted in three cases (P2–T5, P3-T4, P5-T4) when it was placed too close to a critical structure originally (without assistance - Fig. 3/b), which made AP impossible.

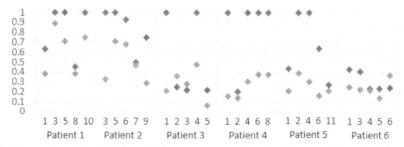

Fig. 7. Comparison of risk. Values in blue represent trajectories that were planned without the AP, while results in orange were acquired using the AP module.

The AP module provided a more feasible angle in all cases, while length of the trajectory was shorter in 57 of the 60 cases. The overall risk was smaller in 57 of the 60 cases using the AP, for the remaining 3 cases the risk was only marginally higher while both angle and length values were better. The general feedback from the surgeon was that the new system provides trajectories that are easier to implement in theatre and a lower risk profile by locating feasible entry points. The required planning time reduced to 2-3min per electrode, which is approximately the time it takes to thoroughly inspect the full length of the planned trajectory.

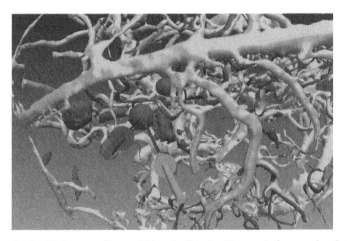

Fig. 8. Change in the Trajectory. Green: Old path; Purple: New path from assisted planning. The increased distance to blood vessels can be observed.

4   Conclusion

We have demonstrated that EpiNav^{TM} finds safer trajectories that are easier to implement and gives the surgeon greater confidence in individual electrode trajectory. The GPU based implementation enables real-time interaction and risk evaluation that reduces planning time and allows a more efficient clinical workflow. One limitation with assisted planning is the reliance on the quality of segmented surfaces that are used. As new imaging and segmentation tools become available, assisted planning will become increasingly reliable. Future work will concentrate on optimising electrode efficiency by segmenting out grey and white matter, and by simulating electrode contacts. The user will then be able to combine safety, feasibility and efficiency scores to select the most appropriate trajectory. The next logical advance on assisted planning is to incorporate electrode arrangements instead of individual electrodes and to add a semi-automatic target placement by employing anatomical parcellation tools.

Acknowledgements. This publication presents independent research supported by the Health Innovation Challenge Fund (HICF-T4-275), a parallel funding partnership between the Department of Health and Wellcome Trust. The views expressed in this publication are those of the author(s) and not necessarily those of the Department of Health or Wellcome Trust.

References

1. Sirven, J.I., Pedley, T.A., Wilterdink, J.L.: Evaluation and management of drug-resistant epilepsy (2011), http://www.uptodate.com/contents/evaluation-and-management-of-drugresistant-epilepsy (accessed November 22, 2013)
2. David, O., Blauwblomme, T., Job, A.-S., Chabardès, S., Hoffmann, D., Minotti, L., Kahane, P.: Imaging the seizure onset zone with stereo-electroencephalography. Brain 134, 2898–2911 (2011)
3. Olivier, A., Boling, W.W., Tanriverdi, T.: Techniques in epilepsy surgery: the MNI approach. Cambridge University Press (2012)
4. Bériault, S., Subaie, F.A., Mok, K., Sadikot, A.F., Pike, G.B.: Automatic trajectory planning of DBS neurosurgery from multi-modal MRI datasets. In: Fichtinger, G., Martel, A., Peters, T. (eds.) MICCAI 2011, Part I. LNCS, vol. 6891, pp. 259–266. Springer, Heidelberg (2011)
5. Essert, C., Haegelen, C., Lalys, F., Abadie, A., Jannin, P.: Automatic computation of electrode trajectories for Deep Brain Stimulation: a hybrid symbolic and numerical approach. International Journal of Computer Assisted Radiology and Surgery 7, 517–532 (2012)
6. De Momi, E., Caborni, C., Cardinale, F., Castana, L., Casaceli, G., Cossu, M., Antiga, L., Ferrigno, G.: Automatic Trajectory Planner for StereoElectroEncephaloGraphy Procedures: A Retrospective Study. IEEE Transactions on Biomedical Engineering 60, 986–993 (2013)
7. Navkar, N.V., Tsekos, N.V., Stafford, J.R., Weinberg, J.S., Deng, Z.: Visualization and planning of neurosurgical interventions with straight access. In: Navab, N., Jannin, P. (eds.) IPCAI 2010. LNCS, vol. 6135, pp. 1–11. Springer, Heidelberg (2010)
8. Shamir, R.R., Tamir, I., Dabool, E., Joskowicz, L., Shoshan, Y., Jonnagaddala, J., Li, J., Ray, P.: A method for planning safe trajectories in image-guided keyhole neurosurgery. In: Jiang, T., Navab, N., Pluim, J.P.W., Viergever, M.A. (eds.) MICCAI 2010, Part III. LNCS, vol. 6363, pp. 457–464. Springer, Heidelberg (2010)
9. Bériault, S., Al Subaie, F., Collins, D.L., Sadikot, A.F., Pike, G.B.: A multi-modal approach to computer-assisted deep brain stimulation trajectory planning. International Journal of Computer Assisted Radiology and Surgery 7, 687–704 (2012)
10. Herghelegiu, P.-C., Manta, V., Perin, R., Bruckner, S., Gröller, E.: Biopsy Planner–Visual Analysis for Needle Pathway Planning in Deep Seated Brain Tumor Biopsy. In: Computer Graphics Forum, pp. 1085–1094. Wiley Online Library (2012)
11. Rincon, M., Navkar, N., Tsekos, N., Deng, Z.: GPU-Accelerated Interactive Visualization and Planning of Neurosurgical Interventions (2013)
12. Rodionov, R., Vollmar, C., Nowell, M., Miserocchi, A., Wehner, T., Micallef, C., Zombori, G., Ourselin, S., Diehl, B., McEvoy, A.W.: Feasibility of multimodal 3D neuroimaging to guide implantation of intracranial EEG electrodes. Epilepsy Research 107, 91–100 (2013)
13. Lauterbach, C., Garland, M., Sengupta, S., Luebke, D., Manocha, D.: Fast BVH construction on GPUs. In: Computer Graphics Forum, pp. 375–384. Wiley Online Library (2009)
14. Karras, T.: Maximizing parallelism in the construction of BVHs, octrees, and k-d trees. In: Proceedings of the Fourth ACM SIGGRAPH/Eurographics conference on High-Performance Graphics, pp. 33–37. Eurographics Association (2012)

Articulated Statistical Shape Model-Based 2D-3D Reconstruction of a Hip Joint

S. Balestra[1], S. Schumann[1], J. Heverhagen[2], L. Nolte[1], and G. Zheng[1]

[1] Institute for Surgical Technology and Biomechanics,
University of Bern, Switzerland
guoyan.zheng@ieee.org, steven.balestra@istb.unibe.ch
[2] Department of Radiology, University of Bern, Switzerland
johannes.heverhagen@insel.ch

Abstract. In this paper, reconstruction of three-dimensional (3D) patient-specific models of a hip joint from two-dimensional (2D) calibrated X-ray images is addressed. Existing 2D-3D reconstruction techniques usually reconstruct a patient-specific model of a single anatomical structure without considering the relationship to its neighboring structures. Thus, when those techniques would be applied to reconstruction of patient-specific models of a hip joint, the reconstructed models may penetrate each other due to narrowness of the hip joint space and hence do not represent a true hip joint of the patient. To address this problem we propose a novel 2D-3D reconstruction framework using an articulated statistical shape model (aSSM). Different from previous work on constructing an aSSM, where the joint posture is modeled as articulation in a training set via statistical analysis, here it is modeled as a parametrized rotation of the femur around the joint center. The exact rotation of the hip joint as well as the patient-specific models of the joint structures, i.e., the proximal femur and the pelvis, are then estimated by optimally fitting the aSSM to a limited number of calibrated X-ray images. Taking models segmented from CT data as the ground truth, we conducted validation experiments on both plastic and cadaveric bones. Qualitatively, the experimental results demonstrated that the proposed 2D-3D reconstruction framework preserved the hip joint structure and no model penetration was found. Quantitatively, average reconstruction errors of 1.9 mm and 1.1 mm were found for the pelvis and the proximal femur, respectively.

Keywords: 2D-3D Reconstruction, articulated statistical shape model, Femoroacetabular Impingement (FAI).

1 Introduction

Femoroacetabular impingement (FAI) is recognized as a cause of early osteoarthritis and has therefore a major impact on a patient's further life [1]. FAI as a clinical diagnosis is estimated to exist within $10 - 15\%$ of the adult population [2]. FAI occurs in the hip joint and specifies the condition of too much friction between the

D. Stoyanov et al. (Eds.): IPCAI 2014, LNCS 8498, pp. 128–137, 2014.

femoral head and the acetabular rims. The abnormal friction will cause damage to the structure on either or both parts of the joint. Computed tomography scans are generally not acquired in FAI patients because of the high radiation. FAI is assessed using two-dimensional (2D) X-ray images in clinical routine, although it is a three-dimensional (3D) problem. Reconstructing of 3D patient-specific models from 2D X-ray images will facilitate the diagnosis and surgical planning of FAI treatment.

Reconstructing patient-specific 3D surface models from 2D x-ray images is a challenging task. *A priori* information is often required to handle this otherwise ill-posed problem [3]. In this paper, we focus on using statistical shape models (SSMs) learned from a given population data as the *A priori* information.

Existing SSM-based 2D-3D reconstruction techniques usually reconstruct a patient-specific model of a single anatomical structure without considering the relationship to its neighboring structures [4] [5] [7] [8] [9]. When those techniques would be applied to reconstruction of patient-specific models of a hip joint, the reconstructed models may penetrate each other due to narrowness of the hip joint space and hence do not represent a true hip joint of the patient. To address this problem we propose a novel 2D-3D reconstruction framework using an articulated statistical shape model (aSSM).

There already exist attempts to use aSSM for 2D-3D reconstruction[10] [11], 3D ultrasound registation [12] and segmentation [13] [14]. Common to all these works is that the postures between neighboring structures are modeled as articulation in a training set via statistical analysis. This may be true for anatomical structures such as spine but it will not hold for structures such as the hip joint as joint posture is usually not a patient-specific anatomical property [15].

Different from previous work on using aSSM for 2D-3D reconstruction, in this paper we construct an aSSM of hip joint by performing statistical shape analysis on a set of aligned training models to capture the pure shape variation, without considering joint posture variation. As the hip joint can be approximately modeled as a ball-and-socket joint, joint posture is then explicitly modeled as a parametrized rotation of the femur around the joint center. The exact rotation of the proximal femur as well as the patient-specific models of the neighboring structures, i.e., the proximal femur and the pelvis, are then estimated by optimally fitting the aSSM to a limited number of calibrated X-ray images. Although a similar strategy in constructing an aSSM of the hip joint has been explored in [15] for 3D image segmentation, this strategy has never been explored for 2D-3D reconstruction. Furthermore, no result was shown in [15] that their segmented surface models had no penetration. In contrast, our experimental results demonstrated that our aSSM-based 2D-3D reconstruction framework had the advantage of preserving join structure and that the reconstructed surface models had no penetration.

The remainder of this paper is arranged as follows. Section 2 will describe how to construct aSSM of the hip joint. Details about our aSSM-based 2D-3D reconstruction framework will be presented in Section 3. Section 4 presents the results of our validation experiments conducted on plastic and cadaveric bones, followed by discussions and conclusions in Section 5.

2   Construction of an aSSM of the Hip Joint

Statistical Model Definition
In order to build a SSM we assume a set of n aligned training shapes s_i, where $i \in \{0, 1, ..., n-1\}$. Each shape s_i is described by a vector containing m vertices: $s_i = \{x_0, y_0, z_0, x_1, y_1, z_1, ..., x_{m-1}, y_{m-1}, z_{m-1}\}$. By performing Principal Component Analysis (PCA) on the training set, the shape varation can be described by a linear model:

$$S(\mathbf{b}) = \bar{s} + \sum_{i=0}^{n-2} b_i p_i \tag{1}$$

where $\bar{s}$ is the mean shape vector, p_i the eigenvectors spanning the principal directions of the shape space and $\mathbf{b} = (b_0, b_1, ..., b_{n-2})$ the shape coefficient vector.

aSSM Model Definition
A compound model was built containing two objects P and F and a rotation center c. Whereas object P and F represents the pelvis- and femur-model respectively. We denote a vertex in a shape instance $S(\mathbf{b})$ as $v_j(\mathbf{b})$, $j \in \{0, 1, ..., m-1\}$. $v_j(\mathbf{b})$ with $j \in \{0, 1, ..., u-1\}$ belong to object P, whereas u denotes the number of vertices of P. Object F's vertices are $v_j(\mathbf{b}); j \in \{u, u_{+1}, ..., m-2\}$ and the joint center is defined as $v_c(\mathbf{b})$ and $c = m - 1$.
As we approximate the relation between the femur and the pelvis as a ball-and-socket joint, the joint posture is explicitly parametrized by a rotation R of object F around the joint center $v_c(\mathbf{b})$ which defines the relative transformation of the femur to the pelvis. Furthermore, assuming a scaled rigid transformation T between the shape space and the input image space, our parametrized aSSM is described as $S(\mathbf{b}, T, R)$:

$$S(\mathbf{b}, T, R) = (T \circ R(v_c(\mathbf{b})))(S(\mathbf{b})) \tag{2}$$

where $R(v_c(\mathbf{b}))$ describes the rotation of all vertices on the proximal femur around the joint center $v_c(\mathbf{b})$ and will be only applied to those vertices $v_j(\mathbf{b}); j \in \{u, u_{+1}, ..., m-2\}$ on the instantiated femoral object and T is the scaled rigid transformation that will be applied to all vertices on the instantiated compound model.

aSSM Model Construction
In order to model the shape variation, the correspondences between the training shapes were established using a templating method [16]. To obtain the same vertex ordering the training shapes were reconstructed from a single template mesh by displacing its vertices to other shapes in the training set with a non-rigid transformation. To build the template mesh, one of the CT volumes was selected as the initial reference. Out of the reference volume data two surface meshes were generated which were smoothed, decimated and remeshed in order to obtain an equally distributed triangular mesh which acted as template mesh for the pelvis and the femur individually. The non-rigid transformation was calculated using the diffeomorphic demons algorithm [17]. For the model generation we used 26

CT scans of the human hip containing the complete pelvis and the proximal femur.

After correspondence establishment, all models, femurs and pelvises, were stored in their original space and are thus still representing the original joint configuration. We denote the unaligned training shapes as s_i, $i \in \{0, 1, ..n - 1\}$. Vertices corresponding to object P are denoted as $p = p_i = v_{ij}; j \in \{0, 1, ..., u-1\}$ and for object F as $f = f_i = v_{ij}; j \in \{u, u_{+1}, ..., m-2\}$. The joint center is defined as $c = c_i = v_{ic}; c = m - 1$. In a first step, we register the shape instances s_i to the reference shape s_{ref}, based on only object P's vertices, which results in the transformation T_i. The equation

$$T_i = argmin_T \|p_{ref} - (T_i \cdot p_i)\|^2 \tag{3}$$

has to be solved. The transformation T_i is applied to the shape instances s_i. In a second step we find a transformation R_i for each shape instance s_i, which only aligns object F's vertices. Therefore we find a rigid transformation B by solving

$$B_i = argmin_B \|f_{ref} - B(T_i \cdot p_i)\|^2 \tag{4}$$

Afterwards the femur is shifted by a translation S in order to keep the joint center $T_i \cdot c_i$ as a fixed point of R_i, $R_i(T_i \cdot c_i) = R_i \cdot c_i$. Thus R_i can be written as $R_i = S \circ B_i$.

In order to obtain the aSSM, PCA is computed on the shape instances $(T_i \cdot p_i, R_i(T_i \cdot f_i), T_i \cdot c_i)$. In order to get a smooth mean model, the pipeline was passed twice. After the first iteration, the resulting mean model was taken as reference for the second iteration. Again, to obtain a homogeneous mesh, the reference surface was remeshed before applying the deformation field to it.

3   aSSM-Based 2D-3D Reconstruction Framework

The articulated 2D-3D reconstruction addresses the problem of reconstructing the pelvis and the femur in 3D out of calibrated 2D X-ray images and at the same time preserving the joint. The initial aSSM is defined by $S(\mathbf{b}, 0, 0)$ where we define object P's vertices belonging to the pelvis and are denoted as $p(\mathbf{b})$. Object F's vertices belong to the femur and are denoted as $f(\mathbf{b})$ whereas the joint center is $v_c(\mathbf{b})$. As a feature-based 2D-3D reconstruction algorithm, we assume that image contours have been extracted from the input X-ray images and all images are calibrated in a common reference coordinate system called target space. The semi-automatic contour extraction method as presented in our previous work [3] is used in this work. 2D-3D correspondences between the 2D image contours and the 3D apparent contours of our aSSM are established using the algorithm introduced by Zheng et al.[7] such that we can convert a 2D-3D reconstruction problem to a 3D-3D one, where each 3D point pair consists of one point on the apparent contour of the instantiated aSSM and the other point calculated as the closest point on the corresponding projection ray to the point on the apparent contour. Assuming that the target points are denoted as $p' = \{p'_i =$

$(x'_i, y'_i, z'_i); i = 0, 1, ..., k - 1\}$ and $f' = \{f'_i = (x'_i, y'_i, z'_i); i = 0, 1, ..., l - 1\}$, for the pelvis and femur, respectively. k and l are the numbers of found correspondences for the pelvis and femur, respectively.

The articulated 2D-3D reconstruction consists of five different steps:

1. Initial landmark based scaled rigid registration
2. Iterative scaled rigid registration of the pelvis
3. Iterative constrained registration of the femur
4. Instantiation of a compound model from the aSSM
5. Thin-Plate-Spline (TPS) based deformation of the instantiated compound model

Initial Landmark Based Scaled Rigid Registration

In the initial step the aSSM is registered to the X-ray scene by a scaled rigid transformation T_0. The transformation is found based on selected and predefined pelvic-landmarks on the X-ray images and on the aSSM, respectively. T_0 is then applied to the current shape instance $S(\mathbf{b}, T_0, 0) = T_0 \cdot S(\mathbf{b}, 0, 0)$.

Iterative Scaled Rigid Pelvis Registration

The scaled rigid registration is performed using an adapted iterative closest point (ICP) algorithm presented in [7]. The transformation T_{j+1} is calculated based on object P's vertices and applied to object P and F, where $j \in \{0, 1, ..., Q\}$ denotes the iteration step and Q is the maximum number of iterations.

The transformation for the pelvis is found minimizing the following function

$$T_{j+1} = argmin_T \|p' - (p(\mathbf{b}, T, 0))\|^2 \tag{5}$$

After the algorithm converges, the scaled rigid transformation T between the shape space $S(\mathbf{b}, 0, 0)$ and the target space is computed.

Iterative Constrained Rigid Femur Registration

After the scaled rigid transformation, a constrained rotation is performed in order to orient object F's vertices to match to the target space. The rotation is constrained around the instantiated joint center $T \cdot v_c(\mathbf{b})$. To reconstruct the femur orientation a transformation is calculated by solving

$$R_{j+1} = argmin_R \|f' - f(\mathbf{b}, T, R(T \cdot v_c(\mathbf{b})))\|^2 \tag{6}$$

After the algorithm converges, the constrained rotation $R(T \cdot v_c(\mathbf{b}))$ between the transformed shape space $S(\mathbf{b}, T, 0)$ and the target space is computed.

Instantiation of a compound model from the aSSM

In order to calculate the shape parameters $\mathbf{b}$ of the aSSM the following equation is solved:

$$b_{j+1} = argmin_b \|S(\mathbf{b}, 0, 0) - Inv(p', f')\|^2 \tag{7}$$

where $Inv(p', f')$ represents all inversely transformed target points. They are transformed from the target space to the aSSM shape space using T and $R(T \cdot$

$v_c(\mathbf{b})$) computed in the last two steps. The instantiated compound model consists of vertices for both pelvis and proximal femur objects.

Regularized Shape Deformation
The regularized shape deformation is adapted from [7] whereas for both models the correspondences are set up individually but the TPS is solved using the information of both point sets.

4   Experiments and Results

To evaluate the accuracy of the reconstructions we conducted three experiments based on calibrated X-ray radiographs. Three bones, i.e., two cadaveric hips (we named them as model #1 and #2 respectively) with each one cadaveric femur and one plastic hip containing two femurs with metallic coating (we named these two as model #3 and #4), are used in our experiment. Three X-ray images (AP, Oblique, Outlet) were acquired for each of the four hip joints and used as input for the reconstruction algorithms. All X-ray images were calibrated with the method that we proposed before [18]. For model #1 we reconstructed the right hip joint and for model #2 the left hip joint. For the plastic bone we did a reconstruction of both left and right hip joints.

To validate the present method and to compare the performance of the present method to our previous work [7] which we denoted as the individual SSM-based 2D-3D reconstruction, we acquired a CT scan for each bone which was then segmented with Amira (VSG, FEI Company, Hillsboro, United States of America). The segmented models were regarded as the ground truth. For both methods, we used statistical shape models that were built from the same population containing 26 human hips.

An example of the complete procedure of the aSSM-based reconstruction is shown in Figure Figure 1.

In order to validate the reconstruction accuracy, the reconstructed models were transformed into the ground truths coordinate system by performing a surface-based rigid registration. For the reconstructed shape models based on the individual SSM reconstruction we observed a mean surface distance error of 1.1mm ±0.04mm and 2.1mm ±0.3mm for the femur and the pelvis, respectively. For the aSSM-based reconstruction we observed a mean surface distance error for the femur of 1.1mm ±0.2mm and 1.9mm ±0.2mm for the pelvis. Figure 2 shows the 5, 25, 75 and 95 percentile errors of both methods for all four hip joints.

Finally, in order to investigate the feasibility of our aSSM-based 2D-3D reconstruction for FAI diagnosis, we visually observed the reconstructed joint in order to check for joint space preservation. In order to observe if the joint spaces were preserved and no penetration of the surfaces was present, we removed parts of the surface and conducted a visual check as shown in Figure 3. For all reconstructions based on the individual SSM penetrating surfaces were observed, while for all articulated SSM-based reconstructions the joint spaces were preserved. Using an in-house developed program, we further computed the femoral head coverage which is regarded as one of the important parameters for FAI diagnosis [19] and is computed as the ratio between the area of the upper femoral head surface covered by the acetabulum and the area of the complete upper femoral head surface. Comparison of the femoral head coverage for the ground truths and for the reconstructions is shown qualitatively in Figure 4 and quantitatively in Table 1. The mean error of the femoral head coverage of the articulated reconstruction is $3.8\% \pm 2.4\%$ when compared to the ground truth.

5   Discussions and Conclusions

In this paper, we presented a novel 2D-3D reconstruction algorithm using articulated statistical shape model and showed its application in reconstruction patient-specific models of a hip joint. Our method has the advantage of preserving hip joint structure and holds the potential to be used in challenging femoroacetbular impingement diagnosis and surgical treatment applications.

One limitations of the present study is the relatively small number of cases used in our validation experiment. Our future work will focus on conducting a thorough investigation of the performance of the present method using clinical datasets.

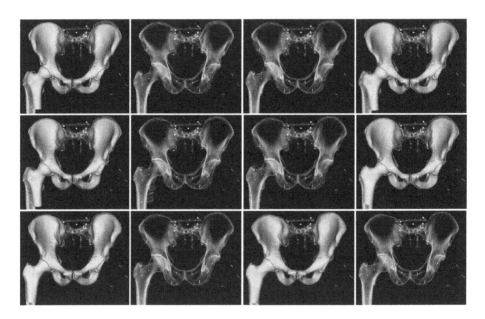

Fig. 1. Stages of the aSSM-based 2D-3D registration. *yellow:* pelvis contour, *purple:*pelvis silhouette,*cyan:*femur contour, *red:* femur silhouette, *green:* correspondence lines. *Top row:* First three iteration steps of the scaled rigid pelvis registration. *Middle row:* First three iteration steps of the constrained femur registration while keeping the pelvis fixed. *Bottom row:* Left two images: Correspondences after instantiation step. Right two images: After first and second TPS-based deformation.

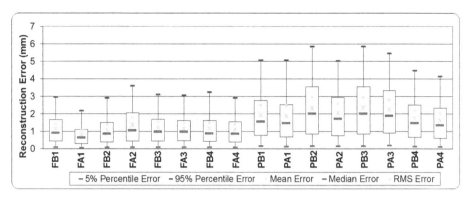

Fig. 2. The reconstructed surface distances from both algorithms compared to the ground truths. F: Femur, P:Pelvis, B: individual SSM-based 2D-3D reconstruction algorithm, A: aSSM-based 2D-3D reconstruction algorithm. For example, FB1 means the boxplot results of the proximal femur of the model #1 when the individual SSM-based 2D-3D reconstruction algorithm is used.

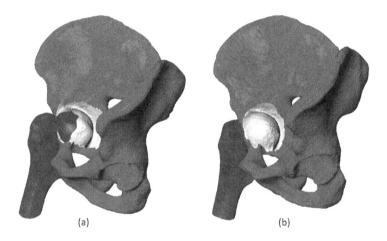

Fig. 3. Penetration verification. (a) Penetrating surfaces observed for the individual SSM-based 2D-3D reconstruction. (b) No penetration can be found for the articulated SSM-based reconstruction.

Table 1. Quantative comparison of femoral head coverage computed on CT segmentation-based ground truth models and on models obtained with the present aSSM-based 2D-3D reconstruction framework

Model	CT [%]	Reconstruction [%]
1	82.6	79.4
2	87.3	85.5
3	82.4	90.3
3	89.1	91.4
Mean	85.4	86.7

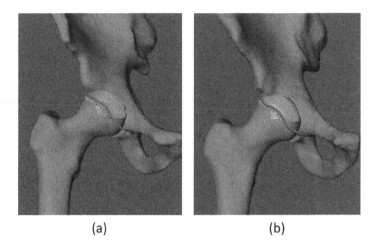

(a)   (b)

Fig. 4. Femoral head coverage comparison. Coverage assessed on ground truth (a) and on models obtained from the aSSM-based 2D-3D reconstruction (b).

References

1. Ganz, R., Parvizi, J., Beck, M., Leunig, M., Notzli, H., Siebenrock, A.: Femoroacetabular impingement: a cause for osteoarthritis of the hip. Clin. Orthop. Relat. Res. 417, 112–120 (2003)
2. Laborie, L.B., Lehmann, T.G., Engester, I., Eastwood, D.M., Engester, L.B., Rosendahl, K.: Prevalence of radiographic findings thought to be associated with femoroacetabular impingement in a population-based cohort of 2081 healthy young adults. Radiology 260(2), 494–502 (2011)
3. Zheng, G.: Statistical shape model-based reconstruction of a scaled, patient-specific surface model of the pelvis from a single standard AP x-ray radiograph. Medical Physics 37(4), 1424–1439 (2010)
4. Fleute, M., Lavallée, S.: Nonrigid 3-D/2-D registration of images using statistical models. In: Taylor, C., Colchester, A. (eds.) MICCAI 1999. LNCS, vol. 1679, pp. 138–147. Springer, Heidelberg (1999)
5. Lamecker, H., Wenckebach, T.H., Hege, H.-C.: Atlas-based 3D-shape reconstruction from X-ray iamges. In: Proceedings of ICPR 2006, pp. 371–374. IEEE Computer Society (2006)
6. Sadowsky, O., Chintalapani, G., Taylor, R.H.: Deformable 2D-3D registration of the pelvis with a limited field of view, suing shape statistics. In: Ayache, N., Ourselin, S., Maeder, A. (eds.) MICCAI 2007, Part II. LNCS, vol. 4792, pp. 519–526. Springer, Heidelberg (2007)
7. Zheng, G., Gollmer, S., Schumann, S., et al.: A 2D/3D correspondence building method for reconstruction of a patient-specific 3D bone surface model using point distribution models and calibrated X-ray images. Medical Image Analysis 13(6), 883–899 (2009)
8. Baka, N., Kaptein, B.L., de Bruijne, M., et al.: 2D-3D shape reconstruction of the distal femur from stereo X-ray imaging using statistical shape models. Medical Image Analysis 15, 840–850 (2011)

9. Zheng, G.: 3D volumetric intensity reconstruction from 2D X-ray images using partial least squares regression. In: Proceedings of ISBI, pp. 1268–1271 (2013)
10. Boisvert, J., Cheriet, F., Pennec, X., Labelle, H., Ayache, N.: Articulated spine models for 3-D reconstruction from partial radiographic data. IEEE Transactions on Biomedical Engineering 55(11), 2565–2574 (2008)
11. Harmouche, R., Cheriet, F., Labelle, H., Dansereau, J.: 3D registration of MR and X-ray spine images using an articulated model. Computerized Medical Imaging and Graphics 36, 410–418 (2012)
12. Khallaghi, S., Mousavi, P., Gong, R.H., Gill, S., Boisvert, J., Fichtinger, G., Pichora, D., Borschneck, D., Abolmaesumi, P.: Registartion of a statistical shape model of the lumbar spine to 3D ultrasound images. In: Jiang, T., Navab, N., Pluim, J.P.W., Viergever, M.A. (eds.) MICCAI 2010, Part II. LNCS, vol. 6362, pp. 68–75. Springer, Heidelberg (2010)
13. Klinder, T., Wolz, R., Lorenz, C., Franz, A., Ostermann, J.: Spine segmentation using articulated shape models. In: Metaxas, D., Axel, L., Fichtinger, G., Székely, G. (eds.) MICCAI 2008, Part I. LNCS, vol. 5241, pp. 227–234. Springer, Heidelberg (2008)
14. Yokota, F., Okada, T., Takao, M., Sugano, N., Tada, Y., Tomiyama, N., Sato, Y.: Automated CT segmentation of diseased hip using hierarchical and condictional statistical shape models. In: Mori, K., Sakuma, I., Sato, Y., Barillot, C., Navab, N. (eds.) MICCAI 2013, Part II. LNCS, vol. 8150, pp. 190–197. Springer, Heidelberg (2013)
15. Kainmueller, D., Lamecker, H., Zachow, S., Hege, H.-C.: An articulated statistical shape model for accurate hip joint segmentation. In: Proceedings of IEEE EMBS 2009, Part II, pp. 6345–6351 (2009)
16. Heitz, G., Rohlfing, T., Maurer Jr., C.R.: Statistical shape model generation using nonrigid deformation of a template mesh. In: Medical Imaging 2005: Image Processing, vol. 5747, pp. 1411–1421 (2005)
17. Vercauteren, T., Pennec, X., Perchant, A., Ayache, N.: Diffeomorphic demons: efficient non-parametric image registration. NeuroImage 45(suppl. 1), S61–S72 (2009)
18. Schumann, S., Liu, L., Tannast, M., Bergmann, M., Nolte, L.-P., Zheng, G.: An integrated system for 3D hip joint reconstruction from 2D X-rays: an preliminary validation study. Annals of Biomedical Engineering 41(10), 2077–2087 (2013)
19. Banerjee, P., Mclean, C.R.: Femoroacetabular impingement: a review of diagnosis and management. Curr. Rev. Musculoskelet Med. 4(1), 23–32 (2011)

Pairwise Comparison-Based Objective Score for Automated Skill Assessment of Segments in a Surgical Task

Anand Malpani[1], S. Swaroop Vedula[1],
Chi Chiung Grace Chen[2], and Gregory D. Hager[1]

[1] Dept. of Computer Science, Johns Hopkins University
[2] Dept. of Gynecology and Obstetrics, Johns Hopkins University School of Medicine

Abstract. Current methods for manual evaluation of surgical skill yield a global score for the entire task. The global score does not inform surgical trainees about where in the task they need to improve. We developed and evaluated a framework to automatically generate an objective score for assessing skill in maneuvers (circumscribed segments) within a surgical task. We used an existing video and kinematic data set (with manual annotation for maneuvers) of a suturing and knot-tying task performed by 18 surgeons on a bench-top model using a da Vinci® Surgical System (Intuitive Surgical, Inc., CA). We collected crowd annotations of preferences, for which of the maneuver in a presented pair appeared to have been performed with greater skill and their confidence in the annotation. We trained a classifier to automatically predict preferences using quantitative metrics of time and motion. We generated an objective percentile score for skill assessment by comparing each maneuver sample to all remaining samples in the data set. Accuracy of the classifier for assigning a preference to pairs of maneuvers was at least 80.06% against a single individual (with a larger training data set) and at least 68.0% against each of the seven individuals (with a smaller training data set). Our reliability analyses indicate that automated preference annotations by the classifier are consistent with those by the seven individuals. Trial-level scores computed from maneuver-level scores generated using our framework were moderately correlated with global rating scores assigned by an experienced surgeon (Spearman correlation = 0.47; P-value < 0.0001).

1 Introduction

Robot-assisted laparoscopic (robotic) surgery is a widely used technique to treat many conditions in several surgical disciplines [1]. Surgeons trained on other techniques, such as laparoscopic or open surgery, experience a learning curve while performing robotic surgery [2]. Thus, training for robotic surgical (technical) skills is essential to ensure that competent surgeons deliver safe and effective patient care.

Robotic surgical skills among trainees are typically assessed for overall performance of a task. For example, the Objective Structured Assessment of Technical Skills (OSATS) [3] and the Global Evaluative Assessment of Robotic Skills

D. Stoyanov et al. (Eds.): IPCAI 2014, LNCS 8498, pp. 138–147, 2014.

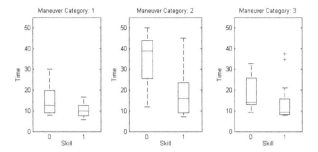

Fig. 1. Time to complete maneuvers in trials with low GRS (≤ 10; marked 0 on the X-axis) and high GRS (≥ 27; marked 1 on the X-axis). Trial-level global scores do not provide information on maneuver-level skill. Note: GRS $\in [5, 30]$.

(GEARS) [4] include manual assessment on a few components to generate a global rating score for the surgeons' skill. Similarly, objective metrics such as time to task completion, motion efficiency, etc., are computed using data from the entire task for an overall assessment of skill [5,6].

Global assessment of skill, in the form of global rating scores, does not necessarily measure performance on the components of the surgical task – referred to as *maneuvers*[1]. For example, Fig. 1 illustrates that objective metrics for maneuvers within a surgical task are similar for trials assigned high and low global rating scores (GRS) using the OSATS approach. Global assessment of skill also does not inform trainees about which part of the task they need to perform better. Although targeted feedback, in the form of individualized coaching, is considered an effective means to teach surgical skills [7], such individualized training with targeted feedback by a supervising surgical educator within academic surgical training programs is inefficient and not feasible. Thus, there is a pressing need for automated, objective measures of surgical skill that also provide targeted feedback for individualized training.

Our goal was to develop and evaluate a framework for automated, objective assessment of skill with which surgeons perform maneuvers. Previous research that attempted skill assessment for segments within a task focused on surgical gestures, which are atomic segments of surgical activity [8,9]. We exploit the inherent structure of surgical activity (comprised of maneuvers, refer Fig. 2) to develop objective measures of surgical skill at a component level, which can be useful for targeted feedback and individualized skill acquisition.

Manual assessment of surgical skill for maneuvers is infeasible and of uncertain validity. Each instance of a surgical task may include multiple maneuvers and manually assigning a skill score to all maneuvers in every instance of a surgical task in a data set can easily become a resource-intensive effort. In addition, our

---

[1] *maneuvers* are components of a surgical task, wherein a series of actions are performed to reach checkpoints on the task roadmap. Figure 2 shows the maneuvers performed during a suturing and knot tying task.

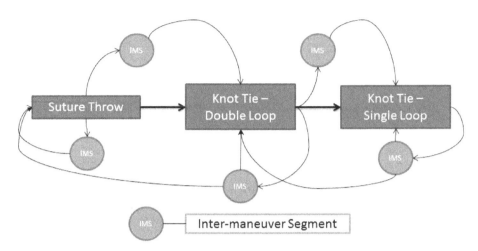

Fig. 2. Maneuver segments in a suturing and knot tying task. The circles indicate inter-maneuver segments, wherein actions are performed to bring the tools into position for starting the next maneuver.

attempts to manually assess surgical skill for maneuvers using GRS indicate that maneuvers may contain insufficient information to make an overall assessment of segment-level skill. To our knowledge, manually assigned GRS for maneuvers are of unproven validity. Skill assessment based on relative rating is an alternative to manual assessment of skill for maneuvers in a task. Ranking and scoring items based on pairwise comparisons has been shown to yield reliable and valid assessment of severity of disease [10], results for information retrieval [11], and recommendations for movies [12,13]. We apply the relative rating approach to generate an objective measure of surgical skill for maneuvers.

2   Methods

2.1   Framework

Our framework to apply relative rating of maneuvers to generate an objective measure for maneuver-level surgical skill consists of the following components: 1) training an automated classification tool to assign preferences for pairs of maneuvers; and 2) generating a quantitative skill score for each maneuver in a task based on pairwise preferences assigned by the automated classification tool. A flow diagram of the framework is shown in Fig. 3. Each of the components of the diagram are described below.

Automated Classification Tool for Pairwise Preferences. To identify which of the two maneuvers in a given pair is preferred, i.e., performed with greater skill, we defined a classifier C as follows:

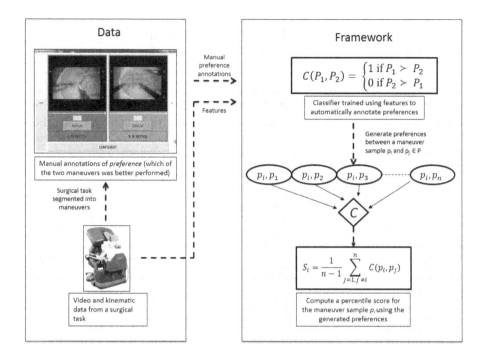

Fig. 3. Our proposed framework to generate objective metrics to measure skill for maneuvers in a surgical task

$$C(P_1, P_2) = \begin{cases} 1 & \text{if } P_1 \succ P_2 \\ 0 & \text{if } P_2 \succ P_1 \end{cases} \quad (1)$$

where $\succ$ indicates *preference* such that $P_1 \succ P_2$ means that the maneuver listed as P_1 was performed with greater skill than the maneuver listed as P_2.

We then computed a set of objective metrics using kinematic data describing surgical tool motion for each maneuver in a pair to generate a feature vector $\mathbf{f}(P)$:

$$\mathbf{f}(P) = [T, PL, RA, MV] \quad (2)$$

where, T = time taken to complete the maneuver, PL = path length traversed by the surgical tools, RA = area swept by the instrument wrist [14,15], and MV = number of movements made by the surgical tools to perform the maneuver. To count the number of movements, we applied a median filter to the speed of surgical tool motion (window size = 9 frames), and used a previously described definition for a movement [16], as an acceleration followed by a deceleration, i.e., a peak in speed. All four features we used have been shown to be a valid measure of skill at the level of the entire surgical task [5,6]. To train the classifier, we provided it with a concatenation of pairs of feature vectors $[\mathbf{f}(P_1), \mathbf{f}(P_2)]$ corresponding to pairwise comparisons of the maneuvers. We used a linear support vector machine (SVM) as the classification tool.

Quantitative Skill Score for Maneuvers. For a given maneuver, we apply the SVM trained as described above to compare it with all corresponding maneuvers in the data set of the same type as the given maneuver. We then compute a percentile score based on the number of maneuver samples that were preferred over the given maneuver as follows:

$$S_i = \frac{1}{n-1} \sum_{\substack{j=1 \\ j \neq i}}^{n} C(P_i, P_j) \tag{3}$$

where S_i is the percentile score for the given maneuver i, n is the total number of maneuvers in the data set of the same type as the given maneuver, P_i is the given maneuver, and P_j is one of the other $n-1$ samples of the same maneuver type. S_i is a measure of relative performance of the given maneuver compared with all corresponding maneuvers in the data set. The score lies between an interval of $[0, 1]$, where a score of 1.0 means the maneuver was rated as having been performed better than all other samples of the same type of maneuvers in the data set.

2.2   Experiments

Data Set. We used kinematic data describing tool motion as 18 (14 novices and 4 experienced) surgeons performed a suturing and knot-tying task on a benchtop model using the da Vinci® Surgical System (dVSS; Intuitive Surgical Inc., Sunnyvale, CA). Each surgeon repeated the task in multiple sessions, performing three instances (trials) of the task during each session. We captured the kinematics for a total of 135 trials from the dVSS [15]. We specified seven maneuvers for the suturing and knot-tying task through consultations with an experienced surgeon.

We annotated the data for skill and maneuver segments. An experienced surgeon, watched a combined video for all three trials of the task for each session, and assigned a GRS using a 5-point Likert scale across 6 criteria from the OSATS [3]. We extrapolated the session-level GRS to each trial in the session. Two individuals, independent of each other, manually annotated video recordings of the trials for start and end of maneuvers within the task, for a total of 1008 maneuvers in the 135 trials in our data set. For our experiments described below, we used 502 maneuvers after omitting all maneuvers that were labeled as incomplete and as inter-maneuver segments. We also grouped the maneuvers into four categories as follows:

– Throw1 - for a suture throw performed in two steps, one for each edge of the incision;

- Throw2 - for a suture throw performed in one step, through both edges of the incision;
- Knot1 - for the first instance of a knot in the task;
- Knot2 - for any knot in the task other than the first one.

We also manually annotated maneuvers for preferences. We randomly sampled a subset of all possible pairwise combinations of maneuvers in our data set. We displayed each pair of maneuvers in the random sample to the annotators and asked them to select the maneuver with the better performance, and whether they were confident in their choice. We did not specify explicit criteria for the crowd to use for the annotation. We used two sources – a group of individuals or a 'crowd' independently annotated 80 pairs of maneuvers (A_C), and a single individual annotated an additional 284 pairs of maneuvers (A_I). We recruited seven colleagues in our laboratory, including an expert surgeon, to provide the crowd annotations (A_C).

Training and Evaluation. As part of our experiment, we evaluated the reliability and validity of automated preferences assigned by the SVM classifier and the validity of objective skill scores generated using our framework. We used the SVM implementation available in MATLAB (version 8.2.0, The Mathworks, Inc., Natick, MA). We first trained a separate SVM classifier for each category of maneuvers using the 364 pairs of maneuvers annotated in A_I and A_C. We used a k-fold cross-validation setup leaving out a randomly selected 30% of the maneuver pairs for testing in each of the 30 folds. Next, we trained a SVM classifier for each category of maneuvers using all 284 pairs of maneuvers in A_I and tested on the 80 pairs of maneuvers annotated in A_C. We assessed reliability of the classifier by computing a Fleiss' kappa [17] as a measure of inter-annotator agreement among all annotators, including and excluding the classifier, along with its 95% confidence interval (95% CI). We examined whether the Fleiss' kappa including the classifier was consistent with the 95% CI for the kappa computed after excluding the classifier. We used only pairs of maneuvers that the individuals marked as being confident about their preference. We assessed validity of preferences assigned by the classifier by computing the accuracy compared against A_C for each member in the crowd.

We also assessed validity of objective skill scores generated using our framework. For this purpose, we used all data from A_I and data from A_C from the same individual whose annotations are part of A_I to yield a larger training data set. Using this approach for our analysis of scores is unlikely to introduce bias in our analyses on scores because the average accuracy for all member-pairs in the crowd was similar to the average accuracy between the individual whose annotations are part of A_I and each member of the crowd.

For each maneuver performance P_i in our data set ($\mathbb{P}$ - set of all maneuver performances), we removed all pairs from $A_I + A_C$ containing P_i. The SVM was trained on this data and used to compare P_i with all other P_j $(j \neq i)$ belonging to the same maneuver category as P_i and marked as a 'confident' annotation by the annotator. A percentile score indicating skill was computed using Eq. (3). We do not have a ground truth for maneuver-level skill, with which we could have correlated objective skill scores generated using our framework. Thus, we adopted an alternative approach, where we used the scores for the individual maneuvers in each trial to compute a score for the entire trial. We then validated the trial-level score against manually assigned GRS for the trial. To compute a score for the entire trial we created a vector of three values for each trial - a combined score for maneuvers in categories 1 & 2 (average), a score for maneuvers in category 3, and a score for maneuvers in category 4. If a trial included multiple maneuvers in categories 3 or 4 then we averaged the scores of maneuvers in each category. We trained a linear regression model where GRS is predicted by the category-level scores in a k-fold cross-validation setup, leaving out one trial in each of 135 folds. We computed a Spearman correlation coefficient between the predicted scores for the trial and manually assigned GRS.

2.3 Results

Our initial k-fold cross-validation revealed that the trained classifier using data from $A_I + A_C$ was able to automatically annotate preferences with an average accuracy of at least 80%.

Table 1. Accuracy of SVMs trained in a 30-fold cross-validation setup

	Throw1	Throw2	Knot1	Knot2
Mean (std. dev.)	85.71 (6.91)	82.92 (6.95)	90.23 (3.52)	80.06 (5.88)

We observed moderate inter-rater agreement among manual preference annotations provided by the crowd. The Fleiss' kappa was 0.88 (95% CI = 0.85 to 0.91) among the crowd members using only preference annotations about which the individuals expressed confidence. Including the classifier as another member of the crowd did not seem to alter the inter-rater agreement; the Fleiss' kappa was 0.89 (95% CI = 0.87 to 0.92). The confidence intervals for the inter-rater agreement among all the annotators, including and excluding the automated classifier trained on A_I indicate that the classifiers we trained for each maneuver category may be considered a representative member of the crowd. Although agreement among manual annotators was lower when we used all preference annotations (those for which the individuals did and did not express confidence) with a Fleiss' kappa of 0.42 (95%CI = 0.40 to 0.43), the classifier's annotations were still consistent with those from the crowd. We observed moderate to high agreement between the single expert and rest of the members of the crowd on average (84.36% for rankings with confidence and 74.38% for all rankings). We also observed moderate accuracy in preferences assigned to pairs of maneuvers between the automated classifier and each member of the crowd (Table 2).

Finally, we found that the overall trial-level score obtained as a linear combination of maneuver-level scores generated using our framework was moderately

Table 2. Accuracy of automated classifier (averaged across the 4 maneuver categories) against each member of the crowd

Crowd Member	1	2	3	4	5	6	7
Accuracy (%)	75.00	85.71	76.36	82.35	68.25	69.23	80.00

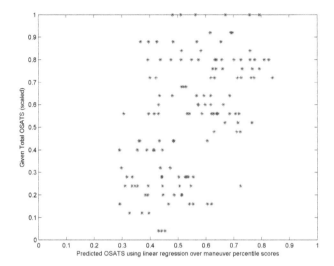

Fig. 4. Plot of predicted GRS for trial using a linear regression over maneuver percentile scores generated using our framework. The manual GRS using OSATS have been scaled to the [0,1] interval.

correlated with manually assigned GRS (Figure 4). The correlation coefficient between the two scores was 0.47 (P-value < 0.0001).

3   Discussion

We developed and evaluated a framework to use relative preferences assigned by manual annotators to pairs of short segments in a surgical task (maneuvers), and compute an objective measure of surgical skill with which the maneuver was performed. Such segment-level skill assessment is necessary to provide automated targeted feedback for individualized training and skill acquisition by surgical trainees. Our analyses based on an existing data set show that a reliable and valid classifier can be trained to automatically annotate the better-performed maneuver in a pair of maneuvers, and can thus be scaled to large data set.

Limitations of findings in our analyses described here pertain to aspects of our data set and study design. Only a small fraction of trials in our data set were performed by experienced surgeons (24/135); the rest were performed by surgeons with none to little experience (111/135). Consequently, the scores generated using our framework are accurate but may not translate into relevant feedback for trainees. The crowd that participated in our study included a single expert surgeon. We are unable to say how the size, member constitution, or other properties of the crowd affect reliability and validity of findings obtained from applying our framework. Manually assigned GRS reflects a global assessment of task performance by an experienced surgeon and includes elements such as knowledge of task, respect for tissue, and forward planning. The objective skill scores generated using our framework did not account for all items considered when a surgeon manually assigns a GRS to a trial because of the few elements in the feature vector $\mathbf{f}$ that we used to train the classifier.

Our work described in this manuscript leads to additional future research. A library of expert maneuver performances is required for our framework to generate scores that provide relevant and meaningful feedback to trainees. Crowdsourcing surgical skill assessment at the task-level is a recent phenomenon [18], and sensitivity of the annotations to constitution and characteristics of the crowd remains an open question. The constitution of the crowd that provides manual preference annotations for the pairs of maneuvers may affect performance of our framework and should be investigated in future research. To apply our framework as part of a system to provide real-time assessment and targeted feedback to trainees, the surgical task must be automatically and accurately segmented into its constituent maneuvers. While previous research on recognition of surgical activity has focused on atomic segments called gestures [9,19,20], our work illustrates the need for reliable and accurate technology for automatic recognition of surgical maneuvers.

Acknowledgments. This work is funded through the NSF-NRI Award 1227277 and the Intuitive Surgical, Inc. Fellowship. We would like to thank individuals who provided anonymous preference annotations as part of the crowd described in our manuscript. Any opinions, findings, conclusions or recommendations expressed in this material are those of the authors and do not necessarily reflect the views of the National Science Foundation.

References

1. Wilson, E.B.: The evolution of robotic general surgery. Scandinavian Journal of Surgery 98, 125–129 (2009)
2. Chang, L., Satava, R.M., Pellegrini, C.A., Sinanan, M.N.: Robotic surgery: identifying the learning curve through objective measurement of skill. Surgical Endoscopy and Other Interventional Techniques 17, 1744–1748 (2003)
3. Martin, J.A., Regehr, G., Reznick, R., MacRae, H., Murnaghan, J., Hutchison, C., Brown, M.: Objective structured assessment of technical skill (OSATS) for surgical residents. The British Journal of Surgery 84, 273–278 (1997)

4. Goh, A.C., Goldfarb, D.W., Sander, J.C., Miles, B.J., Dunkin, B.J.: Global evaluative assessment of robotic skills: validation of a clinical assessment tool to measure robotic surgical skills. The Journal of Urology 187, 247–252 (2012)
5. Kumar, R., Jog, A., Malpani, A., Vagvolgyi, B., Yuh, D., Nguyen, H., Hager, G.D., Chen, C.C.G.: Assessing system operation skills in robotic surgery trainees. The International Journal of Medical Robotics and Computer Assisted Surgery 8, 118–124 (2012)
6. Mason, J.D., Ansell, J., Warren, N., Torkington, J.: Is motion analysis a valid tool for assessing laparoscopic skill? Surgical Endoscopy 27, 1468–1477 (2013)
7. Cole, S.J., Mackenzie, H., Ha, J., Hanna, G.B., Miskovic, D.: Randomized controlled trial on the effect of coaching in simulated laparoscopic training. Surgical Endoscopy, 1–8 (2013)
8. Reiley, C.E., Hager, G.D.: Decomposition of Robotic Surgical Tasks: An Analysis of Subtasks and Their Correlation to Skill. In: Medical Image Computing and Computer-Assisted Intervention M2CAI Workshop (2009)
9. Ahmidi, N., Gao, Y., Béjar, B., Vedula, S.S., Khudanpur, S., Vidal, R., Hager, G.D.: String Motif-Based Description of Tool Motion for Detecting Skill and Gestures in Robotic Surgery. In: Mori, K., Sakuma, I., Sato, Y., Barillot, C., Navab, N. (eds.) MICCAI 2013, Part I. LNCS, vol. 8149, pp. 26–33. Springer, Heidelberg (2013)
10. Kumar, R., Rajan, P., Bejakovic, S., Seshamani, S., Mullin, G., Dassopoulos, T., Hager, G.: Learning disease severity for capsule endoscopy images. In: IEEE International Symposium on Biomedical Imaging: From Nano to Macro, pp. 1314–1317 (2009)
11. Dwork, C., Kumar, R., Naor, M., Sivakumar, D.: Rank Aggregation Methods for the Web. In: Proceedings of the 10th International Conference on World Wide Web, pp. 613–622 (2001)
12. Yoav, F., Raj, I., Schapire Robert, E., Singer, Y.: An Efficient Boosting Algorithm for Combining Preferences. The Journal of Machine Learning Research 4, 933–969 (2013)
13. Kumar, R., Raghavan, P., Rajagopalan, S., Tomkins, A.: Recommendation Systems: A Probabilistic Analysis. In: Proc. IEEE Symp. on Foundations of Computer Science FOCS, pp. 664–673 (1998)
14. Curet, M., Dimaio, S.P., Gao, Y., Hager, G.D., Itkowitz, B., Jog, A.S., Kumar, R., Liu, M.: Method and system for analyzing a task trajectory. Patent, WO2012151585 A2 (2012)
15. Kumar, R., Jog, A., Vagvolgyi, B., Nguyen, H., Hager, G., Chen, C.C.G., Yuh, D.: Objective measures for longitudinal assessment of robotic surgery training. The Journal of Thoracic and Cardiovascular Surgery 143, 528–534 (2012)
16. Dosis, A., Aggarwal, A., Belllo, F., Moorthy, K., Munz, Y., Gillies, D., Darzi, A.: Synchronized video and motion analysis for the assessment of procedures in the operating theater. Archives of Surgery 140, 293–299 (2005)
17. Fleiss, J.L.: Measuring nominal scale agreement among many raters. Psychological Bulletin 76, 378–382 (1971)
18. Chen, C., White, L., Kowalewski, T., Aggarwal, R., Lintott, C., Comstock, B., Kuksenok, K., Aragon, C., Holst, D., Lendvay, T.: Crowd-Sourced Assessment of Technical Skills: a novel method to evaluate surgical performance. Journal of Surgical Research (2013)
19. Varadarajan, B.: Learning and inference algorithms for dynamical system models of dextrous motion. Ph.D. Thesis (2011)
20. Tao, L., Zappella, L., Hager, G.D., Vidal, R.: Surgical gesture segmentation and recognition. In: Mori, K., Sakuma, I., Sato, Y., Barillot, C., Navab, N. (eds.) MICCAI 2013, Part III. LNCS, vol. 8151, pp. 339–346. Springer, Heidelberg (2013)

Random Forests for Phase Detection in Surgical Workflow Analysis

Ralf Stauder[1,*], Aslı Okur[1,*], Loïc Peter[1], Armin Schneider[2],
Michael Kranzfelder[2], Hubertus Feussner[2], and Nassir Navab[1]

[1] Computer Aided Medical Procedures, Technische Universität München, Germany
[2] MITI, Klinikum rechts der Isar, Technische Universität München, Germany
{stauder,okur}@cs.tum.edu

Abstract. Identifying and recognizing the workflow of surgical interventions is a field of growing interest. Several methods have been developed to identify intra-operative activities, detect common phases in the surgical workflow and combine the gained knowledge into Surgical Process Models. Numerous applications of this knowledge are conceivable, from semi-automatic report generation, teaching and objective surgeon evaluation to context-aware operating rooms and simulation of interventions to optimize the operating room layout.

In this work we propose a method to utilize random decision forests to detect surgical workflow phases based on instrument usage data and other, easily obtainable measurements. While decision forests have become a very versatile and popular tool in the field of medical image analysis, this is to the best of our knowledge its first application to surgical workflow analysis.

Our method is in principle suitable for online usage and does not rely on an explicit model or a strict temporal relationship between observations. With their structure, random forests are inherently suited for multi-class detection and therefore for detection of workflow phases. Due to the transparent nature of random forests, additional information may also be obtainable in parallel to the phase detection.

1 Introduction

Nowadays, with the advancements in technology and medicine, the operating room (OR) has become a much more complex working environment and therefore concepts such as *context-aware* ORs appeared. A key component towards context-awareness is the analysis of the surgical workflow [1,2], which is a field of growing interest.

Several methods have been developed to identify intra-operative activities, detect common phases in the surgical workflow and combine the gained knowledge into Surgical Process Models (SPMs) [3]. The signals that can be used for surgical phase determination are manifold, varying from manual annotations by an observer [4], to sensor data such as surgical tool tracking based on video images

---

* Joint first authors.

D. Stoyanov et al. (Eds.): IPCAI 2014, LNCS 8498, pp. 148–157, 2014.

[5,6], intraoperative localization systems [7] or surgical robots [8]. Patient monitoring systems used to acquire the vital signals of the patient during surgeries can also be incorporated [7]. A recent methodological review of the literature focusing on the creation and the analysis of SPMs can be seen by [9].

Many of the works in the literature rely on Dynamic Time Warping (DTW) and derivations of Hidden Markov Model (HMM) algorithms for workflow detection [5,6]. Decision forests are widely utilized in the field of medical image analysis by now, but to the best of our knowledge have not yet been employed for surgical workflow analysis.

We will explain the concept of random forests in section 2, describe our acquired data and the results of our method on them in section 3, and finally discuss our insights in 4.

2 Materials and Methods

2.1 Problem Statement

The phase recognition problem in a surgical workflow is modeled as a classification problem as follows. At a given time point t of an operation, the current setting of the operating room is represented by a set of d real-valued signals $\mathbf{x}(t) = [x_1(t), \ldots, x_d(t)]$. Based on these signals, our goal is to infer the current phase of the worklow among a predefined set Y of possible labels. In other words, we aim at finding a mapping $f : \mathbb{R}^d \to Y$ such that $f(\mathbf{x}(t)) = $ label of the phase at time t. We explicitly avoid usage of temporal models, to enable our method to detect activity outside the regular workflow in the future.

2.2 Random Forest Classifier

Since the number of possible phases is greater than 2, the previously described problem is multi-class. We propose to infer our decision rule *via* a random forest classifier [10] which naturally handles multiple outputs. A decision tree is a hierarchical collection of nodes and a random forest is a set of T decorrelated decision trees. Each tree (indexed by an integer $\tau \in \{1, \ldots, T\}$) performs, given a feature vector $\mathbf{x}$, a prediction $f_\tau(\mathbf{x}) \in Y$. By averaging out the predictions over all trees, one obtains for each label y a classwise posterior probability $P(y|\mathbf{x})$ stating how likely the label y is given the current signals.

$$P(y|\mathbf{x}) = \frac{1}{T} \sum_{\tau=1}^{T} (f_\tau(\mathbf{x}) = y) \tag{1}$$

The final prediction of the ensemble classifier is defined as

$$f(\mathbf{x}) = \operatorname*{argmax}_{y \in Y} P(y|\mathbf{x}) \tag{2}$$

Note that such a combination of tree outputs outperforms each single tree prediction by reducing the risk of overfitting.

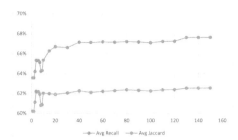

Fig. 1. Performance evaluation over different forest sizes

Training. We expose in this paragraph how the individual decision rule f_τ of each tree can be inferred from a set of labelled examples called *training set*. A training set $S = \{(\mathbf{x}_i, y_i), i = 1 \ldots N\}$ is defined as N feature vectors $\mathbf{x}_i$ for which the label y_i is known. In practice, a training set is obtained by labelling several operation signals and aggregating them independently of their time point. Each node contains an axis-aligned splitting rule $\sigma_{s,\theta} : \mathbb{R}^d \to \{0,1\}$ defined as $\sigma_{s,\theta}(\mathbf{x}) = (x_s \leq \theta)$, where $s \in \{1, \ldots, d\}$ is a signal index and θ a threshold. At a root node, a randomly-chosen subset of splitting rules is drawn and their ability to discriminate the different labels of the training set is evaluated through an information gain criterion. The decision rule with the highest separation capability is retained and the training set samples are sent to the left and right child nodes according to the output of σ. This procedure is recursively repeated, offering thereby a hierarchical series of splitting rules, until a stopping criterion is satisfied. Each terminal node votes for the predominant class label among the training samples that reached it. This defines a local prediction rule on the subset of $\mathbb{R}^d$ defined by the splitting rules of all the parent nodes. More details about random forests and their application to medical image analysis problems can be found in [11].

Implementation and Parameters. We used the random forest implementation of the open-source library OpenCV[1]. Maximal tree depth is an important parameter to influence the forest's tendency to under- or overfit the data, next to the number of randomly chosen features evaluated per node, while a higher number of trees increases generalization. We chose a forest size of 50 trees with a maximal tree depth of 4 nodes to achieve best results. Per node we evaluated a number of features equal to the square root of the total amount of available features (in our case $\sqrt{16} = 4$). The performance improvement usually flattens out after a certain number of trees (as can be seen in Fig. 1), but as our training and testing times were very low (as described in 3.3), we chose a rather high number. In order to counter single, time-consuming phases to dominate the training, we balanced the class sizes by oversampling shorter phases.

---

[1] http://opencv.org/

3 Experiments and Results

3.1 Medical Application

Laparoscopic cholecystectomy (removal of the gallbladder) was selected for this study, because it is a highly standardized surgical operation. It is also previously investigated in many other works of surgical process modeling and recognition of phases, due to the advantages that it has a comparable easy workflow, it is a procedure of short to medium OR time and it is done in large numbers per year all over the world.

The intervention is performed under general anesthesia. Initially a small needle is inserted into the peritoneal cavity for inflating the abdomen with gas. This provides room for easier viewing and for the surgical manipulations to be performed. After that, at the same point, a small incision is made and a trocar, a thin tube for easier exchange of the instruments and ensuring the gas-tightness, is inserted. Via this first port, the telescope is introduced to visualize the interior of the abdomen. After a test insertion with a hypodermic needle, three other trocars are inserted under view of the laparoscopic camera. To get access to the gallbladder, first a retraction device is inserted in the upper right trocar. Then the right liver lobe is elevated. Finally, a grasping forceps is inserted into the right lower and the dissection device in left lower trocar.

The primary step of the surgical procedure is to dissect the Calot's triangle, the area which includes the bile duct and the cystic artery. This is done by blunt dissection with a forceps and cutting and coagulation current. If both structures are clearly visible, each of them is clipped with three clips, followed by cutting both structures between the clips with laparoscopic scissors.

The following step is dissection of the gallbladder, which is done by back and forth touching of the areas between gallbladder and liver and applying cutting and coagulation current.

To remove the dissected gall bladder a salvage bag is inserted into the abdomen, the gallbladder packed up into the bag and the bag extracted together with the trocar. In case of big stones, the bag cannot be extracted through the trocar incision. In that case, the calculi are extracted extracorporally out of the salvage bag. Thus, the content of the bag is adequately reduced to pull it out.

Finally, the surgical area is explored again to detect and take care of bleedings. A drainage is inserted through a trocar hole and all instruments are removed. The trocars are extracted under visual control and the incisions are closed by sutures.

During the procedure, in case of bleedings in the operation field, a device which allows flushing and suction is used. Also controlling for bleedings after extraction of the gallbladder is done with this device.

3.2 Data Acquisition

In order to evaluate the performance of our method, we conducted two experiments. In the integrated OR with augmented sensor equipment [12] in the

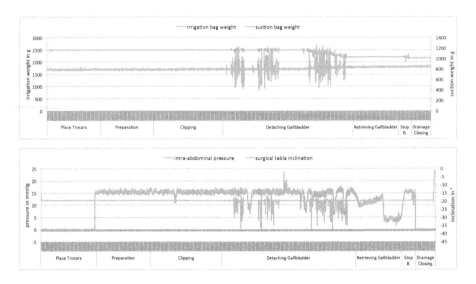

Fig. 2. Synchronized measurements recorded during one surgery

surgical department of our institution, we recorded a total of nine laparoscopic cholecystectomy surgeries as described in 3.1 with synchronised sensor data. Our measurements consisted of the weight of the irrigation and suction bags (Fig. 2(a)), the intra-abdominal CO_2 pressure and the inclination of the surgical table (Fig. 2(b)). Additionally all laparoscopic instruments were marked with RFID tags, so we were able to collect binary usage data for each of the eight available instruments [13]. We also recorded similar binary data for the two possible HF modes (coagulating and cutting) that are available with all laparoscopic instruments, and the state of both the room lights and the surgical lamp (Fig. 3). All this data was collected with an average frequency of 7.6Hz. For four surgeries a medical expert also labeled each sample of the datasets manually with the corresponding surgical workflow phase.

We then used the labeled datasets to train and test the random forests for detection of surgical workflow phases, and all nine datasets in a slightly adjusted manner (as described in 3.4) to detect the states of the OR and surgical lights. In both experiments we only used the raw, unfiltered measurements as features.

3.3   Phase Detection

We collected four surgeries with full sensor data and obtained labels for workflow phases for all samples from a medical expert. We used a total of seven phases, which are in their typical order:

1. Trocar placement
2. Preparation and exposition of duct and artery
3. Clipping and cutting of duct and artery

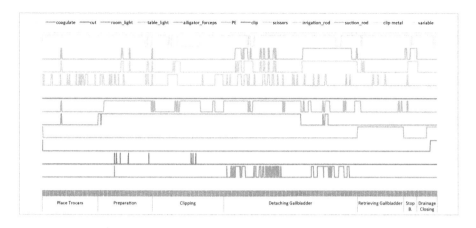

Fig. 3. Synchronized binary signals recorded during one surgery

4. Detaching of gallbladder from liver bed
5. Retrieving gallbladder from body
6. Checking for and stopping of possible bleedings
7. Drainage, trocar removal and closing of wounds

We trained the random forest on all but one of the available datasets and tested it on the remaining one. We did this so that every dataset was used for testing once in leave-one-out-fashion, and calculated evaluation measures over the combined classification results. The training took on average one minute on a common laptop computer[1] for three surgeries with a total of circa 45,000 raw samples, testing of a single surgery with circa 15,000 samples was done in under five seconds. Over all four combinations we achieved an accuracy of 68.78%, an average recall over classes of 73.41% and an average Jaccard index of 58.64%. More detailled performance values are given in table 1.

Table 1. Recognition rates for all seven workflow phases over four labeled surgeries

Phase	Precision	Recall	Jaccard
Trocar placement	99.99%	99.52%	99.51%
Preparation	68.83%	79.36%	58.38%
Clipping	42.54%	40.50%	26.18%
Detaching gallbladder	77.89%	11.34%	10.98%
Retrieving gallbladder	98.06%	99.74%	97.81%
Stop bleeding	18.52%	83.49%	17.87%
Drainage and closing	99.85%	99.89%	99.73%

---

[1] 2.4GHz CPU, 8GB RAM

Recognition rates covered the whole possible range, with over 99% precision and recall for some labels (e.g. drainage and closing), while in some selected surgeries detection of the clipping phase even failed completely (5% recall). But as can be seen in the confusion matrix in table 2, the classification errors happen in a strict subset of all phases.

Table 2. Confusion matrix for the recognition of seven workflow phases. Rows are ground truth, columns are predictions.

	Troc.	Prep.	Clip.	Det.	Retr.	St. bl.	Drng.
Trocar pl.	0.995	0.000	0.005	0.000	0.000	0.000	0.000
Preparation	0.000	0.794	0.093	0.016	0.000	0.098	0.000
Clipping	0.000	0.361	0.405	0.013	0.000	0.221	0.000
Detaching gb.	0.000	0.293	0.201	0.113	0.006	0.387	0.000
Retrieving gb.	0.000	0.000	0.002	0.000	0.997	0.000	0.001
Stop bleeding	0.000	0.012	0.105	0.001	0.047	0.835	0.000
Drainage	0.000	0.000	0.000	0.000	0.000	0.001	0.999

3.4 Light State Detection

As with every laparoscopic surgery, most work is done solely by observing the surgical site indirectly through the laparoscopic camera. In order to avoid distractions and reflections on the monitor, all lights in the OR are turned off after all trocars have been set, and turned on again when they are being removed. As retrieval of the gallbladder is done externally, the surgical lamp is turned on during that phase of the surgery, but turned off again afterwards. Currently the non-sterile circulator nurse has to stop their current activities whenever the lights have to be switched, move in the OR to turn the lights on or off, and return to their work. As a hypothetical future application of our approach, we tried to predict the light state based on the other, available data.

We adjusted all nine datasets by creating a new label for each sample based on the state of both observed lights. As one combination never occured, we used the three new labels:

1. Both room and table lights are on
2. Only the surgical lamp is on
3. No light is on

Then we removed the light signals from the datasets and trained and tested the random forest (with tree depth 10) on the remaining signals. We achieved an overall accuracy of 87.57%, an average recall of 75.44% and an average Jaccard index of 64.20%. The values for each individual state are given in table 3(a), a confusion matrix in table 3(b).

Table 3. a) Recognition rates for light states over nine surgeries. b) Confusion matrix for light states. Rows are ground truth, columns are predictions.

	Prec.	**Recall**	**Jaccard**		**both**	**table**	**none**
both	77.43%	83.45%	67.12%	both	0.835	0.032	0.134
table	66.51%	48.89%	39.23%	table	0.037	0.489	0.474
none	91.29%	93.96%	86.23%	none	0.028	0.033	0.940

4   Discussion

The detection rates given in 3.3 and 3.4 are not optimal, but as the possible signal values have a relatively high variation over different surgeries, more training data is needed to cover this variability. With an accuracy of over 65% for seven labels and an accuracy over 85% for three labels, the method provides very promising first results.

An advantage of random forests over other methods is the fact that they are inherently well suited for multi-class outputs. This combined with the fact that no prior or implicit sequential model is required suggests that random forests have various characteristics that can be exploited for surgical workflow detection. As we calculate our features without temporal information it seems plausible that workflow phases could be detected also in atypical order. It can be a subject of further research to analyze the ability of random forests to do that, as well as detect problems that happened during single surgeries and detect more low-level activities by focusing on the mentioned properties.

While this was not yet employed in this paper, random forests also have the ability to ignore missing features for individual samples by building a second, surrogate criterion based on other features, which can be beneficial for our case. Indeed, some of our input signals (described in more details in 3.2) are based on surgical instruments equipped with RFID tags, and it occasionally happens that a single instrument needs to be replaced during the course of a surgery, in which case the replacement instrument is usually not marked with the same RFID tag. These missing instrument signals can then be ignored to not disturb the remaining classification.

Another interesting aspect of random forests that can be utilized is the possibility to estimate relative feature importance after training the forest. As suggested by Breiman [10], random forests can be used to assess the importance of each feature for classification by performing random permutations of each individual feature value over samples and measuring the resulting loss of accuracy. While attention is required as these numbers do contain a substantial level of randomness, Figure 4 gives an example of this relative feature importance of our trained phase detector. Some of the features with least importance can be skipped to achieve comparable results, but more importantly it can be seen that even features that appear to carry very little information can have a high impact on the classification. Figure 2(b) shows an example: The table inclination itself does not change during the course of a surgery, but during some times the sensor seems to produce severe noise. Closer inspection reveals that this noise happens mainly and reliably during the phase of gallbladder detachment. The actual reason for this correlation has to be investigated in the coming experiments, but is actually secondary to this work. Based on these findings we suggest that an operating room of the future should be generously equipped with various sensors, as apparently even data sources with little obvious information can contribute to other, context-sensitive and integrated systems.

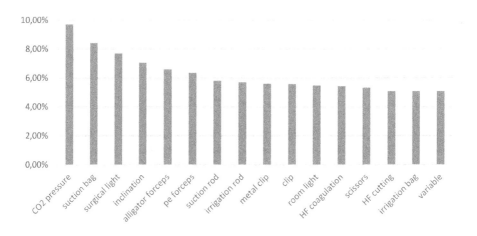

Fig. 4. Relative importance of all available features after training on the fully labeled datasets

5 Conclusion

In this work we trained random forests to detect either workflow phases or OR light states based solely on simple measurements and instrument usage data. Detection rates for both applications were promising. We also pointed out additional ways to exploit the methods and calculations done by random forests to gain knowledge in parallel to the detection of workflow phases. For further steps in this direction we plan to evaluate our method on more datasets with labeled low-level activities, as well as compare it quantitatively with other standard classifiers.

References

1. Lemke, H.U., Ratib, O.M., Horii, S.C.: Workflow in the operating room: A summary review of the arrowhead 2004 seminar on imaging and informatics. International Congress Series, vol. 1281, pp. 862–867 (May 2005)
2. Cleary, K., Kinsella, A., Mun, S.K.: OR 2020 workshop report: Operating room of the future. International Congress Series, vol. 1281, pp. 832–838 (May 2005)

3. Neumuth, T., Strauß, G., Meixensberger, J., Lemke, H.U., Burgert, O.: Acquisition of process descriptions from surgical interventions. In: Bressan, S., Küng, J., Wagner, R. (eds.) DEXA 2006. LNCS, vol. 4080, pp. 602–611. Springer, Heidelberg (2006)
4. Neumuth, T., Jannin, P., Schlomberg, J., Meixensberger, J., Wiedemann, P., Burgert, O.: Analysis of surgical intervention populations using generic surgical process models. Int. J. Comput. Assist. Radiol. Surg. 6(1), 59–71 (2011)
5. Padoy, N., Blum, T., Ahmadi, S.A., Feussner, H., Berger, M.O., Navab, N.: Statistical modeling and recognition of surgical workflow. Med. Image Anal. 16(3), 632–641 (2012)
6. Lalys, F., Riffaud, L., Morandi, X., Jannin, P.: Surgical phases detection from microscope videos by combining SVM and HMM. In: Menze, B., Langs, G., Tu, Z., Criminisi, A. (eds.) MICCAI 2010. LNCS, vol. 6533, pp. 54–62. Springer, Heidelberg (2011)
7. Agarwal, S., Joshi, A., Finin, T., Yesha, Y., Ganous, T.: A pervasive computing system for the operating room of the future. Mobile Networks and Applications 12(2-3), 215–228 (2007)
8. Lin, H.C., Shafran, I., Yuh, D., Hager, G.D.: Towards automatic skill evaluation: Detection and segmentation of robot-assisted surgical motions. Computer Aided Surgery 11(5), 220–230 (2006)
9. Lalys, F., Jannin, P.: Surgical process modelling: a review. International Journal of Computer Assisted Radiology and Surgery, 1–17 (2013)
10. Breiman, L.: Random forests. Machine Learning (2001)
11. Criminisi, A.: Decision forests: A unified framework for classification, regression, density estimation, manifold learning and semi-supervised learning. Foundations and Trends® in Computer Graphics and Vision (2011)
12. Kranzfelder, M., Schneider, A., Gillen, S., Feussner, H.: New technologies for information retrieval to achieve situational awareness and higher patient safety in the surgical operating room: the MRI institutional approach and review of the literature. Surgical Endoscopy 25(3), 696–705 (2011)
13. Kranzfelder, M., Schneider, A., Fiolka, A., Schwan, E., Gillen, S., Wilhelm, D., Schirren, R., Reiser, S., Jensen, B., Feussner, H.: Real-time instrument detection in minimally invasive surgery using radiofrequency identification technology. Journal of Surgical Research 185(2), 704–710 (2013)

Knowledge-Driven Formalization of Laparoscopic Surgeries for Rule-Based Intraoperative Context-Aware Assistance

Darko Katić[1], Anna-Laura Wekerle[2], Fabian Gärtner[1], Hannes Kenngott[2], Beat Peter Müller-Stich[2], Rüdiger Dillmann[1], and Stefanie Speidel[1]

[1] Institute for Anthropomatics (IFA), Humanoids and Intelligence Systems Laboratories (HIS), Karlsruhe Institute of Technology (KIT), Germany,
darko.katic@kit.edu
[2] Department of General, Abdominal and Transplantation Surgery, University of Heidelberg

Abstract. The rise of intraoperatively available information threatens to outpace our abilities to process data and thus cause informational overload. Context-aware systems, filtering information to match the current situation in the OR, will be necessary to reap all benefits of integrated and computerized surgery. To interpret surgical situations, such systems need a robust set of knowledge to make sense of intraoperative measurements. Building on our own ontology for laparoscopy, we formalized the workflow of laparoscopic adrenalectomies, cholecystectomies and pancreatic resections and developed a novel, rule-based situation interpretation algorithm based on OWL and SWRL to recognize phases of these surgeries. The system was evaluated on ground truth data from 19 manually annotated surgeries with an average recognition rate of 89%.

Keywords: Laparoscopic Surgery, Cognitive Surgery, Context-Awareness.

1 Introduction

The large amounts of information, provided by advancements in image guided surgery, have great potential to improve surgical therapy. However, the rise of available information threatens to outpace our capabilities to process and interpret the data [1]. The point where data is "physically available" but "not operationally effective" is quickly reached [2]. This is especially true for surgical interventions where large amounts of pre- and intraoperative information (MRI/CT images, endoscopic data, device states etc.) are available and need to be selectively considered when making decisions [4]. To cope with this, new man-machine interaction techniques are necessary. A solution can be found in context-aware systems which interpret the situation in the OR and display information targeted for the current circumstances, thus picking out the important bits from the wealth of data. The need for such adaptive interfaces in surgery

D. Stoyanov et al. (Eds.): IPCAI 2014, LNCS 8498, pp. 158–167, 2014.

has been emphasized by Kranzfelder et al. [5]. In the instance of laparoscopy, visualizations of tumors, vessels and other information can be selectively displayed only when necessary.

In literature, different approaches to context-awareness can be found. Currently predominant is the use of machine learning techniques, like Hidden Markov Models [6,7], Dynamic Time Warping [8] or statistical analysis [9]. Combinations thereof are also successfully used [10,11]. Another approach is raw signal processing. Blum et al. represent surgeries with snippets of signals [3]. Suzuki et al. quantify motion using video file size and oral conversations in the OR, without speech recognition for surgical phase detection [12]. Both approaches fail to include medical background-knowledge in a standardized, reusable way. Top-down approaches, in contrast, aim to formalize medical knowledge generically [13]. Description Logics (DL) [14] or UML [15] are used to this purpose. Combinations of formalized and machine learning approaches have also emerged [16]. A related field is the area of surgical evaluation, where similar methods are used to assess the performance of the surgeon [17]. Lack of knowledge has been identified as a major obstacle to discovering meaning in data [1]. We therefore believe that a strong foundation of knowledge is key to attain situational awareness in the sense of "knowing what is going on, so you can decide what to do" [18].

Our contribution is the formalization of laparoscopic adreanectomies, cholecystectomies and pancreatic resections, as performed at the University Hospital of Heidelberg, along with a novel mechanism for analyzing the resulting models for intraoperative context-awareness. Based on our ontology for laparoscopy, used as a semantic vocabulary, we formalized phases of the surgeries and identified rules which govern the transitions between them. Lastly we developed a mechanism, which allows rule-based situation interpretation. The system was realized using DLs [19] in OWL (Web Ontology Language) and SWRL (Semantic Web Rule Language)[20]. SWRL and our way of using it has not yet been applied to surgical phase recognition. Furthermore, we showed the effectiveness of our approach for situation interpretation on 19 annotated surgeries. In contrast to our previous work in context-awareness [21,22], we are no longer restricted to reasoning over distance-based relations between instruments and anatomical structures. Given input at the level of activities, the analysis is now performed on all surgical activities, with the benefit of detecting all medically relevant phases. Currently, this input is provided by manual annotation. The integration of the widely recognized SWRL standard is also a great step towards future interoperability and knowledge exchange with other systems.

2   Methods

We use DL to represent medical knowledge, inspired Neumann et al. [23]. According to the levels of granularity, as presented in [16], our system takes input of surgical activities and interprets them to infer the current phase of the surgery. In its intended use, the input is to be provided by intraoperative sensor analysis [24]. Similar to [25], we define activities as a triple of the used instrument, the performed action and the organ acted upon. For instance, the grasping of the splenic vein with a grasper is expressed as $(Grasper, grasp, SplenicVein)$. Activity triplets offer great insight in the current situation and are very expressive. It has been shown that reduction to, for instance, the currently used instrument can suffice to recognize certain phases. Yet complex scenarios require more detailed situation features. Early tests on our data showed that restricting the recognition to just the instrument is inadequate. Situations are described as the set of activities currently occurring in the OR. The phase to be recognized, in the case of a adrenalectomy for instance $Resection$ or $PortPlacement$, is a set of situations similar in the medical sense and in need of a common type of assistance, e.g. a specific visualization. We call a description of the possible sequences in which phases can occur chronologically a surgery plan. The result of the situation interpretation is the recognized phase and we therefore use the terms situation interpretation and phase recognition synonymously.

2.1 Formalization of Laparoscopic Adreanectomies, Cholecystectomies and Pancreatic Resections

To formalize adreanectomies, cholecystectomies and pancreatic resections, we devised a way to represent the surgery plan and intraoperative situations. It is based on the ontology for laparoscopy, the foundational vocabulary for the representation of the models. The approach is detailed in the following.

Ontology for Laparascopic Surgery. The purpose of the ontology is to represent all information necessary to interpret situations in a medically sound way. At the activity level, this includes instruments, actions and anatomical structures. Additionally, we model phases of the surgeries. In accordance to the ABox/TBox paradigm of DL our TBox represents time-invariant, taxonomical knowledge about objects and their relations, whereas the ABox represents dynamic knowledge about specific, real-world occurances. In other words, the TBox represent the terminology, whereas the ABox contains instances of these terms. The TBox is a hierarchy of concepts connected with the $is - a$ relation, denoted by $\sqsubseteq$. The main branches for medical knowledge are $Fluid$, $Organ$ and $Instrument$. All other concepts are nested there. For instance the left renal artery is integrated via $LeftRenalArtery \sqsubseteq Artery \sqsubseteq Vessel \sqsubseteq Organ$. Similarly, instruments are handeled. The l-hook cauter is expressed by $LHookCcauter \sqsubseteq ElectricInstrument \sqsubseteq SharpInstrument \sqsubseteq Instrument$. This way semantic information, like organ types (blood vessel) and instument properties (sharpness) are represented. The main branch for actions is $surgicalAction$. Actions, like $clip$, cut or $grasp$, are subrelations of this concept. They are organized in a meaningful, hierarchical structure. For instance, $coagulate$, cut and $resect$ are subsumed by $cuttingAction$. Overall, the ontology contains 26 relations and 130 concepts. All modeled knowledge is accessible to logical reasoning. The knowledge acquisition technique we used to create the ontology is the "Teach-Back Method" [26]. The basic idea is to first let the medical experts explain the domain to the engineer, who then in turn teaches the information back, as he

Pancreatic Resection

Phase	Description
Start	Beginning of the intervention
Port placement	Insertion of surgical instruments and the endoscope
Mobilisation	Transsection of the gastrocolic ligament access the pancreas.
Dissection	Dissection of the parietal peritoneum to mobilize the pancreas
Resection	Removal of pathologic tissue of the pancreas (e.g. IPMN, benign tumor or cyst)
Closure	Removal of resected tissue in a specimen bag
Drain	Drainage for early indication of pancreatic fistula or bleeding

Cholecystectomy

Phase	Description
Start	Begin of the surgery
Port placement	Insertion of surgical instruments and the endoscope
Mobilisation	Exposure of the gallbladder
Dissection	Prepationduring of the triangle of calot
Resection cystic artery	Resection of the the cystic artery
Resection cystic duct	Resection of the cystic duct
Resection gallbladder	Removal of the gallbladder from the liverbed
Closure	Removal of the gallbladder in a specimen bag
Drain	Drainage of infectious liquid or for early indication of bleeding

Adrenalectomy

Phase	Description
Start	Begin of the surgery
Port placement	Insertion of surgical instruments and the endoscope
Mobilisation	Mobilization of adjacent adhesions and the colon to access gerota's fascia
Dissection	Cutting of gerota's fascia to get direct access to the adrenal gland
Resection	Resection of the adrenal gland
Closure	Removal of adrenal gland in a specimen bag
Drain	Drainage for an early indication of bleeding

Fig. 1. Surgical phases for the laparoscopic interventions

understood it. Possible misconceptions and gaps in understanding are filled and mutual understanding is assured. As the ontology editor, Protege [27] was used.

Formalization of the Surgery Plan. The relevant phases we identified are shown in Fig.1, and the possible transitions between them in Fig.2. This informal description is translated to OWL as follows. Phases are represented as subconcepts of *Phase*, another branch of the ontology. To represent the order in which phases can occur, i.e. the surgery plan, we use the relation *nextPossiblePhase* and its inverse *previousPhase*. We call a transition between phases p_1 and p_1 valid, if *nextPossiblePhase*(p_1, p_2) is asserted. Essentially, *nextPossiblePhase*(p_1, p_2) encapsulates the knowledge, that p_2 can occur right after p_1, representing a predecessor relationship. The surgery plan is then implemented by creating instances of all phases of the surgery in the ABox and connecting them with the *nextPossiblePhase* relation.

Formalization of Surgical Situations. To model the current situation in the OR, the formalization of the surgery plan is augmented with new activities as they occur. Activities are expressed by creating instances and asserting relations between them. For example, the occurrence of a ligasure cutting the gastrocolic ligament is expressed with $Ligasure(aLigasure) \wedge GastrocolicLigament(aGl) \wedge cut(aLigasure, aGl)$. Thereby the notation $C(a)$ denotes that a is an instance of concept C, and $r(a, b)$ that relation r holds between instances a and b. Once the

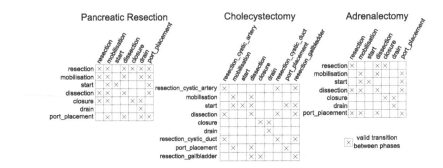

Fig. 2. Display of valid phase transistions

activity is over, it is removed from the ABox. Entire situations are expressed in the ABox as sets of activities currently occurring in the OR.

2.2   Rules and their Application for Situation Interpretation

The idea behind our situation interpretation is to execute rules for each phase whose condition is true once the phase is currently occurring in the OR. The interpretation cycle is triggered at each beginning and end of an activity. The rules check for two transition conditions. The first one, the validness, is about whether the phase is possible considering the surgery plan, i.e. whether there is a valid transition from the current phase. The second one, the phase specific, checks whether the current situation contains an event typical for the phase, a so called triggering event. These events are shown in Fig. 3. If both conditions apply, the corresponding phase is assumed to be the current one.

To formalize these conditions, we use SWRL, an established standard for rule-based reasoning, with a wealth of available tools for editing and execution. The rules consist of an antecedent (body) and consequent (head). The head is asserted in the ABox, given that the body is fulfilled. The body of all rules checks whether both transition conditions are fulfilled, the head asserts that the phase under consideration is occurring. The validness condition in SWRL is: $Phase(?p) \wedge CurrentPhase(?current) \wedge nextPossiblePhase(?current, ?p)$. Intuitively this means that the variable p must refer to an instance of $Phase$ and $current$ to an instance of $CurrentPhase$. Furthermore, $nextPossiblePhase$ must be asserted between them. In other words, p refers to all phases for which the validness condition is fulfilled. To check the second condition, we need to see whether one of the triggering events is present. In the case of the phase of port placement in a pancreatic resection, this would be: $Port(?instrument) \wedge Abdomen(?structure) \wedge place(?instrument, ?structure)$. In other words, we check whether there are instances $instrument$ of $Port$ being placed on a $structure$ of concept $Abdomen$. The other phase specific conditions are translated into SWRL syntax in the same way. The overall body of a rule is the conjunction of both expressions.

The naive choice for the head of each rule would be $CurrentPhase(?p)$. However, the expressivity of SWRL is limited. Particularly, the monotonicity

Pancreatic Resection

Phase	Triggering Activities
Start	-
Port placement	(Port, place, Abdomen)
Mobilisation	(AtraumaticGrasper, grasp, GastrocolicLigament), (Instr, surgicalAction, splenocolicLigament),
	(AtraumaticGrasper, grasp, GreaterOmentum), (SharpInstr, cuttingAction, GastrocolicLigament),
	(SharpInstr, cuttingAction, Adhesion)
Dissection	(SharpInstr, cuttingAction, DorsalParietalPeritoneum), (Instrument, bluntDissect, DorsalParietalPeritoneum),
	(AtraumaticGrasper grasp DorsalParietalPeritoneum), (BluntInstr, bluntDissect, SplenicArtery),
	(SharpInstr, dissect, SplenicArtery), (Clip, clipping, SplenicArtery),
	(Instr, knot, SplenicArtery), (BluntInstr, bluntDissect, SplenicVein),
	(SharpInstr, dissect, SplenicVein), (Clip, clipping, SplenicVein), (Instr, knot, SplenicVein)
Resection	(SharpInstr, cuttingAction, Pancreas), (SharpInstr, cuttingAction, RetropancreaticTissue),
	(SharpInstr, dissect, Pancreas), (SharpInstr, cuttingAction, Tumor),
	(SharpInstr, cuttingAction, Cyst), (Stapler, resect, Pancreas), (NeedleHolder, suture, Pancreas),
	(NeedleHolder, suture, Stomach), (SharpInstr, cuttingAction, SplenicArtery),
	(SharpInstr, cuttingAction, SplenicVein)
Closure	(SpecimenBag, surgicalAction, Organ)
Drain	(Drainage, surgicalAction, organ)

Cholecystectomy

Phase	Triggering Activities
Start	-
Port placement	(Port, place, Abdomen)
Mobilisation	(AtraumaticGrasper, grasp, GallbladderFundus), (AtraumaticGrasper, grasp, GastrocolicLigament)
Dissection	(AtraumaticGrasper, grasp ,HepatoduodenalLigament),
	(AtraumaticGrasper, lift , HepatoduodenalLigament), (Instr, surgicalAction, CalotTriangle),
	(SharpInstr, cuttingAction, HepatoduodenalLigament)
Resection cystic artery	(SharpInstr, cut, CysticArtery), (Clip, clipping, CysticArtery)
Resection cystic duct	(SharpInstr, cuttingAction, CysticDuct), (Clip, clipping, CysticDuct)
Resection gallbladder	(SharpInstr, cuttingAction, GallbladderSerosa), (SharpInstr, dissect, GallbladderSerosa),
	(SharpInstr, cuttingAction, Gallbladder), (SharpInstr, cuttingAction, GallbladderLiverbed)
Closure	(SpecimenBag, surgicalAction, Organ)
Drain	(Drainage, surgicalAction, organ)

Adrenalectomy

Phase	Triggering Activities
Start	-
Port placement	(port, place, abdomen)
Mobilisation	(SharpInstr, cuttingAction, Adhesion), (SharpInstr, mobilize, Liver),
	(AtraumaticGrasper, lift, Liver), (AtraumaticGrasper, grasp, Adhesion),
	(AtraumaticGrasper, grasp, GreaterOmentum),
	(SharpInstr, cuttingAction, SplenoralLigament), (SharpInstr, mobilize, Colon)
Dissection	(SharpInstr, cuttingAction, GerotasFascia), (Instr, surgicalAction, DorsalParietalPeritoneum)
Resection	(SharpInstr, cuttingAction, AdrenalGland), (Instr, surgicalAction, PerirenalFatTissue)
Closure	(SpecimenBag, surgicalAction, organ), (AtraumaticGrasper, puttingAction, ResectedTissue)
Drain	(Drainage, surgicalAction, organ)

Fig. 3. List of typical activties for phases (trigger activities)

of DL and SWRL requires that adding more information does not invalidate previous reasoning results. Therefore, once a phase has been inferred to be a *CurrentPhase*, no SWRL rules can change this. To counter this problem we set the head of each rule to *DetectedPhase*(?p). After each interpretation cycle the model is "cleaned up" with means outside of SWRL. In the case of a *DetectedPhase* being asserted, we use an outside program to remove the assertion *CurrentPhase* of the current phase and make it a *VisitedPhase* to mark that it did occur. Then, the *DetectedPhase* is asserted to be no longer a *DetectedPhase* but of type *CurrentPhase*. This way, the representation is set up for the next interpretation cycle. We take all phases of type *CurrentPhase* as the result of the interpretation. Initially, we mark *Start* as a *CurrentPhase*. The process is illustrated in Fig. 4. As the technical solution for ABox representation, reasoning and rule execution we use HermiT [28].

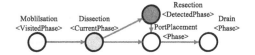

Fig. 4. Classification of phases with SWRL rules

3   Evaluation and Results

The evaluation of the system is based on ground truth data, i.e. manually annotated videos of surgeries with SWAN-Suite [29]. We recorded 11 pancreatic resections, 3 cholecystectomies and 5 adrenalectomies surgeries and annotated them with experienced clinicians who did not participate in the surgery. The annotations consist of timed activities and phase transitions (Fig. 5). For the evaluation, the annotations are played back in real-time to simulate results of sensors. The situations are interpreted as described above and the recognized phase is compared to the ground-truth. We consider two quality measures, the recognition rate and confusion matrices (Fig. 6). We define the recognition rate as the fraction of time, in which the system's assessment is correct, i.e. matches the ground truth. This is computed by comparing the interpretation result to the ground truth at a frequency of over 100Hz. By design, the measure not only represents if the situation was interpreted correctly, but also whether it happened in time. As for the confusion matrix, each element colorcodes the number of times the phase in the row was recognized as the one in the column. Incidentally, the diagonal entries represent the number of correct recognitions. Note that absolute numbers without normalization are used.

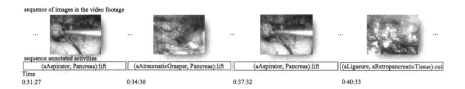

Fig. 5. Annotation of surgical recordings

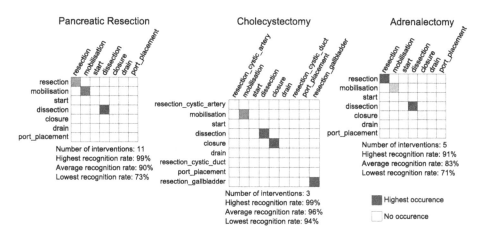

Fig. 6. Confusion matrices and recognition rates

4   Discussion

The results show that our system is capable of providing context-awareness in complex, realistic and medically relevant scenarios, given input at the level of activities. The recognition rate is a valuable quality measure since it considers timing and is indicative of the ability to reasonably asses the situation. This is fundamental to bringing context-aware systems in the OR, where the medical benefits can be evaluated. The confusion matrices show that situations are reliably, yet not perfectly, detected. Mistakes occur when an interrupted phase is resumed. For instances, after a port is placed, the system, correctly recognizing the port placement, waits for a triggering activity to fall back to the previous phase. Also, sometimes the triggering activities are not specific enough and occur in several phases. Yet mostly, as shown by the recognition rates, correct interpretations are given. Future work will include the comparison of our result to related work. The major obstacle to this is high fragmentation in the field. The use of different quality measures, surgery types and phase partitions as well as closed-sourced implementation makes unbiased comparison difficult.

Also, the formalization of laparoscopic adreanectomies, cholecystectomies and pancreatic resections is an important step toward semantification of surgical workflows. For context-aware system, it is vital to have a robust set of knowledge, as emphasized in [5]. In contrast to other sciences, such as physics where mathematics has emerged as the main means of representation, the medical science still lacks a generally agreed on formal method to represent knowledge. Most surgical knowledge is contained in literature or passed down informally from experienced surgeons to novice ones. It is commonly inaccessible to computation. Ontologies can be part of a solution in this regard. The formalization also helps in a practical way. The encoding is human readable and can be verified directly.

This along with the evaluation results and evidence for rule-based deduction in human cognition [30] shows that rules are likely to play an important role in context-aware systems. Yet knowledge acquisition can be difficult since numerous rules must be formulated for rich scenarios. Also, the surgery needs to be sufficiently standardized with few anomalies to expect. Furthermore, for practical application, inputs at the level of activities need to be generated by sensor analysis. This is a difficult task for which systems like [24] are planned to be used. However, it is likey that this will result in noisy data. To counter these problems, a combination of the top-down approach with machine learning seems promising. Future work will therefore focus on evaluating the robustness of the rule-based approach and its combination with machine learning.

Acknowledgements. The present research was supported by the "SFB TRR 125" funded by the DFG and the ESF of Baden-Wuerttemberg.

References

1. Woods, D.D., Patterson, E.S., Roth, E.M.: Can We Ever Escape from Data Overload? A Cognitive Systems Diagnosis Cognition, Technology and Work 4(1), 22–36 (2002)
2. Joyce, J.P., Lapinski, G.W.: A history and overview of the safety parameter display system concept. IEEE Nuclear Science NS-30 (1983)
3. Blum, T., Feußner, H., Navab, N.: Modeling and Segmentation of Surgical Workflow from Laparoscopic Video. In: Jiang, T., Navab, N., Pluim, J.P.W., Viergever, M.A. (eds.) MICCAI 2010, Part III. LNCS, vol. 6363, pp. 400–407. Springer, Heidelberg (2010)
4. Cleary, K., Chung, H., Mun, S.: Or 2020: The operating room of the future. Laparoendoscopic and Advanced Surgical Techniques (2005)
5. Kranzfelder, M., Staub, C., Fiolka, A., Schneider, A., Gillen, S., Wilhelm, D., Friess, H., Knoll, A., Feussner, H.: Toward increased autonomy in the surgical OR: needs, requests, and expectations. Surg. Endosc. 27(5), 1681–1688 (2013)
6. Blum, T., Padoy, N., Feussner, H., Navab, N.: Workflow mining for visualization and analysis of surgeries. Int. J. Comput. Assisted. Radiol. Surg. 3(5), 379–386 (2008)
7. Bouarfa, L., Jonker, P.P., Dankelman, J.: Discovery of high-level tasks in the operating room. J. Biomed. Inform. 44(3), 455–462 (2010)
8. Ahmadi, S.-A., Sielhorst, T., Stauder, R., Horn, M., Feussner, H., Navab, N.: Recovery of surgical workflow without explicit models. In: Larsen, R., Nielsen, M., Sporring, J. (eds.) MICCAI 2006. LNCS, vol. 4190, pp. 420–428. Springer, Heidelberg (2006)
9. Reiley, C., Lin, H., Varadarajan, B., Vagolgyi, B., Khudanpur, S., Yuh, D., Hager, G.: Automatic Recognition of Surgical Motions Using Statistical Modeling for Capturing Variability Medicine Meets Virtual Reality (2008)
10. Lalys, F., Riffaud, L., Morandi, X., Jannin, P.: Surgical phases detection from microscope videos by combining SVM and HMM. In: Menze, B., Langs, G., Tu, Z., Criminisi, A. (eds.) MICCAI 2010. LNCS, vol. 6533, pp. 54–62. Springer, Heidelberg (2011)
11. Padoy, N., Blum, T., Ahmadi, S.A., Feussner, H., Berger, M.O., Navab, N.: Statistical modeling and recognition of surgical workflow. Med. Image Anal. 16(3), 632–641 (2010)
12. Suzuki, T., Sakurai, Y., Yoshimitsu, K., Nambu, K., Muragaki, Y.: Iseki. H.: Intraoperative multichannel audio-visual information recording and automatic surgical phase and incident detection. In: 32nd Annual International Conference of the IEEE EMBS, pp. 1190–1193 (2010)

13. Neumuth, T., Jannin, P., Schlomberg, J., Meixensberger, J., Wiedemann, P., Burgert, O.: Analysis of Surgical Intervention Populations Using Generic Surgical Process Models. International Journal of CARS (2010)
14. Burgert, O., Neumuth, T., Lempp, F., Mudunuri, R., Meixensberger, J., Strauss, G., Dietz, A., Jannin, P., Lemke, H.U.: Linking top-level ontologies and surgical workflows. Int. J. Comput. Assisted. Radiol. Surg. 1(1), 437–438 (2006)
15. Jannin, P., Morandi, X.: Surgical models for computer-assisted neurosurgery. Neuroimage 37(3), 783–791 (2007)
16. Lalys, F., Bouget, B., Riffaud, R., Jannin, P.: Automatic knowledge-based recognition of low-level tasks in ophthalmological procedures. Int. J. CARS 8, 39–49 (2013)
17. Oropesa, I., Sánchez-González, P., Lamata, P., Chmarra, M.K., Pagador, J.B., Sánchez-Margallo, J.A., Sánchez-Margallo, F.M., Gómez, E.: Methods and tools for objective assessment of psychomotor skills in laparoscopic surgery. J. Surg. Res. 171(1), 81–95 (2011)
18. Adam, E.C.: Fighter cockpits of the future. In: Proceedings of 12th IEEE/AIAA Digital Avionics Systems Conference (DASC), pp. 318–323 (1993)
19. Baader, F., Calvanese, D., McGuiness, D.L., Nardi, D., Patel-Schneider, P.F.: The Description Logic Handbook: Theory, Implementation, Applications. Cambridge University Press, Cambridge (2003) ISBN 0-521-78176-0
20. SWRL: A Semantic Web Rule Language Combining OWL and RuleML W3C Member Submission (2004)
21. Katic, D., Sudra, G., Speidel, S., Castrillon-Oberndorfer, G., Eggers, G., Dillmann, R.: Knowledge-based Situation Interpretation for Context-aware Augmented Reality in Dental Implant Surgery. In: Proc. Medical Imaging and Augmented Reality (2010)
22. Katic, D., Wekerle, A.L., Görtler, J., Spengler, P., Bodenstedt, S., Röhl, S., Suwelack, S., Kenngott, H.G., Wagner, M., Mueller-Stich, B.P., Dillmann, R., Speidel, S.: Context-aware Augmented Reality in laparoscopic surgery. Comp. Med. Imag. and Graph. 37(2), 174–182 (2013)
23. Neumann, B., Moeller, R.: On scene interpretation with description logics. Image and Vision Computing 26 (2008)
24. Speidel, S., Benzko, J., Sudra, G., Azad, P., Mütich, B.P., Gutt, C., Dillmann, R.: Automatic classification of minimally invasive instruments based on endoscopic image sequences. In: SPIE Medical Imaging, vol. 7261 (2009)
25. Neumuth, T., Strauß, G., Meixensberger, J., Lemke, H.U., Burgert, O.: Acquisition of process descriptions from surgical interventions. In: Bressan, S., Küng, J., Wagner, R. (eds.) DEXA 2006. LNCS, vol. 4080, pp. 602–611. Springer, Heidelberg (2006)
26. Kripalani, S., Bengtzen, R., Henderson, L., Jacobson, T.: Clinical Research in Low-Literacy Populations: Using Teach-Back to Assess Comprehension of Informed Consent and Privacy Information IRB: Ethics and Human Research (2008)
27. http://protege.stanford.edu/
28. Shearer, R., Motik, B., Horrocks, I.: HermiT: A Highly-Efficient OWL Reasoner. In: 5th Int. Workshop on OWL: Experiences and Directions (2008)
29. Neumuth, T., Jannin, P., Strauss, G., Meixensberger, J., Burgert, O.: Validation of knowledge acquisition for surgical process models. J. Am. Med. Inform. Assoc. (2009)
30. Smith, E.E., Langston, C., Nisbett, R.E.: The case for rules in reasoning. Cognitive Science 16(1), 1–40 (1992)

Temporally Consistent 3D Pose Estimation in the Interventional Room Using Discrete MRF Optimization over RGBD Sequences

Abdolrahim Kadkhodamohammadi[1], Afshin Gangi[2],
Michel de Mathelin[1], and Nicolas Padoy[1]

[1] ICube, University of Strasbourg, CNRS, France
{kadkhodamohammad,demathelin,npadoy}@unistra.fr
[2] Radiology Department, University Hospital of Strasbourg, France
gangi@unistra.fr

Abstract. Tracking and body pose estimation of clinical staff have several applications in the analysis of surgical workflow, such as radiation monitoring, surgical activity recognition and the study of ergonomics. The operating room is, however, a very complex environment for visual tracking due to frequent illumination changes, clutter, similar color of clinicians' scrubs and limited sensor positioning. Furthermore, several applications, such as radiation monitoring, require consistent and accurate body part tracking over defined periods of time, which is a challenging task in the aforementioned conditions. In this paper, we tackle the problem of pose estimation in the interventional room. We also propose a method to consistently track upper body parts in short sequences by using RGBD data and discrete Markov Random Field (MRF) optimization over the complete set of frames. The proposed MRF energy formulation enforces both body kinematic and temporal constraints in order to cope with the natural ambiguities of tracking and with the frequent failure of the underlying depth-based body part detector in such conditions. We evaluate our approach quantitatively on seven manually-annotated sequences recorded in the interventional room and show that it can consistently track the upper-body of persons present in the room.

Keywords: Body pose estimation, clinician tracking, surgical workflow analysis, Markov random field, RGBD images.

1   Introduction

Reliable pose estimation and tracking of clinical staff can benefit many applications for the interventional room, such as context-aware user interfaces [1, 2], real-time recognition and monitoring of medical activities [3, 4], performance assessment of the surgical team [5], radiation safety monitoring [6] and ergonomics analysis [7].

Few approaches have been proposed for person tracking in the interventional room due to the numerous difficulties impeding the installation of computer

D. Stoyanov et al. (Eds.): IPCAI 2014, LNCS 8498, pp. 168–177, 2014.

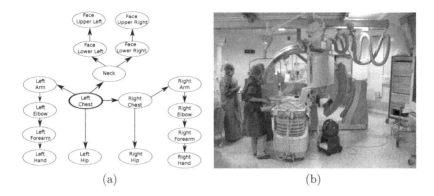

(a)   (b)

Fig. 1. (a) Upper body kinematic tree consisting of 17 parts and rooted at the left chest. (b) A typical interventional radiology room.

vision systems in such an environment (see figure 1(b)). First of all, because of safety requirements and the presence of many articulated arms mounted on the ceiling of the room, the options for camera positioning are very limited. Second, the frequent changes of illumination, similar color of clothes and equipments and the numerous occlusions present in the room make pose estimation and tracking very challenging.

The current work is motivated by the increasing need for radiation monitoring during X-ray based interventional procedures. A recent large consortium-based study [8] showed that radiation exposure differs at different locations of the staff's bodies. Hence, the current practice of using a single dosimeter for radiation monitoring does not provide accurate information about the radiation exposure of different body parts. Since it would be impractical for the staff to wear a multitude of dosimeters on a regular basis, especially on their head and arms, there exists a need to complement these devices with a radiation awareness system combining vision-based pose estimation with radiation simulation, as presented in [6]. Computation of the radiation risk for each body part can be used to generate exposure warnings and to perform statistical analysis in correlation with the different activities performed during the procedure.

To make the aforementioned application possible, a pose estimation approach yielding temporally consistent results during the short bursts of emission from the X-ray device is necessary in order to accurately estimate accumulated radiation per body part over time. We therefore focus, in this paper, on consistent upper-body tracking of persons present in the interventional room during such short sequences. Since the lower-body is generally less susceptible to movement and is occluded by the apron or by the patient table, we exclude it from the tracking approach. Because the light is often turned off during the use of the X-ray device for better visualization of the X-ray images, we propose to use the depth channel of an RGBD camera to capture the scene and perform the pose estimation. This is in contrast to [6] who uses a 16 camera multi-view reconstruction system, based on background subtraction and shape from silhouette, that is difficult to introduce into the interventional room.

There exists a large body of work on 2D and 3D human pose estimation and person tracking in the computer vision community, targeting various applications such as activity recognition, human-machine interactions, video surveillance or virtual character animation. They rely on one or more visual sensors, such as RGB, infrared or time-of-flight cameras. The interested reader is referred to [9] for a more complete presentation of the literature. State-of-the-art human pose estimation in RGB images is mainly addressed by part-based methods [10–12], which combine various image cues, such as gradient, motion or color to detect body parts. The part detector responses are then used to infer single frame body pose according to an underlying body model. Temporal tracking addresses on-line scenarios and makes use of previous frames and of models of dynamics for better temporal estimation [12]. Few works however address the body pose estimation problem as an optimization over the complete sequence. In [13], the 3D pose estimation is refined on a complete multi-camera sequence by iteratively using action recognition for retrieving motion priors to restrict the space of possible poses. In [11], a framework for 2D multiple person tracking in RGB images is proposed to stitch short body trajectories to track pedestrians and their body parts.

With the recent introduction of affordable RGB-Depth sensors, such as the Microsoft Kinect, very successful approaches for 3D part detection and tracking have been proposed using the depth channel of the camera. [14] propose to use random forests on depth images for either body part classification or direct body joint regression after a background subtraction step. [15] uses an approach inspired by [14] to classify the body parts without background subtraction. It relies on an intermediate blob segmentation step and parses the detected parts using dynamic programming for body skeleton estimation. The aforementioned works focus on single-frame body pose estimation and do not enforce any temporal consistency. Due to noise, motion, occlusions and camera positioning, part detection and pose estimation are often inconsistent in consecutive frames.

In this paper, motivated by our radiation monitoring application which requires consistent tracking during the short bursts of X-ray emission, we propose to formulate the pose estimation problem as an optimization over the entire sequence using Markov Random Fields (MRF). We propose a robust cost function that drives the skeleton towards the body parts using the part detector [15] and also simultaneously enforces kinematic and temporal constraints in the sequences. The cost function is then optimized using efficient discrete optimization on the multi-label MRF. The approach is evaluated quantitatively on seven manually-annotated videos recorded in two different interventional rooms.

2   Method

We define the upper body pose of a person using the positions of 17 body parts as shown in figure 1(a). We follow the body kinematics to define a skeleton tree

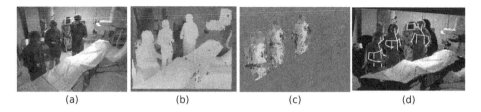

(a)	(b)	(c)	(d)

Fig. 2. (a,b,c) Example of data used in this paper: RGB image, depth image, BPD response. (d) Overlay of the 3D upper-body skeletons on the reconstructed point cloud.

over these parts, rooted at the left chest. This is the same skeleton as the one defined in [15], but restricted to the upper body and rooted at the left chest instead of the neck.

Given a set of consecutive RGBD frames and upper body poses for the persons in the first and last frames, our goal is to consistently estimate the pose of the persons in the whole set of frames. We propose to cast the problem in a multi-label MRF optimization framework: consistent pose estimation over the complete set of frames is defined as an optimization problem in a MRF whose nodes represent the body parts and whose labels encode 3D displacements. The MRF graph $\mathbf{G}$ is constructed by connecting the upper body skeleton tree of each person in consecutive frames, as shown in figure 3. $\mathbf{G} = (\mathcal{P}, \mathcal{E})$, where $\mathcal{P}$ is the set of nodes representing the upper body parts and $\mathcal{E}$ is the set of edges defining the connection between each person's body parts. Two types of edges are to be considered: kinematic edges ($\mathcal{E}^k$), connecting body parts in each frame, and temporal edges ($\mathcal{E}^t$), connecting the same body parts in consecutive frames. As a result, each person has a connected graph over the sequence. The pose is then estimated by optimizing iteratively an energy function that models the different constraints by using discrete optimization. This provides the final 3D displacements of the parts from their initial positions.

A depth body part detector is used to compute the initial position and also to drive the MRF optimization. The detector [15] is used and hereafter referred to as BPD (body part detector). It computes part detections for each depth pixel using random decision forests (see figure 2) and clusters the resulting detections into blobs representing either body parts or background. This results in a list of blobs per body part and frame. We associate a confidence value for each blob by counting the number of pixels voting for the part within the blob and by normalizing the values with the size of the largest blob in the frame corresponding to the same part. This gives low confidence to the small blobs that occur frequently in noisy data.

The blob list corresponding to left chest detections in all frames and the left chest positions in the first frame are used to construct initial 3D trajectories for all persons present in the video. A person trajectory is specified by the 3D positions of the left chest in the frames. It is initialized at the position of the left chest in the first frame. For the rest of the frames, the left chest blob with

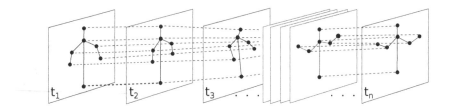

Fig. 3. MRF graph with kinematic and temporal edges over body parts

highest confidence in a sphere of radius θ centered at the previous position is selected. If no chest is found, the previous position is considered for the frame. The parameter θ is chosen to be the average 3D radius of the body trunk, so that the 3D trajectories of different persons do not get mixed.

2.1 Part Position Initialization

The trajectories mentioned in the previous section only determine the positions of the left chests in the frames. They are used together with the list of detected parts in each frame to initialize the positions of all parts. In case the part detector fails and does not provide any detection for some parts, we follow a default kinematic model to initialize these positions. The positions of the upper body parts corresponding to a person standing in an upright position with the arms by the side of the body is used.

Given the detected parts and the position of the root part, two different situations arise for each part: (1) *one or more blobs are available*: the blob with highest confidence value within a neighborhood around the parent position is used to set the position. As in the previous section, the average part size is used to define the neighborhood; (2) *no blob is available*: its position is predicted relative to its parent according to the default kinematic model. Parts are associated following this procedure for each person in a greedy manner.

2.2 Optimization

The optimization is performed over the graph $\mathbf{G} = (\mathcal{P}, \mathcal{E})$ defined over a complete sequence of video frames. The proposed energy is defined as:

$$E(D) = \sum_{p \in \mathcal{P}} V_p(d_p) + \lambda^k \sum_{(p,q) \in \mathcal{E}^k} V_{p,q}^k(d_p, d_q) + \lambda^t \sum_{(p,q) \in \mathcal{E}^t} V_{p,q}^t(d_p, d_q), \quad (1)$$

where $D = \{d_p\}_{p \in \mathcal{P}}$ is a global labelling indicating the displacement for each node, d_p is the 3D displacement offset for node p encoded as a discrete label, $V_p(.)$ are the unary potentials representing the data term, $V_{pq}^k(.,.)$ and $V_{pq}^t(.,.)$ are the pairwise potentials and smoothness terms defined respectively on kinematic and temporal edges and λ^k and λ^t are weighting coefficients. The superscripts k and t refer to kinematic and temporal edges. The two smoothness terms force the parts to follow body kinematics and to move smoothly along the frames. The data term incorporates the image evidence.

Due to the large search space in 3D, two different methods are compared to sample the search space and define the label set L: dense sampling and sparse sampling. $L = L(n, s)$ depends on two parameters: n the number of samples in each 3D direction and s the step size. In dense sampling, we sample the whole cube, while in sparse sampling we only sample along seven 3D directions, namely top-down, left-right, front-back and the four main cube diagonals [16].

Data Term. As mentioned above, the part detector clusters the depth image into body parts and background blobs. This blob segmentation is used to define the data term:

$$V_p(d_p) = \begin{cases} M(C(d_p)) & \text{if } \#(blobs(frame(p), label(p))) > 0 \\ \beta & otherwise \end{cases}, \quad (2)$$

where $frame(p)$ returns the frame number of node p, $label(p)$ is the part label associated with the node, $blobs(f, l)$ returns the list of blobs in frame f labelled as part l, $\#(.)$ is the cardinality operator, $C(d_p)$ is the minimum cost defined below, β is a constant cost for parts without detection, and $M(.)$ is a robust error function (ROEF) chosen as

$$M(x) = \frac{x^2}{x^2 + \alpha^2}. \quad (3)$$

The function $C(d_p)$ computes the minimum cost of a 3D displacement d_p:

$$C(d_p) = \min_{b \in blobs(frame(p), label(p))} \|P(d_p) - Centroid(b)\| * (\gamma - Conf(b)), \quad (4)$$

where $P(d_p)$ is the 3D position of node p moved by an offset d_p, $\|.\|$ is the ℓ_2-norm, and $Centroid(b)$ and $Conf(b)$ are respectively the centroid and the confidence value of blob b. Since $Conf(b)$ is between 0 and 1, to penalize larger distance to the blob centroid, we avoid making this term zero by choosing $\gamma > 1$.

In eq. (2), the cost of moving a node by a specified offset is computed according to the part detector's response. If no detection is available for the part, a constant cost is used. As a result, undetected parts are only adjusted by the kinematic and temporal constraints.

Kinematic Term. The kinematic term defines the geometrical relationships between parts:

$$V_{p,q}^k(d_p, d_q) = |\|P(d_p) - P(d_q)\| - \mu_{pq}|, \quad (5)$$

where $(p, q) \in \mathcal{E}^k$, $|.|$ is the absolute value operator and μ_{pq} is the mean distance between the parts p and q in the kinematic model. This term encodes the kinematic dependency between parts. Since the positions are in 3D, it penalises variations with respect to an average kinematic model.

Table 1. Presentation of the dataset (sequence IDs, number of frames, BPD misdetection rates and room IDs)

ID	#Frames	#Pers.	Misdet.(%)	Room
S1	50	2	28	IR1
S2	100	2	29	IR2
S3	100	3	27	IR2
S4	110	3	32	IR2
S5	200	2	27	IR2
S6	200	2	47	IR1
S7	200	3	29	IR1

Table 2. Noisy initialization experiment. Mean error in meter with std before and after optimization for right hip and all parts.

	ID	Initial	Optim.
Right hip	S1	1.02 ± 0.36	0.11 ± 0.05
All parts	S1	1.86 ± 1.17	0.32 ± 0.31
Right hip	S2	0.91 ± 0.36	0.16 ± 0.14
All parts	S2	1.81 ± 1.21	0.31 ± 0.33
Right hip	S3	0.94 ± 0.38	0.13 ± 0.13
All parts	S3	1.87 ± 1.25	0.36 ± 0.38

Temporal Term. Temporal consistency of the body parts is enforced by

$$V_{p,q}^t(d_p, d_q) = \|P(d_p) - P(d_q)\|, \tag{6}$$

where $(p, q) \in \mathcal{E}^t$. Here we assume that parts do not move very fast compared to the acquisition rate of the camera. It would however be possible to incorporate other types of dynamics if needed.

Optimization. Optimization is performed in several rounds by varying the parameters of the label set $L(n, s)$ to cover a smaller search space at each iteration, using the result of the previous optimization as new initialization. During optimization, the nodes in the first and last frames are kept constant using the provided upper body poses for the persons in the first and last frames. The FastPD algorithm [17] is used to perform the optimization in this paper.

3   Experiments

We evaluate our approach on seven RGBD sequences recorded in two different interventional rooms using an *Asus Xtion Pro Live* camera. The sequences have been recorded with a frame rate of 15fps and each sequence has a duration between 3 and 13 seconds. Two to three persons are present per recording. All sequences have been manually annotated to provide ground truth positions for the skeleton body parts. Parts that are not visible due to occlusions have been annotated too, using positions predicted by the annotator. This is an easy task in case of self-occlusions that occur frequently for the arms. Annotation during inter-person occlusions was also possible in these datasets because they do not happen for long periods. The dataset is summarized in table 1. The *BPD misdetection rate* is an indicator of the failure of the part detector. It indicates the ratio of parts in the skeletons, for all persons and in the complete sequence, that cannot be associated with any blob detection.

The proposed approach is evaluated using three experiments. The first experiment compares the two 3D space sampling methods described in section 2.2.

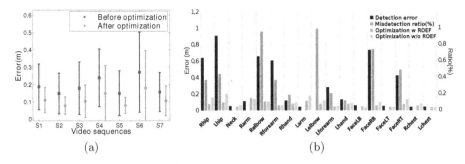

Fig. 4. Pose estimation error. (a) average error per sequence at initialization and after optimization; (b) errors per part for sequence S2 (at initialization and after optimization with and without robust error function) along with BPD misdetection rate.

The second experiment quantitatively evaluates the approach using the seven annotated datasets. The third experiment assesses the impact of noise during trajectory initialization by randomly drifting the parts away.

In all experiments, the discrete optimization step is iterated by shrinking the sampling step size by 20% at each iteration until the radius of the 3D search space covered by the labels becomes smaller than 5 centimeters. The initial radius of the 3D search space is chosen to be 60 centimeters. The parameters used in all experiments are $\theta = 0.4, \lambda^k = \lambda^t = 3, \beta = 5, \alpha = 0.1, \gamma = 1.01$. They have been determined using grid search over a complete sequence (S1). Errors and positions are expressed in meter. The accuracy is evaluated by computing the mean and standard deviation of the 3D Euclidean distances between the optimized body parts and the ground truth body parts in all frames.

Sampling Methods. The performance of the two 3D space sampling methods was compared and evaluated on the sequences using different spatial step sizes and iterative optimization as described above. The number of discrete labels per direction was chosen so that the initial 3D space covered has a radius of 60 centimeters. These preliminary experiments yielded better results for the dense sampling approach but no significant improvement for larger sets of labels. Consequently, we choose to use the dense sampling $L(1, 0.5)$ for the experiments below. This corresponds to a set of 27 labels.

Quantitative Evaluation. The approach is evaluated on all annotated sequences. Results are displayed in Fig. 4(a). Mean and standard deviation of the part localization errors are shown for each sequence before and after optimization. The results are optimal for sequence S1 in the sense that the parameters have been selected using grid search for this particular sequence. We see that the optimization performs equally well on the other sequences using the same parameters. In general, the mean error has decreased by over 30 percent and the standard deviation (STD) is lowered. Even though sequences S4 and S6 have the highest misdetection rate (see table 1), the optimization still reduces their mean error and std significantly. This implies that the optimization has correctly guided the detected and undetected parts toward their correct positions by using the image evidence and the kinematic and temporal constraints.

The mean error for each part is displayed in Fig. 4(b), for sequence S2, before and after optimization along with the part misdetection ratio. The optimization reduces the error considerably, especially for the parts with high misdetection rates. The figure also compares the influence of the robust error function (ROEF) used in the data term V_p. The ROEF largely reduces the error for parts with high misdetection rates. The ROEF is steep in the interval $[0, 2 * \alpha]$ and is almost flat in $[4 * \alpha, \infty]$. Therefore, detections strongly attract close nodes but have a negligible impact on far nodes. This is crucial to avoid misleading the undetected parts, considering the high part misdetection rate in our multi-person scenarios.

Noise. The impact of noisy initialization is studied by adding random 3D displacements to the initial part positions in all frames. The random displacements are sampled from a uniform distribution with a magnitude of 50 centimeters. Two cases are considered: noise is added to a single part (right hip) or to all parts at the same time. Table 2 shows the mean and std of the error before and after optimization. When noise is only added to the right hip, the results are reported for this single part. Results are reported on sequences S1,S2 and S3 that have little BPD noise to better identify the performance of our approach against initial noise. The results show that the approach can recover from a large amount of noise.

4   Conclusions

In this paper, we propose an approach to track consistently the upper-body parts of persons present in an interventional room over short RGBD sequences. Due to the visual challenges posed by the interventional room, body part detectors often fail to detect the body parts in individual frames. Consequently, we propose an approach based on optimization over the complete set of frames to improve tracking. Our approach uses discrete optimization in an MRF framework. We propose an energy function that incorporates both kinematic and temporal constraints in addition to the image evidence. We evaluated this approach quantitatively on seven manually-annotated RGBD sequences captured in two different interventional rooms. In this data, the part tracking error is reduced in average by half. The experiments also show robust results in the presence of multiple persons and occlusions, even when the number of part misdetections is high.

Future work will focus on tracking the persons in longer sequences and on improving the body part detectors. One approach in this direction will be to train the detectors for the camera setup specific to this environment. We also plan to incorporate an occlusion model and to use multiple RGBD cameras in order to deal with challenging multi-person scenarios.

Acknowledgements. This work was supported by French state funds managed by the ANR within the Investissements d'Avenir program under references ANR-11-LABX-0004 (Labex CAMI), ANR-10-IDEX-0002-02 (IdEx Unistra) and ANR-10-IAHU-02 (IHU Strasbourg). The authors would like to thank Laurent Goffin and Nicolas Loy Rodas for their help in recording the dataset used in this paper.

References

1. Schwarz, L.A., Bigdelou, A., Navab, N.: Learning gestures for customizable human-computer interaction in the operating room. In: Fichtinger, G., Martel, A., Peters, T. (eds.) MICCAI 2011, Part I. LNCS, vol. 6891, pp. 129–136. Springer, Heidelberg (2011)

2. Noonan, D.P., Mylonas, G.P., Darzi, A., Yang, G.Z.: Gaze contingent articulated robot control for robot assisted min. invasive surgery. In: IROS (2008)

3. Padoy, N., Mateus, D., Weinland, D., Berger, M.O., Navab, N.: Workflow Monitoring based on 3D Motion Features. In: VOEC-ICCV, pp. 585–592 (2009)

4. Lea, C., Facker, J.C., Hager, G.D., Taylor, R.H., Saria, S.: 3d sensing algorithms towards building an intelligent intensive care unit. In: AMIA CRI (2013)

5. Gentric, J.C., Trelhu, B., Jannin, P., Riffaud, L., Ferré, J.C., Gauvrit, J.Y.: Development of workflow task analysis during cerebral diagnostic angiographies: Time-based comparison of junior and senior tasks. Journal of Neuroradiology (2013)

6. Ladikos, A., Cagniart, C., Ghotbi, R., Reiser, M., Navab, N.: Estimating radiation exposure in interventional environments. In: Jiang, T., Navab, N., Pluim, J.P.W., Viergever, M.A. (eds.) MICCAI 2010, Part III. LNCS, vol. 6363, pp. 237–244. Springer, Heidelberg (2010)

7. Nara, A., Izumi, K., Iseki, H., Suzuki, T., Nambu, K., Sakurai, Y.: Surgical workflow monitoring based on trajectory data mining. In: Bekki, D. (ed.) JSAI-isAI 2010. LNCS, vol. 6797, pp. 283–291. Springer, Heidelberg (2011)

8. Carinou, E., Brodecki, M., Domienik, J., Donadille, L., Koukorava, C., Krim, S., Nikodemová, D., Ruiz-Lopez, N., Sans-Mercé, M., Struelens, L., Vanhavere, F.: Recommendations to reduce extremity and eye lens doses in interventional radiology and cardiology. Radiation Measurements (May 2011)

9. Holte, M., Tran, C., Trivedi, M., Moeslund, T.: Human pose estimation and activity recognition from multi-view videos. IEEE Journal of Selected Topics in Signal Processing 6(5), 538–552 (2012)

10. Felzenszwalb, P.F., Girshick, R., McAllester, D., Ramanan, D.: Object detection with discriminatively trained part based models. PAMI 32(9), 1627–1645 (2010)

11. Izadinia, H., Saleemi, I., Li, W., Shah, M. (MP)2T: Multiple people multiple parts tracker. In: Fitzgibbon, A., Lazebnik, S., Perona, P., Sato, Y., Schmid, C. (eds.) ECCV 2012, Part VI. LNCS, vol. 7577, pp. 100–114. Springer, Heidelberg (2012)

12. Choi, W., Pantofaru, C., Savarese, S.: A general framework for tracking multiple people from a moving camera. PAMI 35(7), 1577–1591 (2013)

13. Baak, A., Rosenhahn, B., Mueller, M., Seidel, H.P.: Stabilizing motion tracking using retrieved motion priors. In: ICCV, pp. 1428–1435 (2009)

14. Shotton, J., Girshick, R., Fitzgibbon, A., Sharp, T., Cook, M., Finocchio, M., Moore, R., Kohli, P., Criminisi, A., Kipman, A., Blake, A.: Efficient human pose estimation from single depth images. PAMI 35(12), 2821–2840 (2012)

15. Buys, K., Cagniart, C., Baksheev, A., Laet, T.D., Schutter, J.D., Pantofaru, C.: An adaptable system for rgb-d based human body detection and pose estimation. Journal of Visual Communication and Image Representation (2013)

16. Padoy, N., Hager, G.D.: 3d thread tracking for robotic assistance in tele-surgery. In: IROS, pp. 2102–2107. IEEE (2011)

17. Wang, C., Komodakis, N., Paragios, N.: Markov random field modeling, inference & learning in computer vision & image understanding: A survey. CVIU 117(11), 1610–1627 (2013)

Relevance-Based Visualization to Improve Surgeon Perception

Olivier Pauly[1], Benoît Diotte[1], Séverine Habert[1], Simon Weidert[2],
Ekkehard Euler[2], Pascal Fallavollita[1,*], and Nassir Navab[1]

[1] Chair for Computer Aided Medical Procedures,
Technische Univ. München, Germany
[2] Chirurgische Klinik und Poliklinik Innenstadt, München, Germany
`fallavol@in.tum.de`

Abstract. In computer-aided interventions, the visual feedback of the
doctor is vital. Enhancing the relevant object will help for the perception
of this feedback. In this paper, we present a learning-based labeling of
the surgical scene using a depth camera (comprised of RGB and depth
range sensors). The depth sensor is used for background extraction and
Random Forests are used for segmenting color images. The end result
is a labeled scene consisting of surgeon hands, surgical instruments and
background labels. We evaluated the method by conducting 10 simulated
surgeries with 5 clinicians and demonstrated that the approach provides
surgeons a dissected surgical scene, enhanced visualization, and upgraded
depth perception.

Keywords: visualization, medical augmented reality, machine learning,
multimodal image fusion, operating room.

1 Introduction

Humans boast a sophisticated cognitive system which takes approximately 15-
20 different psychological stimuli into account in order to perceive spatial relationships between objects [1]. Nevertheless, in complex settings, such as the
operating room theatre, the cognitive system is challenged as clinicians are confronted with information stemming from multiple sources when making surgical
decisions. Presenting all of the information in an effective manner is a difficult
task. Consequently, improving the understanding and perception of clinicians
towards their surgical environment becomes an important feedback for the success of computer-assisted intervention applications (e.g. labeling the surgeons
action helps in workflow analysis [2], or improving surgeon visualization of fused
modalities helps successful patient outcomes).

This feedback can be provided by mixed and augmented reality (AR) visualizations for use in computer-assisted interventions. However, few of these systems
have been introduced for daily use into the operating room (OR). This may be

---

* Corresponding author.

D. Stoyanov et al. (Eds.): IPCAI 2014, LNCS 8498, pp. 178–185, 2014.

the result of several factors: the systems are developed from a technical perspective, are rarely evaluated in the field, and/or lack consideration of the clinician and the constraints of the OR [3].

As of late, the community did achieve success in deploying the first medical augmented reality technology (an AR mobile fluoroscope) within orthopedic and trauma surgery rooms, and this recent introduction promises to support surgeons in their understanding of the spatial relationships between anatomy, implants and their surgical tools [4,5]. The output overlay of such a technology is a uniform alpha-blending between the X-ray and optical images. The issue with this blending type is that the understanding of the scene can be altered when the field of view of the scene becomes highly cluttered (e.g. with surgical tools and implants). It becomes increasingly difficult to rapidly recognize and differentiate different structures in the fused image. Moreover, the clinicians depth perception is altered as (i) the X-ray anatomy appears floating on top of the scene in the optical image, (ii) hands and surgical instruments occlude the visualization, and (iii) there is no correct ordering between structures in the fused images.

With these issues in mind, we note that all pixels in X-ray and optical images do not have the same importance and contribution to the final blending (e.g. the background is not important compared to the surgical tool). This observation suggests extracting only relevant-based data according to pixels belonging to background, tools and clinician hands [6]. The labeling of the surgical scene by a precise segmentation and differentiation of its different parts allows a relevant blending respecting the desired ordering of structures. A few attempts have been endeavored, such as in [7]. In these early works, a Naive Bayes classification approach based on color and radiodensity is applied to recognize the different objects in X-ray and color images. Depending on the pair of pixels it belongs to, each pixel is associated to a mixing value to create a relevant-based fused image. While authors showed promising results, recognizing each object on their color distribution is very challenging and not robust to changes in illumination.

Contribution: We introduce a surgical scene labeling paradigm based on machine learning and having as input both an optical and depth camera in a medical AR setting. In our application, the depth is a useful hint for the segmentation and ordering of hands and tools with respect to anatomy since the clinician performs surgery over the patient. Thus, our visualization paradigm is founded on segmentation consisting in modeling the background via depth data. We perform in parallel color image segmentation via the state-of-the-art Random Forests. To refine our segmentation method we use the GrabCut algorithm. Lastly, we combine our background modeling and color segmentation in order to identify the objects of interests in the color images and achieve successfully ordering of structures. We conducted 10 simulated surgeries with 5 clinicians to showcase our visualization results.

2   Methods

A depth camera with an integrated optical camera (Asus Xtion Pro Live) is affixed to a mobile C-arm fluoroscope above of the surgery workspace, giving a general overview of clinician gestures and surgical tool manipulations. The depth camera is positioned at its fabricated optimal visual focal length (70cm) of the patient table. Since the camera has a visual view of the surgical scene it is reasonable to assume that the hands and surgical instruments are on top of or at the same level as the patient. The depth image is built-in registered to the RGB camera therefore the image I and depth image D are defined on the same domain $\Omega \in \mathbb{R}^2$ with I and D being defined respectively as $I : \sigma \to \mathbb{R}^3$ and $D : \sigma \to \mathbb{R}$.

2.1   Identifying Objects of Interest in RGB-D

The objective is to dissect the surgical scene using the images from the RGB and depth camera. We divide the scene into 3 classes $C = \{tool, hands, background\}$. The surgeon actions via tools and hands are combined to form the foreground class (closer to the camera). We use the depth image to create a background model that will, for every frame, give a probability at a given pixel x, $P_D(f^c|x)$ of belonging to the background (f^c, complement class of the foreground). With the RGB images, the probabilities $P_I(c|x)$ of belonging to the tools, the surgeon hand or the background is obtained using Random Forests. Then, since the modalities RGB and depth are independent (the color is not interfering on the depth), we can decompose the joint distribution of a pixel belonging to the foreground and to an object c $P_{I,D}(f,c|x)$ as

$$P_{I,D}(f,c|x) = (1 - P_D(f^c|x))P_I(c|x) \tag{1}$$

Background Extraction Using Depth Images. Background modeling has been widely studied for performing background subtraction in color images in tracking applications. In a fixed camera setup, the key idea is to learn a color distribution for each pixel from a set of background images. As reported in [8], several approaches have been proposed within the last decade for adaptive real-time background subtraction based on running Gaussian averages, mixture models, kernel density estimation or the so-called Eigenbackground. In the present work, we propose to learn a fixed background model using the depth image and based solely on a set of acquired depth frames at the beginning of the surgery. A fixed model is more suitable to our application since adaptive models presume that foreground objects are moving fast, while in surgery, the object of interest (hands or tools) may stay immobile the majority of the time. Formally, we consider a set of N depth frames D accumulated at the beginning of the surgical sequence, when no objects of interest are present in the scene. We consider the background model at each pixel $x \in \Omega$ as a univariate gaussian model where the mean and variance of this distribution are the values measured over the set of frames D at the pixel $x \in \Omega$. Lastly, in the remaining images of the sequence (objects of interests enter the scene), a background probability image is created for each individual frame.

Segmentation by Random Forest of RGB Images. As reported in [9], random forests have found a wide variety of applications in medical image analysis such as anatomy localization, segmentation or lesion detection. As an ensemble of decision trees, they provide piecewise approximations of any distribution in high-dimensional space. In our case, we model the probability $P_I(c|x)$ $x \in \Omega$ to belong to a class $c \in C = \{tool, hands, background\}$. The visual content of a pixel x is defined by a feature vector $\mathbf{X} \in \mathbb{R}^d$. $\mathbf{X}$ encodes the mean intensity value computed in d rectangular regions of different sizes in the neighborhood of x in the color channels of the CIELab color space. Following a "divide" and "conquer" strategy, each tree t, $t \in \{1, T\}$, first partitions the feature space in a hierarchical fashion and then estimates the posterior probabilities in each "cell" of this space. Given a training set of pixels from different color images and their corresponding labels, a tree t aims at subdividing these data by using axis-aligned splits in $\mathbb{R}^d$ so that consistent subsets are created in its "leaves" in terms of their visual context and class information c. Each leaf of a tree models "locally" the posterior probability $P_I^t(c|x)$, encoded as a class histogram, computed from the set of observations reaching the leaf. At test time, the output of the trees can be combined by using posterior averaging: $P_I(c|x) = \sum_{t=1}^{T} P_I^t(c|x)$.

Object Extraction. For each frame, the joint probability can be calculated by multiplying the probability of belonging to the foreground $P_D(f|x)$ with the probability of belonging to any class c $P_I(c|x)$. Finally, the class label $\hat{c}$ of a pixel is estimated by finding the class whose probability $P_{I,D}(f, c|x)$ is higher, such as $\hat{c} = argmax_{c \in C} P_{I,D}(f, c|x)$.

Refinement Using GrabCut. Since the class estimations might be noisy, we choose to refine the current extraction of interest objects by a segmentation algorithm [10]. Known as GrabCut, this algorithm is an extension of the graph-cut framework that uses an efficient iterative estimation and handles incomplete labelling. GrabCut permits decreasing the labelling burden as it integrates 4 possible label classes: foreground, probably foreground, probably background, background. For more details, we refer the reader to [10]. In our case, to refine the extraction of tools in the frame, the pixels classified as tool by the Random Forest are labelled as possible foreground, the rest is labelled as background. GrabCut is then performed on the corresponding color frame using that labelling to provide a finer extraction of the tool. The same step is renewed also for the clinician's actions. Even though this step requires additional computations, it is fast and efficient, and permits to filter out some false positives or catch false negatives that comes from missing depth values. At this step, the different parts (background, clinician's hands and tools) have been classified in the image. This process is repeated for every frame of the video.

2.2   Application Using an Augmented Reality Fluoroscopy

Identifying Object of Interest in X-ray. We consider an X-ray image J that is co-registered to the color and depth images, with $J : \Omega \to \mathbb{R}$. To improve the alpha-blendings developed in [5,4], the segmentation in different clusters as previously described is used. However, to further improve the visualization, we also extract from the X-ray image J the objects of interest to the clinician (e.g. bones, implants). This classification task will assign a label $r \in \{0, 1\}$ for each pixel x, where $r = 1$ if x belongs to a relevant structure or $r = 0$ if not. In a probabilistic framework, we model the posterior distribution $P_J(r|x)$ by using a random forest. Similarly, the visual context of each pixel x is described by a feature vector $X \in \mathbb{R}^t$, encoding mean radiodensity values computed in t rectangular regions in its neighborhood. Once the forest has been trained by using a set of annotated images, a new incoming X-ray can be labelled by using $\hat{r} = argmax_{r \in \{0,1\}} P_J(r|x)$. Once the labelling is done, we refine with Grab-Cut the current segmentation. All the pixels classified as belonging as relevant structure $(r = 1)$ are labeled as possible foreground and the rest is labeled as background.

Relevance-Based Image Fusion. The AR fluoroscopy technologies use an uniform alpha-blending to overlay the color images and the X-ray where the blending coefficient α is constant for all pixels. In this paper, we introduce a pixel dependant α parameter that changes values according to its belonging to an object of interest in the color image or in the X-ray image. Our new mixing paradigm is:

$$I_{overlay}(x) = \alpha(x)I(x) + (1 - \alpha(x))J'(x) \tag{2}$$

where J' is the 3-channels grayscale image corresponding to J such $J' = [J, J, J]$. Note that those values can be changed on the fly according to the will of the clinician, the type of clinician and also the different phases of the surgery workflow. For example, the value for the hands and tools can be decreased to allow the clinician to see the anatomy on the X-ray when performing distal locking on an intramedullary nail.

3   Experiments and Results

3.1   Evaluation of the Objects Identification

To evaluate the object identification algorithm for color images, 10 different orthopedic surgery simulations using a surgical phantom have been performed. Each simulation involves various clinician tasks and tools (clamps, screwdrivers, hammer, radiolucent drill, and scalpel). Each surgical simulation acquisition consisted of an average of 1000 frames. For the background modelling, the first 30 images ($\sim$ 1 second) of each sequence have been used to compute the background model.

Object Identification Using Color Images. In each of the 10 sequences, 4 video frames have been annotated. To describe the visual context of each pixel in the color image, 50 context features are extracted per CIElab channel. To tackle the task of object identification, a random forest classifier consisting in 20 trees of depth 15 is trained. After the first identification step, the GrabCut algorithm is executed using 2 iterations to refine the classifier results. The medium- to larger-sized surgical instruments are segmented very well. Minor segmentation errors occur specifically for the tip of the clamp allowing us to conclude that the segmentation algorithm needs further improvement to handle thin structures. The clinician's hands are globally well segmented over the various examples however we observe in some cases a wrong segmentation for the fingers primarily due to an aggressive GrabCut algorithm step that withdraws false positives, but also considers as background the pixels where the probability classes are too ambiguous to be considered as possible foreground. For quantitative results, we measure the accuracy of the classification into a class c thanks to the precision $\mathcal{P}$ and recall $\mathcal{R}$ measures over the annotated frames. We also calculate the DICE score $\mathcal{D}$, a similarity measure between the segmented class pixels and the annotated class pixels. The precision is over 0.8 for the hand, foreground and background classes, with a high score of 0.98 for the background, signifying that we have a good classification of most of the pixels belonging to those classes. Regarding the surgical tools, we achieve average precision with a value of 0.53 and a high standard deviation of 0.3. However, this global precision value can be decomposed to tool sizes as seen in Figure 3. As previously mentioned, medium to larger sized tools are generally well segmented. After further investigating our algorithm, the tools precision results can be explained by the amount of images used for the training of the Random Forest. Over the 38 training frames, each surgical tool appears in 5 images maximum and globally the presence of smaller tools in the training frames were much lower than the medium to larger sized tools. Resolving these issues will undoubtedly increase the precision values. Lastly, the recall values are really good for hand, foreground and background classes with values over 0.95, meaning that almost every annotated pixels have been recovered in those classes. The recall is good also for the surgical tool class. As a final note, a a clinician had their watch on and due to its black color, this structure was classified as a tool. In surgery and under sterile conditions, this issue would be resolved as the watch would be withdrawn. The computation time is 1.5 seconds per frame.

3.2 Fusion with X-ray Images

For the classification, 20 X-ray shots have been annotated. 50 context features are extracted by pixel, and the classifier consists in a random forest of 20 trees with depth 15. Then, the GrabCut algorithm is performed using 2 iterations to refine the segmentation of the object of interests.

Evaluation of Identification in X-ray Images. We use the same metrics (precision and recall) as with the RGB images. The recall and precision of both background and foreground are close to 1, showing a good performance of the segmentation algorithm.

Evaluation of Fusion Results. The visualization results of the fused X-ray and RGB images are depicted in Figure 1. A qualitative evaluation of the relevance-based blending visualization compared to the uniform blending is performed. In total, 5 clinicians (3 experts surgeons and 2 last year medical students) provide their feedback using the traditional 5-pt Likert scale questionnaire (1- strongly disagree, 2-disagree, 3-neutral, 4-agree, and 5-strongly agree). Participants strongly agreed (4.6 ± 0.5) that the depth ordering is resolved using our approach (e.g. hands/tools first followed by patient/X-ray). Concerning the visibility of the instrument tip or the implants in X-ray, the feedback is respectively neutral (3.0 ± 1.4) and slightly positive (3.4 ± 1.1). Participants agreed

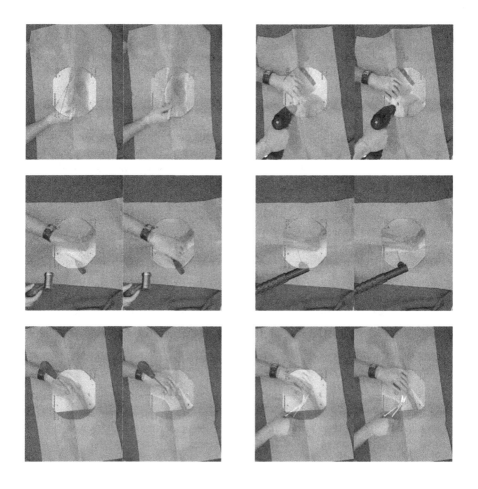

Fig. 1. Uniform and content-based visualizations over 6 frames

(4.0 ± 1.4) that the overall perception of the visualization is improved. Finally, all participants strongly agreed (4.6 ± 0.9) on the fact that they would prefer our new visualization compared to classical alpha blending found in the majority of registration algorithms in our community.

4   Conclusion

In this paper, we proposed a learning-based surgical scene labeling allowing the improved understanding and perception of various tasks when compared to the traditional alpha blending schemes. Our algorithm can detect the position and shape of the surgeon hands as well as the used tools. Our results are very promising for almost all objects, except smaller tools, but a more extended training phase should resolve this issue. We have demonstrated the applicability of our visualization framework in the context of existing medical augmented reality technologies. In future, our method can be extended to further applications such as 3D tool template matching, tool tracking and workflow analysis. Lastly, together with the IPCAI community, we hope to catalyze discussions on possible ways in improving visualization schemes that enable algorithms to "learn" what the surgeon wants to see during the surgical workflow phases.

References

1. Goldstein, B.E.: Sensation and perception. Cengage Learning (2013)
2. Padoy, N., Mateus, D., Weinland, D., Berger, M.O., Navab, N.: Workflow monitoring based on 3d motion features. In: IEEE 12th International Conference on Computer Vision Workshops (ICCV Workshops), pp. 585–592. IEEE (2009)
3. Kersten-Oertel, M., Jannin, P., Collins, D.L.: Dvv: a taxonomy for mixed reality visualization in image guided surgery. IEEE Transactions on Visualization and Computer Graphics 18, 332–352 (2012)
4. Nicolau, S., Lee, P., Wu, H., Huang, M., Lukang, R., Soler, L., Marescaux, J.: Fusion of c-arm x-ray image on video view to reduce radiation exposure and improve orthopedic surgery planning: first in-vivo evaluation. In: 15th Annual Conference of the International Society for Computer Aided Surgery (2011)
5. Navab, N., Heining, S.M., Traub, J.: Camera augmented mobile c-arm (camc): Calibration, accuracy study, and clinical applications. IEEE Transactions on Medical Imaging 29, 1412–1423 (2010)
6. Pauly, O., Katouzian, A., Eslami, A., Fallavollita, P., Navab, N.: Supervised classification for customized intraoperative augmented reality visualization. In: IEEE International Symposium on Mixed and Augmented Reality (ISMAR), pp. 311–312 (2012)
7. Erat, O., Pauly, O., Weidert, S., Thaller, P., Euler, E., Mutschler, W., Navab, N., Fallavollita, P.: How a surgeon becomes superman by visualization of intelligently fused multi-modalities. In: SPIE Medical Imaging, pp. 86710L–86710L (2013)
8. Elgammal, A.: Background Subtraction: Theory and Practice. Springer (2013)
9. Criminisi, A., Shotton, J.: Decision Forests for Computer Vision and Medical Image Analysis. Springer (2013)
10. Rother, C., Kolmogorov, V., Blake, A.: Grabcut: Interactive foreground extraction using iterated graph cuts. ACM Transactions on Graphics (TOG) 23, 309–314 (2004)

Towards Better Laparoscopic Video Database Organization by Automatic Surgery Classification

Andru P. Twinanda[1], Jacques Marescaux[2],
Michel De Mathelin[1], and Nicolas Padoy[1]

[1] ICube, University of Strasbourg, CNRS, France
{twinanda,demathelin,npadoy}@unistra.fr
[2] IRCAD & University Hospital of Strasbourg, France
jacques.marescaux@ircad.fr

Abstract. Minimally invasive surgery is an important breakthrough in the domain of medicine. Not only does it improve the quality of surgery, but the underlying digitization also provides invaluable information that opens up many possibilities for teaching, assistance during difficult cases, and quality evaluation. For instance, with a well-organized database, professors are one click away from showing and comparing various surgical procedures in their classes; surgeons can also retrieve and observe a video segment of a specific surgical task performed by another surgeon in varying conditions. However, to the best of our knowledge, database organization is done manually by experts. Considering the large number of surgical videos recorded, manual annotation is a tedious task. In this paper, we take the first step towards automatic surgical database organization by introducing the laparoscopic video classification problem, which consists of automatically identifying the type of abdominal surgery performed in a video. In spite of the visual challenges of such videos, such as blank frames, rapid movement, and sometimes incomplete recording, we show that we can rely on visual features alone to classify the videos with high accuracy. We use kernel Support Vector Machines (SVMs) for this classification task and compare their performance on different types of visual features. We also show that the result can be improved by combining the visual features using Multiple Kernel Learning approach. The classification pipeline demonstrates a classification accuracy of 91.39% on a database of 151 abdominal videos totaling over 200 hours of 8 different kinds of surgeries performed by 10 surgeons.

Keywords: Minimally invasive surgery, laparoscopic video classification, support vector machine, multiple kernel learning.

1 Introduction

The domain of medicine has been radically improved by concurrent developments in technology. One of the most important innovations in medicine is minimally invasive surgery (MIS). Introducing a camera to the procedure makes

D. Stoyanov et al. (Eds.): IPCAI 2014, LNCS 8498, pp. 186–195, 2014.

it easy to record performed actions during the surgery in close-up view. These recordings result in a rich video database with invaluable information about the execution of surgeries in various configurations. Subsequently, there is a high interest in incorporating this database into many applications. Here, we focus on a database of abdominal surgical videos. With an automatic database organization, laparoscopic video retrieval systems can allow fellow surgeons to observe different techniques for performing specific surgical tasks (e.g. intestinal stitching) in different surgical and/or patient conditions. For example, WebSurg [1], a website that enables the users to browse various surgical videos, provides an intuitive navigation system that permits the selection of the videos based on multiple categories, such as the type of surgery and the operated organ. It also offers an intra-video navigation that allows users (e.g. surgeons) to go directly to the surgical step that they want to observe in detail. All the videos in such systems are typically annotated manually during the surgeries by an expert observer. Yet, the rapid growth in the amount of the data overwhelms the feasibility of manual annotation and thus demands a fully automatic system. In this paper, as the first step towards a fully automatic system, we present an approach to automatically classify laparoscopic videos into multiple types of surgeries.

Automatic laparoscopic video classification is not a trivial problem because of various challenges. Visual challenges, such as the presence of smoke, specular reflection, motion blur, and impurity on the lens are inevitable because they typically appear as the direct consequence of the surgical procedure. Furthermore, the laparoscopic videos look very similar to one another since all of them are from abdominal surgeries. In addition to these challenges, the system also has to deal with massive amounts of data. For example, training centers, such as the IRCAD, record about 70 surgeries per month. In this paper, we use 151 laparoscopic videos of 8 different kinds of surgeries (see Table 1). In terms of duration, most of the laparoscopic videos are over an hour long on average, accumulating to more than 14 million frames in our dataset.

Due to the nature of MIS, the camera is often taken out of the patient's body, typically due to impurity on the lens. Undeniably, this part of the recording gives irrelevant, if not misleading, information about the surgery. Moreover, the action of taking the camera out of the body is recurrent, so the amount of irrelevant frames can build up to a very high number and impede the meaningful representation of the video. In addition, the videos often contain blank frames when the camera is disconnected. Thus, a notion of frame relevance needs to be incorporated in the process to reject such video frames. In a recent work, Atasoy et. al. [2] presented an approach to label informative frames for gastro-intestinal endoscopy. They performed K-means clustering on the energy histogram from the frequency domain and asked an expert to label the clusters. In more recent work [3], a supervised method using color-based features to identify relevant frames from laparoscopic videos is presented. However, both of these methods use supervised approaches to solve the problem. We argue that this problem can be tackled with a simpler approach and propose a simple RGB histogram thresholding to reject irrelevant frames before the feature extraction process.

In various visual-based classification tasks, many features have been repeatedly explored, such as color information, image gradients, and optical flow. In this paper, we focus on several of them which we see as most suitable to the characteristics of our data. Quite recently, the bag-of-visual-words (BoVW) approach has been used in most of whole-image categorization tasks and video classification problems. Zapella et. al. [4] used BoVW to classify three surgical gestures from short sequences (∼6-10 sec. per sequence) performed on suturing pods. The success of BoVW approach in various tasks inspires us to apply the same approach to solve laparoscopic video classification.

Along with the growth in computer-assisted intervention, the amount of work directed to the processing of surgical videos is also increasing. However, most works are directed to the recognition of surgical tasks in one kind of surgery [5,6,7] and to the best of our knowledge, this paper is the first work to address the laparoscopic video classification problem. Blum et. al. [6] presented a method combining the visual information from laparoscopic videos and the signal from surgical tools to train the classification model for segmenting cholecystectomy surgical videos. Just by using the visual information on testing, they were able to segment 7 videos of one type of abdominal surgery. More recently, Lalys et. al. [7] proposed a framework that extracts multiple features to segment high-level surgical tasks from video images of cataract surgeries. The features are categorized into four different groups: shape, color, texture, and mixed information. It is shown that the combination of the extracted features can carry out the surgical task segmentation on 20 cataract surgery videos. In this paper, we propose a state-of-the-art pipeline to classify laparoscopic videos using visual features only.

To carry out the classification, we use non-linear kernel Support Vector Machines (SVMs). In a recent work on surgical gesture classification, Zapella et. al. [4] proposed a system that combines visual and kinematic features using multiple kernel learning (MKL). It was shown that the classification over the combination of features gave better results compared to the classifications over individual features. These results motivated us to combine our features using MKL.

In summary, the contribution of this paper is three-fold: (1) we introduce the problem of laparoscopic video classification; this is the first milestone in surgical video database organization; (2) we investigate various visual features to propose a state-of-the-art pipeline based on MKL to automatically classify laparoscopic videos; (3) we present the classification results over a large database of abdominal surgeries.

2   Automatic Laparoscopic Video Classification

In this section, the laparoscopic video classification pipeline is described. It consists of four main steps: frame rejection, feature extraction, BoVW histogram representation, and MKL-based classification.

2.1   Frame Rejection

The frame rejection is carried out by exploiting the properties of the RGB histogram. It is observed that when the camera is inside the patient's abdomen, the red color channel is particularly more dominant compared to the other color channels. With that observation, a scalar value will then be computed to represent each color channel histogram in such a way that when the red scalar value is in a certain range, the frame will be accepted and later on processed. Three thresholds are set to perform the task: the minimum threshold for the level of "redness", and the lower and upper bounds of the brightness level. These thresholds are set empirically based on our preliminary observations on a few videos.

2.2   Feature Extraction

We extract several features that can be categorized into three groups: color information, salient points and image gradients.

Color Information. We choose color histograms in particular since they offer a simple solution as image descriptors. Especially in laparoscopic videos, there exists significant contrast between human organs, surgical tools, and other objects which contain discriminative information for surgery classification. Here, we extract two separate histograms as our features: Red-Green-Blue (RGB) (3×16 bins) from RGB space and Hue-Saturation (HS) (2×36 bins) from HSV space.

Salient Points. In the topic of salient point detection, scale-invariant feature transform (SIFT) [8] is undeniably the most successful keypoint detectors in the computer vision community. The scale and rotation invariant characteristics of the SIFT descriptor make it very robust in performing image matching tasks. In addition, we also observed that SIFT could detect similar salient points from video frames of the same surgery. Considering these facts, we include the SIFT descriptor in our feature extraction process.

Image Gradients. Here, we focus on Histogram of Gradients (HOG) [9]. It is similar to SIFT since they both compute image gradients. However, SIFT computes the gradient on salient points, while HOG counts occurrences of gradient orientation in a dense grid of uniformly spaced cells on the image and normalizes them based on overlapping local block contrast. We are particularly interested in this feature since SIFT only captures salient points on the frames which might not include all the important information. A global descriptor, like HOG, is required to extract all the possible information from the video frames. In our method, the video frames are divided into 16 cells; a block is defined to contain 2×2 cells and a 8-bin histogram of local gradients is computed from every block; thus a frame is represented with a HOG feature vector of dimension 288.

2.3   Bag-of-Visual-Word Approach

In this paper, we propose to use the bag-of-visual-words (BoVW) model to represent the laparoscopic videos where every feature (mentioned in Subsection 2.2) has its own dictionary containing visual words. The idea of BoVW in our case is to treat the video as a histogram of occurrence counts of the visual words. Various algorithms have been explored to learn the best dictionary, such as K-means clustering and K-SVD [10]. During our preliminary experiments, the results showed that BoVW with K-means gives the best result in terms of classification accuracy. In K-means clustering, every feature vector $\mathbf{f} \in \mathbb{R}^n$ will be expressed in a sparse representation $\mathbf{s} \in \mathbb{R}^K$ that is computed using the learnt dictionary $\mathbf{D} \in \mathbb{R}^{n \times K}$ by solving

$$\mathbf{s}^* = \arg\min_{\mathbf{s}} \|\mathbf{f} - \mathbf{D}\mathbf{s}\|_2 \text{ s.t. } \|\mathbf{s}\|_0 = 1, \|\mathbf{s}\|_1 = 1, \tag{1}$$

where $\|.\|_p$ computes the l_p-norm of the vector. Ultimately for all features, a video is represented by a normalized histogram $\mathbf{x} = \frac{\sum_{i=1}^N \mathbf{s}_i}{\left\|\sum_{i=1}^N \mathbf{s}_i\right\|_2}$.

2.4 Classification

Since laparoscopic video classification is a multi-class problem, we are using a one-against-all SVM. With training instances $\mathbf{X} = [\mathbf{x}_1, \ldots, \mathbf{x}_M]$, where $\mathbf{x}_i$ is a K-dimensional input vector and $y_i \in \{-1, +1\}$ is its corresponding class label, a SVM finds the linear discriminant with the maximum margin which can be expressed as

$$f(\mathbf{x}) = \sum_{i=1}^N \alpha_i y_i k(\mathbf{x}_i, \mathbf{x}) + b, \tag{2}$$

where α is the Langrangian multiplier, b is the bias term of the separating hyperplane, and $k(\cdot, \cdot)$ is the kernel function.

To combine all features, we build a single classification model by using Multiple Kernel Learning (MKL) [11]. Given base kernels $\{k_m(\cdot, \cdot)\}_{m=1}^P$ for P features, the goal of MKL is to compute an optimal combination

$$k_\eta(\tilde{\mathbf{x}}_i, \tilde{\mathbf{x}}_j) = f_\eta\left(\{k_m(\mathbf{x}_i^m, \mathbf{x}_j^m)\}_{m=1}^P \mid \eta\right), \tag{3}$$

where f_η is the function that combines the base kernels and is parameterized by η, and $\tilde{\mathbf{x}}_i = \{\mathbf{x}_i^m\}_{m=1}^P$ are the data instances containing all feature representations, so that $\mathbf{x}_i^m \in \mathbb{R}^{K_m}$ is the i-th data for feature m.

In this paper, we use the VLFeat implementation [12] to compute the kernel SVMs combined with the generalization of MKL approaches (GMKL) proposed by Varma et. al. [13]. The GMKL is particularly interesting because it can learn every possible combination that yields a positive definite kernel, instead of the traditional MKL approaches that focus on learning a linear combination of the base kernels.

Table 1. Experimental setup: (a) list of the abdominal surgery classes in our dataset along with their corresponding number of videos and average video length ($\pm std$) in minutes; and (b) the configuration of dictionary learning for every feature

Surgery	# Vid	Length (min.)
Sigmoidectomy	18	106 ± 44
Eventration	21	79 ± 57
Bypass	21	120 ± 37
Hernia	34	53 ± 29
Cholecystectomy	25	$68 + 42$
Nissen Gerd	17	80 ± 31
Adrenalectomy	7	117 ± 43
Sleeve Gastrectomy	8	89 ± 15

(a)

Feature	Dim.	# Words
SIFT	128	500, 1K, 1.5K
HOG	288	
RGB	48	100, 300, 500
HS	72	

(b)

3 Experimental Results

To test our method, we conducted an experiment with 8 different types of surgeries, consisting of 151 laparoscopic videos by 10 surgeons with a frame rate of 25 frames per second (fps). The detail of our dataset is shown in Table 1-a. Here, we sampled the videos at 1 fps due to redundant information. To build the dictionaries for each feature, we took one video randomly from every class. Since the SIFT feature gives many feature vectors for one frame while the other features (i.e. HOG, RGB, and HS) give only one, we sampled 750 frames per video (i.e. one frame every ~6-10 seconds) to get the training data for SIFT dictionary learning and used all frames to build the other dictionaries. We built 3 overcomplete dictionaries for each feature with different numbers of words, as shown in Table 1-b.

Later, we compute our histogram representations of the videos for all features and build classification models using SVM with the histogram intersection (HI) and chi-square (χ^2) kernels. All classification models are evaluated using leave-one-out cross-validation, i.e. one video for testing and the rest for training.

Effect of Frame Rejection. In this experiment, we trained 6 dictionaries for the SIFT feature. Three (i.e. 500-, 1K-, and 1.5K-word) of them incorporate frame rejection and the rest do not. From Fig. 1-a, it can be seen that with frame rejection, the number of frames that have to be processed decreases for more than 1K frames in average, which is equivalent to over 15 minutes of recording. The frame rejection mechanism falsely identified frames as outside of the body when they are too dark or too bright (bottom row of Fig. 1-c) and falsely identified frames as inside of the body when the image satisfies the red tendency (bottom-right of Fig. 1-d). However, the false negatives do not pose a problem since frames with low or high brightness do not contain important information and the false positives happen rarely thus will not hurt the performance of the classifiers. We can see in Fig. 1-b that the performance of classification with frame rejection

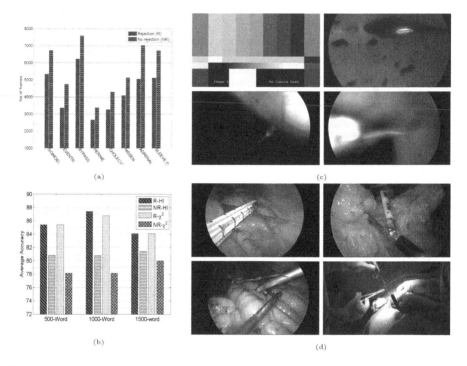

Fig. 1. Frame rejection results: (a) comparison of the average number of processed frames for every surgery type; (b) comparison of the classifier accuracies, in percent (%), with various rejection-kernel-word configurations; (c,d) frames that are classified as (c) irrelevant and (d) relevant

outperforms the performance without frame rejection. The smallest and biggest accuracy gaps (2.7% and 8.7%) are respectively given by the configuration of 1.5k words with HI kernel and the configuration of 1k words with χ^2 kernel. In all classification configurations, the frame rejection mechanism increases the accuracy of the system, thus is used for the rest of the experiments.

Performance on Different Features. The accuracy of various classification model configurations are shown in Fig. 2-a and confusion matrices corresponding to the best word-kernel configuration for each feature independently are shown in Fig. 2-(b-e). It can be seen that RGB and HS perform significantly worse than SIFT and HOG. Despite their ability to capture the color information of the video frames, RGB and HS fail to classify the videos correctly due to the highly similar color information in all the videos. As shown in the confusion matrices of the best case for classification using RGB and HS, the classification is scattered all over the classes. However, we can say that they still contain discriminative information since the accuracies from HS and RGB are better than chance.

In contrast, SIFT and HOG show good results with 87.41% accuracy in their best word-kernel configuration. These features perform really well because they

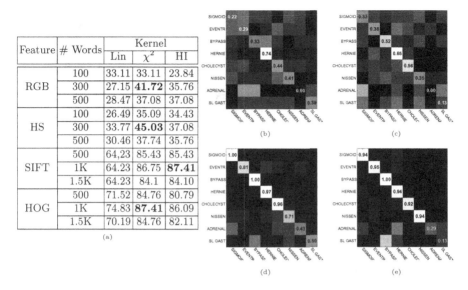

Fig. 2. Classification results: (a) accuracies, in percent (%), using visual features with various word-kernel configurations; (b-e) confusion matrices from the word-kernel configurations that give the highest accuracy for (b) RGB, (c) HS, (d) SIFT, and (e) HOG. The numbers on the diagonal indicate the recall for each class.

capture more essential and higher level information, which gives a better representation of the video frames compared to color histograms.

From the confusion matrices, it can also be seen that the classification accuracies for adrenalectomy and sleeve gastrectomy are lower compared to other classes. This is expected due to the imbalanced dataset.

Effect of Kernel and Number of Words. In Fig. 2-a, it is shown that the non-linear kernel performs significantly better than the linear one, which confirms the claim stated in [14]. More specifically, SIFT performs the best when combined with HI kernel, while the other features with χ^2 kernel. We also investigated the effect of number of words with respect to the performance of classification. It is obvious that there is an optimal number of words for every feature which is the middle value in our number of word ranges. Intuitively, if the dictionary size is too small, the histogram loses its discriminative power; if the dictionary size is too large, the histograms of videos from the same surgery type will not match.

Performance of MKL. In this experiment, we tested two feature combinations: SIFT-HOG and all four features. We constructed this scenario to see the effect of incorporating color information into SIFT and HOG features, which individually perform significantly better than the color histograms. For every feature, we took the kernels from the classification configurations that give the

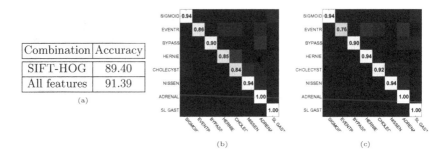

Combination	Accuracy
SIFT-HOG	89.40
All features	91.39

(a)

(b)   (c)

Fig. 3. MKL classification results: (a) accuracy, in percent (%), of the classifiers; and (b,c) confusion matrices from classification using (b) SIFT-HOG combination and (c) all-feature combination

highest accuracy, as shown in bold in Fig. 2-a. Later, we input them as the base kernels for the MKL approach.

By using the combination of SIFT and HOG features, the average accuracy is increased to 89.4% and the recall for every class is more uniformly spread out, i.e. all classes have above 80% recall. With the combination of all features, the accuracy is increased by almost 2%. This may appear surprising since, individually, the color histograms did not perform up to par. However, as previously stated, their performance is still better than chance, so they contain discriminative information that complement the SIFT and HOG features.

4 Conclusions

In this paper, we introduced the surgical video classification problem, which consists of automatically identifying the type of a surgery solely based on the endoscopic video. We proposed a state-of-the-art classification pipeline based on Multiple Kernel Learning (MKL) and have shown that it can solve the problem with high accuracy in spite of the various visual challenges present in the videos. By combining all visual features using MKL, we demonstrated that an accuracy of 91.39% can be reached on a dataset of 151 videos from 8 classes of abdominal surgery.

These surgeries were performed by 10 different surgeons from the same surgical department. Further work should evaluate how the approach scales to larger datasets by including surgeries from different hospitals. For classification, it would also be particularly interesting to combine the video data with additional signals that can be recorded from the surgical equipment.

Acknowledgements. This work was supported by French state funds managed by the ANR within the Investissements d'Avenir program under references ANR-11-LABX-0004 (Labex CAMI), ANR-10-IDEX-0002-02 (IdEx Unistra) and ANR-10-IAHU-02 (IHU Strasbourg). The authors would like to thank the IRCAD audio-visual team and especially David Hiltenbrand for their help in generating the dataset used in this paper.

References

1. WebSurg: the e-surgical reference, `http://www.websurg.com/` (last access: November 21, 2013)
2. Atasoy, S., Mateus, D., Meining, A., Yang, G.Z., Navab, N.: Endoscopic video manifolds for targeted optical biopsy. IEEE Trans. Med. Imaging 31(3), 637–653 (2012)
3. Munzer, B., Schoeffmann, K., Boszormenyi, L.: Relevance segmentation of laparoscopic videos. In: IEEE International Symposium on Multimedia, pp. 84–91 (2013)
4. Zappella, L., Bejar, B., Hager, G., Vidal, R.: Surgical gesture classification from video and kinematic data. Medical Image Analysis 17(7), 732–745 (2013)
5. Padoy, N., Blum, T., Ahmadi, S.A., Feussner, H., Berger, M.O., Navab, N.: Statistical modeling and recognition of surgical workflow. Medical Image Analysis 16(3), 632–641 (2012)
6. Blum, T., Feußner, H., Navab, N.: Modeling and segmentation of surgical workflow from laparoscopic video. In: Jiang, T., Navab, N., Pluim, J.P.W., Viergever, M.A. (eds.) MICCAI 2010, Part III. LNCS, vol. 6363, pp. 400–407. Springer, Heidelberg (2010)
7. Lalys, F., Riffaud, L., Bouget, D., Jannin, P.: A framework for the recognition of high-level surgical tasks from video images for cataract surgeries. IEEE Trans. Biomed. Engineering 59(4), 966–976 (2012)
8. Lowe, D.: Distinctive image features from scale-invariant keypoints. International Journal of Computer Vision 60, 91–110 (2004)
9. Dalal, N., Triggs, B.: Histograms of oriented gradients for human detection. In: International Conference on Computer Vision & Pattern Recognition, pp. 886–893 (2005)
10. Aharon, M., Elad, M., Bruckstein, A.: K-SVD: An Algorithm for Designing Overcomplete Dictionaries for Sparse Representation. IEEE Transactions on Signal Processing 54(11), 4311–4322 (2006)
11. Gonen, M., Alpaydin, E.: Multiple kernel learning algorithms. Journal of Machine Learning Research 12, 2211–2268 (2011)
12. Vedaldi, A., Fulkerson, B.: Vlfeat: An open and portable library of computer vision algorithms. In: Proceedings of the International Conference on Multimedia, pp. 1469–1472. ACM (2010)
13. Varma, M., Babu, R.B.: More generality in efficient multiple kernel learning. In: Proceedings of the International Conference on Machine Learning, pp. 1065–1072. ACM (2009)
14. Yang, J., Yu, K., Gong, Y., Huang, T.: Linear spatial pyramid matching using sparse coding for image classification. In: International Conference on Computer Vision & Pattern Recognition, pp. 1794–1801. IEEE (2009)

Model-Based Identification of Anatomical Boundary Conditions in Living Tissues

Igor Peterlik[1,2,4], Hadrien Courtecuisse[1,2,3],
Christian Duriez[2], and Stéphane Cotin[1,2]

[1] Institut Hospitalo-Universitaire, Strasbourg, France
[2] SHACRA Team, Inria, France
[3] AVR Team, CNRS, France
[4] Institute of Computer Science, Masaryk University, Czech Republic

Abstract. In this paper, we present a novel method dealing with the identification of boundary conditions of a deformable organ, a particularly important step for the creation of patient-specific biomechanical models of the anatomy. As an input, the method requires a set of scans acquired in different body positions. Using constraint-based finite element simulation, the method registers the two data sets by solving an optimization problem minimizing the energy of the deformable body while satisfying the constraints located on the surface of the registered organ. Once the equilibrium of the simulation is attained (i.e. the organ registration is computed), the surface forces needed to satisfy the constraints provide a reliable estimation of location, direction and magnitude of boundary conditions applied to the object in the deformed position. The method is evaluated on two abdominal CT scans of a pig acquired in flank and supine positions. We demonstrate that while computing a physically admissible registration of the liver, the resulting constraint forces applied to the surface of the liver strongly correlate with the location of the anatomical boundary conditions (such as contacts with bones and other organs) that are visually identified in the CT images.

1 Introduction

In the last decade the role of computer medical simulation in surgical training, pre-operative planning and intra-operative guidance has increased considerably. A key factor to the successful use of numerical simulation in medicine is the ability to reproduce the complex behavior of anatomical structures. For soft tissues, the models are usually based on elasticity theory, which provides powerful means of modeling the behavior of soft tissues often displaying complex characteristics such as incompressibility or viscoelasticity. Since the equations derived in the theory of elasticity can be solved analytically only for extremely simple scenarios, numerical methods such as the finite element (FE) method must be employed to solve the problem over a discretized domain.

While an interesting body of research exists regarding domain discretization and appropriate formulation of the physical behavior of living tissues, much

D. Stoyanov et al. (Eds.): IPCAI 2014, LNCS 8498, pp. 196–205, 2014.

less attention has been paid to correct modeling of boundary conditions which influence the model significantly, as they directly determine the particular solution to the overall physical problem. In the domain of patient-specific medical simulations, an attempt to fill this gap becomes really challenging: while the geometrical and physical properties of the living tissues can be obtained either via medical imaging or rheology experiments, it is usually very difficult to obtain reliable data describing the interactions between different regions of living tissues, since these can be given by a complex combination of bilateral constraints (represented for example by ligaments and connective tissues) or unilateral contacts induced by tissue motion (such as respiratory motion, application of external forces or displacements of organs during the surgery).

In this paper, we focus on identification of boundary conditions from medical image data. We propose a method which, given two (or more) different configurations of the same three-dimensional deformable structure, is capable of (i) registering the two volumes using a physically-admissible transformation, (ii) providing a set of surface forces which correspond to the boundary conditions of the object in the target configurations. Although our method requires a construction of a FE model (usually obtained via segmentation and mesh generation), to our best knowledge, it is the first technique allowing for automatic identification of boundary conditions from image data.

2   Related Work

The identification of boundary conditions (BCs) has been studied in the area of structural analysis and computer-aided design. For example, in [1] BCs are identified using a boundary stiffness matrix which is obtained as a solution of characteristic equations formulated for different modes of the object. The characteristic equations are non-linear and their number corresponds to the number of boundary degrees of freedom. Nevertheless, it is supposed that the object is modeled using linear elasticity and the BCs also behave linearly. In [2], accurate determination of BCs including non-linear effects as friction and slip is presented for 2D circular plate. In [3], the non-linear effects are also taken into account in a method based on non-linear normal modes allowing also object with non-linear response; the method is validated using a simple beam. While these methods allow for a very accurate identification of BCs, they can be employed only in the scenario where the objects have a simple and well-defined boundaries. Although the non-linear effects are considered, the type of interactions is usually limited to bilateral constraints with micro-slip. However, this is usually not the case in medical simulations where objects having complex boundaries are involved in different types of interactions including both bilateral and unilateral constraints with and without friction (for example simulatio of abdominal organs).

In the case of soft-tissues, the currently used imaging modalities such as CT, MRI and ultrasound allows for reconstruction of the geometry of the bodies in the scanned volume. However, in order to obtain more information about the motion of the tissues, at least two scans acquired in two different configurations are needed. Nevertheless, in this case, a registration has to be performed in order to find a transformation between the two configurations. In the following we briefly survey relevant methods presented in the area of deformable registration, usually in context of preoperative planning and intra-operative guidance [4]. A 3D registration of intra-operative MR brain images is proposed in [5]: the model is based on linear elasticity discretized by the finite element method. The method is driven by active surface matching which deforms the boundary of brain in one acquired image towards the boundary in the following scan. The image warping based on finite element method is developed in [6]. The hyperelastic formulation is employed and the warping is applied in several domains, e.g. to measure strain in coronal artery or quantify morphology changes in mouse brain. A multi-organ deformable image registration based on mechanical model simulated with finite elements is developed in [7]. The model driven by surface deformation and displacements of landmarks is used to analyze and predict the motion of abdominal organ during respiration. Minimization of landmark displacements is used to drive the deformable registration of mouse brain in [8]: several regularization terms based on finite element formulation are compared including diffusion, linear and non-linear elasticity. In [9], the BCs are estimated by solving an inverse problem optimizing for different explicitly chosen factors causing the brain shift. While in this scenario, different *a priori* chosen distributions of various BCs are evaluated as independent model solutions using the cost function, our method is based on a direct solution of the constrained system where no assumptions about the type and distribution of the BCs are made.

In [10], a model-based method using iterative closest point was presented for registration of muscular structures. In [11] preoperative 3D CT images are registered to either 3D or 2D intra-operative scans. While the registration is driven by optimization of similarity metrics (squared differences, mutual information and correlation ratio are considered), the mechanical model based on linear elasticity is used to regularize the solution. The method is tested on breast phantom. Multi-modality registration for image-guided prostate intervention is described in [12]: in the preoperative phase, a finite element patient specific model is built using the preoperative MR data and a set of deformations corresponding to different BCs and randomly sampled material properties are computed and evaluated statistically using PCA.

Although the referenced methods often provide accurate and physically-admissible transformation between the registered domains, to our best knowledge, none of the methods allows for reliable identification of BCs without any *a priori* assumptions about the BC type and placement.

3 Methodology

Our approach is based on the technique presented in [13] where the method is used to compute a model-based registration between pre-operative data acquired by 3D CT and intraoperative 2D MRI slices. The main contribution of this paper is a generalization of the method so that given a discrete representation of the

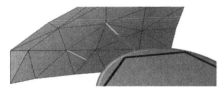

Fig. 1. The control points (grey) are associated to the closest point of the cubic interpolation (blue) of the FE surface (black). Constraints (red) are define along the direction of the the segment connecting the two models (green).

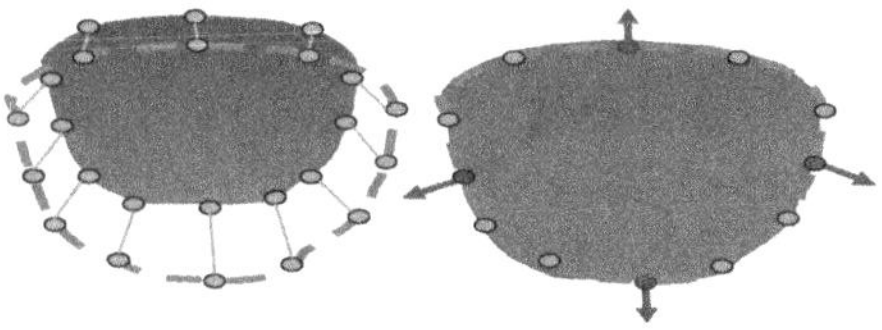

Fig. 2. Binding process (left) and constraint force evaluation (right) to register a deformable object (blue) with the control surface (brown). The Gauss-Seidel algorithm iteratively activates (red) or deactivates (gray) the constraints according to the actual respective violations.

registered object in both configurations, the method provides automatically i) physically-valid registration of the object in the two different configurations and ii) identification of bilateral and unilateral boundary conditions applied to the object in the target configuration.

3.1 Binding Process and Constraints Definitions

The method takes on one side the triangulated surface of the target and on the other side the FE mesh in a different position. The *iterative closest point* (ICP) method [14] is used to associate the set of control point (from the target surface) with their respective closest points on the surface of the simulated FE. The method is improved by using a cubic Bézier interpolation of the FE surface as described in [15]. It provides a smooth description of the triangulation allowing for a continuous sliding of the constraints between edges and triangles (see Fig. 1), which helps to stabilize the registration. The barycentric coordinates of the closest point on the cubic interpolation of the triangles are determined with the Newton-Raphson algorithm.

At each time step, the control points $\mathbf{q}_i$ are associated to their respective closest points $\mathbf{q}_s$ on the Bézier path. For each point $\mathbf{q}_s$, the normal $\boldsymbol{n}_s$ is evaluated on the Bézier interpolation. A set of bilateral constraints is defined so that the constraints be satisfied for $\mathbf{q}_i$ located on the tangential plane given by $\boldsymbol{n}_s$. This formulation allows the control points to "slide" on the surface of the FE mesh in order to stabilize around the configuration minimizing the energy and satisfying the constraints. Since the proximity-based information is formulated in the contact space, it has to be mapped to the standard 3D space of the FE mesh via a mapping matrix $\mathbf{J}$ linking the positions in the contacts space to the 3D space of the object (see [16]). For the violation of the constraints $\boldsymbol{\delta}$ it holds:

$$\boldsymbol{\delta} = dot(\mathbf{q}_i - \mathbf{J}\mathbf{q}_s, \mathbf{n}_c). \tag{1}$$

3.2   Constraint-Based Simulation

The deformation of the tissue is modeled with linear tetrahedral finite elements employing the co-rotational formulation [17]. While handling large displacements properly, it is restricted to small strains. Constraints are imposed using the Lagrange multipliers. Denoting the time as t, the governing differential equation in a quasi-static scenario is given by:

$$f(\mathbf{q}_t) + \mathbf{f} + \mathbf{J}^T \boldsymbol{\lambda} = 0 \tag{2}$$

where $\mathbf{f}$ are external forces (such as gravity), $f(\mathbf{q}_t)$ are the internal volume forces at a given position $\mathbf{q}$. $\mathbf{J}^T$ and $\boldsymbol{\lambda}$ are respectively the Jacobian of the constraints and the force used to drive the registration. This equation is solved with the *Schur complement* method (see [16] for details). It involves mainly two steps: i) during the *free motion*, a step of the simulation is computed without imposing any constraints. This operation requires the solution of a sparse linear system of equations which is done using conjugate gradients. ii) During the *corrective motion*, the control points are binded to the closest surface and constraint forces are evaluated to correct the *free motion*. The constraint forces are obtained by solving a constrained problem $\mathbf{W}\,\boldsymbol{\lambda} + \boldsymbol{\delta} = 0$ where $\mathbf{W}$ is the *Delassus operator* [16], which defines the coupling of the constraints given by the domain of the deformable body. The resulting contact forces $\boldsymbol{\lambda}$ are obtained with an iterative approach based on the Gauss-Seidel method where constraints are treated sequentially one at the time. Depending on the violation of the constraints, each equation is either activated with a non-zero force or deactivated if the violation is zero (see Fig. 2). As a result, only the constraints necessary to suppress the violation are active, and $\boldsymbol{\lambda}$ minimizes the energy required to cancel the constraint violation $\boldsymbol{\delta}$. Therefore, when comparing to the penalty-based methods, the actual approach employing the compliance (encoded in $\mathbf{W}$) minimizes the forces needed to impose the constraints, which in turn leads to a more accurate identification of the boundary conditions.

4   Results

We now evaluate our method in several scenarios: first, we investigate two academic examples to demonstrate the efficiency and the accuracy of the method. In the second part of the section we apply the method to a CT data of a female pig liver in other to show an important match between the predicted surface loads and real boundary conditions induced by the surrounding tissues.

4.1   Accuracy and Efficiency of the Method

For the sake of validation, the method is evaluated using data generated by a simulation (denoted as *direct*) which takes an *initial* configuration of a simple-shaped beam object and computes a *target* configuration induced by gravity and interaction with other solid bodies. Beside the shape of the deformed object in

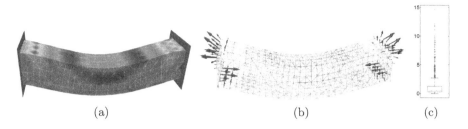

(a)   (b)   (c)

Fig. 3. Deformable beam attached at both extremities under gravity: (a) von Mises stress in the target configuration, (b) surface constraint forces corresponding to target configuration (red) and registered configuration (green). (c) box-and-whisker plot showing the statistics of the von Mises stress error.

target configuration, the constraint forces computed by the direct simulation are stored for the validation step. Next, the initial configuration of the beam is registered to the target configuration using the method presented in section 3. It should be emphasized that in this step, no information about the applied forces and loads, boundary conditions and other solid objects involved in the direct simulation is used and the only input of the procedure is the geometric representation of the beam in initial and target configurations and its physical parameters used in the direct simulation. As soon as the dynamic equilibrium is achieved, the resulting *registered* configuration is stored together with the constraint forces.

The validation consists of comparing (i) von Mises stress computed in the nodes of the mesh and (ii) surface constraint forces obtained in the target configuration and registered configuration. While the forces are compared visually, the von Mises stress is evaluated for node n using a relative error $E_\sigma^n = \frac{|\sigma_r^n - \sigma_t^n|}{\sigma_t^n}$ where σ_t^n is the nodal stress in target configuration and σ_r^n is the nodal stress in the registered configuration. The vector of errors for each case is statistically evaluated over the set of nodes, computing the mean $\bar{E}_\sigma$ and maximum $\hat{E}_\sigma$ value and displaying the standard box-and-whisker plot where values exceeding the error given by $q_3 + 1.5(q_3 - q_1)$, q_1 and q_3 being first and the third quartiles, are considered as the outliers.

In the first scenario depicted in Fig. 3(a), the beam composed of 4350 elements and 1080 nodes is deformed under gravity, being attached at both extremities with fixed constraints which prevent the motion of all nodes located on the corresponding faces of the object. The visualization of the constraint forces (Fig. 3(b) shows a good match between the target and registered configuration. As for von Mises stress error, $\bar{E}_\sigma = 0.1\%$, $\hat{E}_\sigma = 14.6\%$ and Fig. 3 shows 139 outliers (among the 1080 nodes) with error exceeding 2.7%.

In the second scenario, the same beam is also subjected to the gravity, however, only one extremity is fixed. Moreover, the bottom face of the beam collides with a supporting plane and a solid cube falls on its top face as shown in Fig. 4a. Thus, the target configuration is a result of a complex set of bilateral

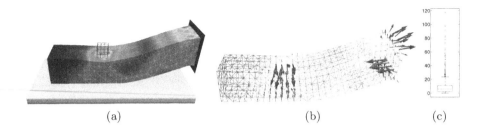

(a)	(b)	(c)

Fig. 4. Deformable beam under gravity in interaction with supporting plane and the cube: (a) von Mises stress in the target configuration, (b) surface constraint forces corresponding to target configuration (red) and registered configuration (green), (c) box-and-whisker plot showing the statistics of the von Mises stress error

and unilateral constraints. The visualization of surface forces reconstructed by the registration method is shown in Fig. 4b. The statistical evaluation of von Mises stress results in $\bar{E}_\sigma = 8.5\%$, $\hat{E}_\sigma = 117.3\%$ and Fig. 3c shows 62 outliers (among 1080 nodes) with error exceeding 23.8%. Although the statistics of the von Mises error shows worse results in the seconds case, the location of the surface loads is predicted quite accurately and we assume that the differences in the von Mises stress rather reflect different orientations of the loads, as indicated by the arrows shown in Fig. 4c.

4.2 Estimation of Boundary Conditions of Living Tissues

The CT scans of a female pig in flank and supine positions were acquired with SOMATOM® Definition AS 128 device. Semi-automatic segmentation of liver were performed in both volumes using ITKSnap. In both volumes, surface mesh was extracted from the segmented maps and in the case of supine data, also the volume mesh was generated using CGAL library resulting in 6506 elements. The method described in section 3 was applied to the discretized data to register the shape of the liver from supine (source) to the flank (target) configuration and to identify the boundary conditions once the equilibrium of the simulation was attained. The deformation field given by the difference of source and registered meshes was then used to warp the source image in order to perform the evaluation of the registration. The surface forces were displayed to asses the method visually as no ground truth exists in the case of medical data.

First, the visual comparison of one slide showing the source, warped and target images is presented in Fig. 5. Moreover, the deformation field was used to warp also the segmented maps, which enabled us to evaluate the segmentation using Dice metric describing the overlap between two binary images. While the Dice coefficient of 47% was computed for the overlap between the source (non-registered) and target data, the coefficient attained 87% when registered and target data were compared. Given the magnitude of initial deformation, the registration clearly gives very good result both in term of quantitative and visual comparison.

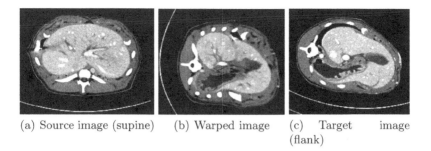

(a) Source image (supine)   (b) Warped image   (c) Target   image
(flank)

Fig. 5. Illustration of the accuracy of the registration for a cut in the source, warped and target volume

The supine and flank configurations are displayed on Fig. 6ab showing an important deformation of the liver and surrounding tissues due to the important deformation of the rib cage. The overall image of the predicted surface loads is given in Fig. 6b. First, it should be recalled that unlike the case in the previous section, neither supine nor flank data provide the configuration which corresponds to the rest position of the liver. In fact, this position is not known, since in both supine and flank configuration, the liver is subjected to gravity and

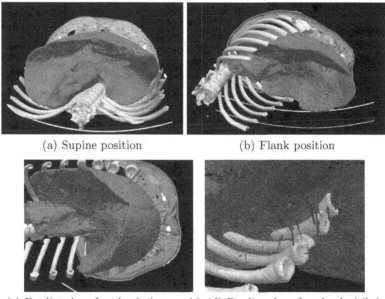

(a) Supine position   (b) Flank position

(c) Predicted surface loads (stomach) (d) Predicted surface loads (ribs)

Fig. 6. Evaluation of the method on porcine liver deformation induced by re-positioning the pig from supine to flank positions (a,b). Details of predicted surface loads (c,d).

to the surface loads induced by the surrounding objects. Therefore, rather than identifying the absolute surface loads in the target configurations, a relative difference in loads applied in supine and flank configurations is obtained indicating the change in boundary conditions. We believe that the estimation of absolute surface loads could be obtained by comparing several different configurations, where the influence of the applied loads and forces could be filtered.

Two details of predicted surface loads are shown in Fig. 6c and 6d. In the first case, the loads that appeared due to the contact with stomach (visceral surface) and diaphragm (diaphragmatic surface), in the other case, interaction between the liver and stiff bodies of ribs are clearly indicated. Apparently, all these loads can be logically justified due to the rotational movement of the liver which occurred during the change of the pig's position from supine to flank configuration: while in the supine position, the lateral surfaces of the liver lobes are not subjected to important contact loads, since the mass is pressing mainly the posterior part of the organ against the spine, in the flank position, important contacts occurs between the left part of the liver and the ribs.

5   Discussion and Conclusion

The precise estimation of boundary conditions in soft tissues plays a crucial role in computer simulation-based planning and guidance. For example, in the case of surgical navigation based on augmented reality, a biomechanical model can be used to predict the actual position of the tumor inside the tissue. In this paper, we propose a model-based method allowing for joint registration and prediction of surface loads in the deformed configuration which can be directly used to identify boundary conditions. The method was validated employing two scenarios with a beam object, where the deformations were computed via simulation in order to have both the deformed shape and surface loads in the target deformation. The data was used as a ground truth and compared to the von Mises stress and surface loads obtained in the registration process. The method was demonstrated on a real medical data of female pig scanned in supine and flank positions in order to induce important deformations of the abdominal cavity. To our best knowledge, no attempt has been made so far to predict the surface loads inside a living body using only the scanned images without any a priori assumption. The evaluation has proven that the method is capable of predicting the difference in surface loads applied to the liver and this data can be straightforwardly used to identify boundary conditions in the target configuration.

We are aware of the fact that while different loading scenarios would further increase the accuracy of our method, it requires multiple acquisitions which are usually not available in humans. Nevertheless, while keeping in mind the patient specific scenario, we would also like to employ an intra-patient evaluation based on atlas, which could provide a base for the BC estimations (e.g. placement of the ligaments and other connective tissues with lower intra-subject variance).

References

1. Ahmadian, H., Mottershead, J., Friswell, M.: Boundary condition identification by solving characteristic equations. J. of Sound and Vibration 247(5), 755–763 (2001)
2. Suzuki, A., Kamiya, K., Yasuda, K.: Identification technique for nonlinear boundary conditions of a circular plate. J. of Sound and Vibration 289(1-2), 130–147 (2006)
3. Ahmadian, H., Zamani, A.: Identification of nonlinear boundary effects using nonlinear normal modes. Mechanical Systems and Signal Processing 23(6), 2008–2018 (2009); Special Issue: Inverse Problems
4. Carter, T.J., Sermesant, M., Cash, D.M., Barratt, D.C., Tanner, C., Hawkes, D.J.: Application of soft tissue modelling to image-guided surgery. Medical Engineering & Physics 27(10), 893–909 (2005)
5. Ferrant, M., Nabavi, A., Macq, B., Jolesz, F.A., Kikinis, R., Warfield, S.K.: Registration of 3-D intraoperative MR images of the brain using a finite-element biomechanical model. IEEE Trans. on Medical Imaging 20(12), 1384–1397 (2001)
6. Veress, A.I., Phatak, N., Weiss, J.A.: Deformable image registration with Hyperelastic Warping. In: Handbook of Biomedical Image Analysis, pp. 487–533 (2005)
7. Brock, K.K., Sharpe, M.B., Dawson, L.A., Kim, S.M., Jaffray, D.A.: Accuracy of finite element model-based multi-organ deformable image registration. Medical Physics 32(6), 1647 (2005)
8. Lin, T., Guyader, C.L., Dinov, I., Thompson, P., Toga, A., Vese, L.: A Landmark-Based Image Registration Model using a Nonlinear Elasticity Smoother for Mapping Mouse Atlas to Gene Expression Data. Sciences-New York (2009)
9. Dumpuri, P., Thompson, R.C., Dawant, B.M., Cao, A., Miga, M.I.: An atlas-based method to compensate for brain shift: Preliminary results. Medical Image Analysis 11(2), 128–145 (2007)
10. Gilles, B., Pai, D.K.: Fast musculoskeletal registration based on shape matching. In: Metaxas, D., Axel, L., Fichtinger, G., Székely, G. (eds.) MICCAI 2008, Part II. LNCS, vol. 5242, pp. 822–829. Springer, Heidelberg (2008)
11. Marami, B., Sirouspour, S., Capson, D.: Model-based deformable registration of preoperative 3D to intraoperative low-resolution 3D and 2D sequences of MR images. In: Fichtinger, G., Martel, A., Peters, T. (eds.) MICCAI 2011, Part I. LNCS, vol. 6891, pp. 460–467. Springer, Heidelberg (2011)
12. Hu, Y., Ahmed, H.U., Taylor, Z., Allen, C., Emberton, M., Hawkes, D., Barratt, D.: MR to ultrasound registration for image-guided prostate interventions. Medical Image Analysis 16(3), 687–703 (2012)
13. Courtecuisse, H., Peterlik, I., Trivisonne, R., Duriez, C., Cotin, S.: Constraint-based simulation for non-rigid real-time registration. In: Medicine Meets Virtual Reality, MMVR21, California, US (to appear, February 2014)
14. Rusinkiewicz, S., Levoy, M.: Efficient variants of the ICP algorithm. In: Proc. of 3rd Conf. on 3D Digital Imaging and Modeling, pp. 145–152 (2001)
15. Vlachos, A., Peters, J., Boyd, C., Mitchell, J.L.: Curved PN triangles. In: Symposium on Interactive 3D Graphics, pp. 159–166 (2001)
16. Duriez, C., Dubois, F., Kheddar, A., Andriot, C.: Realistic haptic rendering of interacting deformable objects in virtual environments. IEEE Transactions on Visualization and Computer Graphics 12(1), 36–47 (2006)
17. Müller, M., Gross, M.: Interactive virtual materials. In: GI 2004: Proc. of Graphics Interface 2004, School of Computer Science, University of Waterloo, Ontario, Canada, pp. 239–246. Canadian Human-Computer Communications Society (2004)

Fast Semi-dense Surface Reconstruction from Stereoscopic Video in Laparoscopic Surgery

Johannes Totz[1], Stephen Thompson[1], Danail Stoyanov[1], Kurinchi Gurusamy[2],
Brian R. Davidson[2], David J. Hawkes[1], and Matthew J. Clarkson[1]

[1] Centre for Medical Image Computing
University College London, UK
[2] Royal Free Hospital
London, UK
{j.totz,s.thompson,danail.stoyanov,k.gurusamy,b.davidson,d.hawkes,
m.clarkson}@ucl.ac.uk

Abstract. Liver resection is the main curative option for liver meta-
stases. While this offers a 5-year survival rate of 50%, only about 20% of
all patients are suitable for laparoscopic resection and thus being able to
take advantage of minimally invasive surgery. One underlying difficulty
is the establishment of a safe resection margin while avoiding critical
structures. Intra-operative registration of patient scan data may provide
a solution. However, this relies on fast and accurate reconstruction methods to obtain the current shape of the liver. Therefore, this paper presents
a method for high-resolution stereoscopic surface reconstruction at interactive rates. To this end, a feature-matching propagation method is
adapted to multi-resolution processing to enable parallelisation, remove
global synchronisation issues and hence become amenable to a GPU-
based implementation. Experiments are conducted on a planar target
for reconstruction noise estimation and a visually realistic silicone liver
phantom. Results highlight an average reconstruction error of 0.6 mm
on the planar target, 2.4–5.7 mm on the phantom and processing times
averaging around 370 milliseconds for input images of size 1920 x 540.

1   Introduction

Resection of a segment or lobe of the liver in metastatic or primary liver cancer
is the main curative option. This is traditionally done in an open procedure,
resulting in a large wound on the patient's abdomen to allow access for the
surgeon to palpate and identify important structures within the liver and distinguish normal liver from tumour. A minimally invasive approach instead might
reduce trauma, infection risk, post-operative pain and cosmetic issues. However,
difficulties in estimating a safe resection margin, proximity to blood vessels and
tumour size, etc deny more than 80% of patients this option. In order to increase suitability for the laparoscopic approach, improved surgical guidance and
navigation is required.

To this end, robust registration methods are necessary that need as input a
physically-based deformable model of the liver [1] and an up-to-date estimate

D. Stoyanov et al. (Eds.): IPCAI 2014, LNCS 8498, pp. 206–215, 2014.

of the organ's surface geometry serving as a deformation target [2,3]. Reconstructing the organ surface in real-time and in sufficient detail is a challenging problem due to view-dependent specular highlights and the relatively uniform appearance of the liver. This also complicates registration because only a small part of it is visible. Existing methods [4,5] use natural features like the falciform ligament and inferior edges along liver segments. As the laparoscope is relatively easy to navigate looking at these features, recovering their position and shape from video should be possible using stereoscopic reconstruction methods.

In building a stereo-matching algorithm, a popular choice is to perform a pyramidal search, reducing the necessary disparity search range. This is because larger features are captured in lower-resolution pyramid levels without increasing the disparity range on that level [6]. A common approach is to filter and subsample the images into Gaussian pyramids first. Then find disparity on low-resolution levels, upscale these to the next level and refine with higher-resolution image data. This, however, easily breaks object boundaries and special care must be taken to consider the effects of down-sampling [7]. Also, while this approach appears to be easily parallelisable, the output degrades quickly. Other recent methods allow real-time reconstruction from either low-resolution [8,9,10] or high-definition video [11].

This paper proposes a stereo-matching strategy based on a coarse-to-fine pyramidal approach, adapted from sequential local match-propagation [12]. Contrary to other approaches that process image pyramid levels in sequence and upscale the results of a lower-resolution level to the next one, the proposed novel approach traverses the pyramid vertically by starting on the pyramid tip and traces out left-right matches to increasing image resolution. This vertical propagation thereby enables correspondence search window sizes to be kept small as a large high-resolution window is equivalent to a small low-resolution one, similar to existing coarse-to-fine approaches. However, vertical propagation also enables bounding of hot-loop data structures in size. This is a prerequisite to efficient GPU-implementation where low-latency on-chip memory is scarce. Multi-threaded operation follows naturally, allowing stereoscopic surface reconstruction at interactive rates from high-resolution video. Recovering the shape of the liver anatomy can then be used to register a deformable liver model, reducing the time required for an initial registration, or updating an existing registration during the procedure.

2   Method

Figure 1 depicts the processing pipeline of the proposed method for an integrated system. After initial transfer of the laparoscopic video frames to GPU memory, left and right channels are prepared for processing, followed by a matching kernel. Highlighted core steps are described in more detail in the following sections. Disparity filtering and triangulation follow standard procedures and are thus not described further.

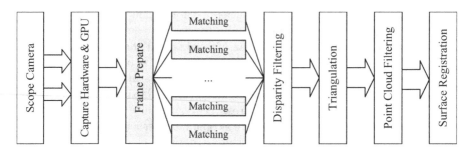

Fig. 1. Pipeline of the proposed method in context for this application. The incoming video frames are captured and transferred to GPU memory for stereoscopic matching and other processing. The highlighted core steps are presented in this paper.

2.1 Frame Preparation

Prior to matching, frame preparation is necessary. Input images left I_0 and right I_1 are cropped to a size that is a multiple of 32. This is necessary to ensure a well-formed 2:1 image pyramid with sufficient levels. Cropping is centred so that only a few pixels along the border, which rarely contain usable features, are lost. Afterwards, the cropped RGBA images are converted to greyscale and each resampled with a box filter into an image pyramid, P_0 and P_1 respectively, at successively lower resolutions. For each level l of each pyramid P^l, quantities required for fixed-window-size zero-mean normalised cross correlation (ZNCC) are precomputed. In addition, a bit mask is computed for textureless areas by checking for a non-zero horizontal and vertical pixel gradient, preventing gross mismatches in the correspondence propagation.

2.2 Match Propagation – Single-Threaded

While the proposed method is motivated by a multi-threaded GPU-amenable design and implementation, it appears reasonable to describe the matching process for a single thread first.

The overall left-to-right matching strategy takes advantage of an existing match and propagates more matches around this initial "seed" position, avoiding a large amount of false matches that could occur otherwise. Matching starts from the lowest-resolution pyramid level l that is large enough to contain the various pixel windows described below. At this resolution, the disparity for intended stereoscopic cameras is sufficiently close to 1 or 2 pixels, removing the need for explicit feature match initialisation between left and right views for the initial seed. Thus, at the very beginning, an initial seed $k := \{x_0, y_0, x_1, y_1\}$ is set to the image centres. Figure 2 illustrates key elements.

Broadly speaking, each iteration of matching performs:

1. Generation of a list of candidate matches around the current seed.
2. Establishment of global uniqueness per level.

3. Initialisation of a new seed for pyramid level $l+1$ from the established matches and jump to $l+1$, starting at (1).
4. On the highest-resolution level, keep matching horizontally.
5. Once the list of candidate matches is exhausted, jump back to previous level $l-1$ and continue at (1).

More specifically, for step (1): Around each seed k, compute ZNCC [13] for a $c \times c$ pixel sized correlation window C in P_0 and P_1, shifted by the neighbourhood window N of up to $n \times n$ pixels in either dimension (allowing matching to skip across poorly defined areas) in both left and right image simultaneously. In the right image only, the correlation window is shifted by an additional search window S of $s \times s$ pixels (this adapts the computed disparity to changes with perspective). This produces a list of up to $n \times n \times s \times s$ left-right coordinate pairs $q := \{x_0, y_0, x_1, y_1, b\} \in Q_0^l$, each with a corresponding correlation b. If b is smaller than a certain threshold $b_<$ then that entry is dropped.

Entries in Q^l are sorted according to numerical value b, highest first. Each entry is read, and its left-right-coordinates written to the disparity map $d := \{x_0, y_0, x_1, y_1\} \in D^l$ (implemented as a 2-channel image, storing x_1, y_1 at each x_0, y_0) for level l if no other match has been recorded for either x_0, y_0 or x_1, y_1 already. If instead an entry already exists in D^l then that particular q is removed from Q^l. Once Q^l has been processed (leaving its entries intact; these will serve as new seeds later), its top entry is used to initialise a new seed for level $l+1$ by multiplying its coordinates by two (step (3) in the list above). Processing then continues with step (1) again at the next level.

Once the highest-resolution level is reached, match propagation continues horizontally (step (4)). Eventually, the processing in step (1) will not add new entries to Q^l due to poor correlation between left and right pixel patches. At this point, propagation stops at the current level and returns to $l-1$, continuing with Q^{l-1} at step (1) where it left off (step (5) in the list above).

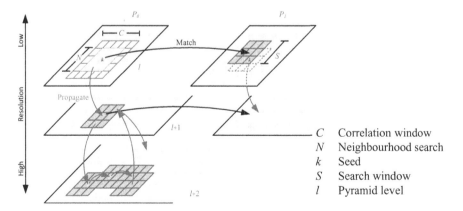

	C	Correlation window
	N	Neighbourhood search
	k	Seed
	S	Search window
	l	Pyramid level

Fig. 2. Illustration of how match propagation proceeds vertically across the pyramid. Symbols are further explained in the text of Sec. 2.2.

2.3 Multi-threaded Matching

The matching strategy described above can easily be run multi-threaded. Instead of a single starting position, many are chosen with pseudo-random offsets. Each thread processes P_0 and P_1 from its assigned seed, independently of other threads. However, as many threads would start off from effectively the same starting conditions they would also produce exactly the same result yielding no improvement in performance or match coverage. Therefore, divergence is triggered by employing a "permissible thread map" T, a bitmap the size of the input images, labelling each pixel for which thread is allowed to process it. The map T is generated once at start-up time representing a simple block structure of 4×2 partitions, yielding 8 different blocks that map onto an 8-bit thread-ID bit pattern. It is then filtered and downsampled into the remaining pyramid levels T^l by OR-ing thread-ID bits from the higher-resolution level, effectively blurring the boundaries between blocks as the pyramid level resolution decreases.

A potential performance bottleneck is the priority queue Q used to store match candidates. While each thread has its own instance per level, it is initially unbounded in size, posing a challenge for an efficient GPU implementation where access patterns to memory are critical. With the proposed method however, it turns out that maximum observed queue sizes are short in practice, only slightly larger than the number of newly arriving candidates in match-step (1). Therefore, constraining the size of Q for each thread allows the fitting of hot data in performance-critical shared memory and registers.

3 Experiments and Results

For all experiments described below, Table 1 lists the parameter values used for the propagation. All experiments are performed on an NVIDIA Quadro K5000 card. Stereo-pairs were recorded with a Viking 3DHD Vision System Dual Channel 30° laparoscope (formerly Viking Systems, Inc., USA). It provides two SDI outputs at 1080i at 59.9 Hz. The bottom field was discarded from both channels as interlacing interferes heavily with matching. Intrinsic and extrinsic camera calibration were determined using functions implemented in OpenCV. Video frames were then undistorted. No further preprocessing was performed.

Table 1. Propagation parameters used for experimental results. They were determined empirically.

Parameter	Symbol(s)	Value	Units
Search window size	$S: s \times s$	$s = 3$	pixels
Correlation window size	$C: c \times c$	$c = 5$	pixels
Neighbourhood window size	$N: n \times n$	$n = 3$	pixels
Correlation threshold	$b_<$	$b_< = 0.6$	—

3.1   Plane Experiment

In stereo-matching, small errors can be amplified easily by the stereo-rig geometry. This manifests in large spread in the z-coordinate. To assess this effect in combination with the above mentioned laparoscope, a flat piece of paper was printed with a noise pattern and filmed at an angle of approximately 30 degrees by pointing the laparoscope straight down. The distance from lens to surface was in the range of 4–7 cm. The resulting stereo-pair was then processed by sequential matching [12] (with a correlation window 19 x 19 pixels) and the proposed method (with parameters in Table 1), yielding two disparity maps. Figure 3 illustrates these. The disparity maps were triangulated into a point cloud using previously obtained camera parameters, and a plane was fitted through each. These planes serve as a silver standard regarding reconstruction noise: computing an RMS distance of reconstructed points to estimated plane yields 0.42 mm for sequential and 0.67 mm for the proposed method.

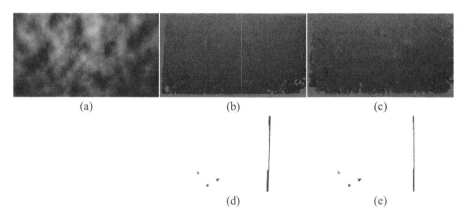

(a)   (b)   (c)

(d)   (e)

Fig. 3. Textured plane imaged at a 30 degree angle for estimating reconstruction noise. (a) shows the left channel of the stereo pair used to reconstruct the disparity maps for (b) the sequential method and (c) the proposed method. Brighter colour corresponds to higher disparity. The corresponding point clouds and fitted planes are shown in (d) and (e), respectively. The axis icon signifies the camera location.

3.2   Phantom Experiment

To evaluate the proposed method in a more realistic scenario, a flexible visually realistic human liver phantom (Healthcuts, London, UK) was custom-made. It consists of a deformable main organ body made of silicone and a rigid carbon fibre base with nine rigid "prongs" holding the body in place, allowing it to be taken off and put back on repeatably (Fig. 4a-b). The phantom was CT-scanned at 0.98 x 0.98 x 0.6 mm voxel resolution, an ISO-intensity surface extracted using Marching Cubes, and edited to remove irrelevant geometry.

The endoscope was positioned at a surface distance of 4–7 cm, making sure at least three prong tips were visible. The tips were marked in the left and right images, triangulated to 3D and aligned to the CT-scan with a least-squares optimisation. This registration was used as the gold standard location of the phantom relative to the camera lens. The corresponding fiducial registration error (FRE) for this alignment is reported in Table 2. The silicone phantom was then replaced onto the prongs and imaged. The left and right image were undistorted, and processed by the sequential method and the proposed one, yielding a point cloud. For each point in the output point cloud, the closest distance to the phantom surface was computed and aggregated into a root-mean-squared error (RMSE) for each method. These steps were repeated for three individual data sets, taken from different angles of the same phantom. Table 2 shows that the proposed method produces slightly higher errors compared to the sequential method, however at a fraction of the run time. Figure 4c-d show unfiltered reconstructed point clouds, overlaying the two methods for comparison. The red point cloud is the sequential method, and the yellow cloud the proposed method. As can be seen, the latter is slightly more noisy. Most of these mismatches are caused by view-dependent specular highlights, which the sequential method can match around more easily as its propagation queue has a global view on all possible match candidates.

All runtime measurements in Table 2 & 3 were conducted on a PC running Windows 7, 16 GB RAM, NVIDIA Quadro K5000 with 4 GB RAM and Intel Xeon E5-2609 at 2.4 GHz dual socket, four cores each.

Table 2. Reconstruction error on the liver phantom, using RMSE between reconstructed points and CT phantom surface as the metric. Input stereo pairs have a resolution of 1920 x 540 pixels. The data set number refers to Fig. 4.

Data set	Fiducial Registration Error	Proposed GPU	Sequential CPU [12]
1	1.3 mm	2.4 mm, 330 ms	1.8 mm, 2855 ms
2	2.1 mm	5.3 mm, 409 ms	4.5 mm, 3333 ms
3	2.6 mm	5.7 mm, 397 ms	2.5 mm, 2875 ms

Existing literature [11,8] compares reconstruction results on the Hamlyn Heart phantom data set [12]. The proposed method reconstructs the surface with an RMSE of 3.2 mm and an average error of 2.1 mm. In comparison, the sequential method, as implemented, reconstructs an RMSE of 3.0 mm and an average error of 2.1 mm (compared to 3.9 and 2.4 mm respectively, as reported previously [8]).

3.3   Runtime Evaluation

The proposed method has been integrated with the NVIDIA Digital Video Pipeline, allowing direct transfer of SDI-supplied high resolution video to GPU memory. Once stereoscopic video frames have arrived in texture memory as

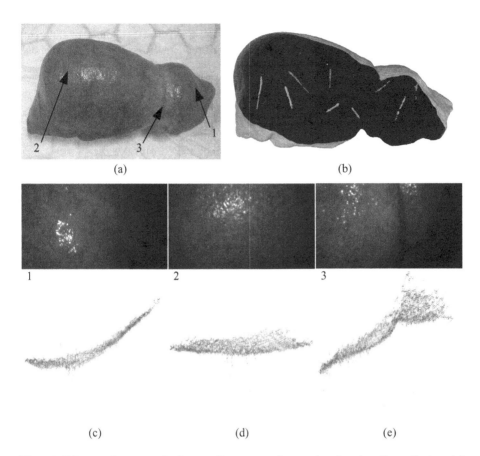

Fig. 4. Silicone phantom of a human liver, manufactured to be visually realistic, with carbon fibre prongs holding the deformable main body in position. (a) shows the main body, mounted on its base; (b) shows the mesh derived from a CT-scan including the prongs inside it. (c)-(d) show laparoscope images and corresponding unfiltered reconstructions for three different view points, overlaying both sequential and parallel method, displayed top-down.

RGBA arrays, the frame preparation process is started, followed by the matching kernel described above. Table 3 shows average processing times on a NVIDIA Quadro K5000 at different input resolutions. Timing resolution is in the order of one millisecond. The frame preparation step is dependent only on image resolution, image content has no impact on timing, hence variation is effectively zero given the timer resolution. The actual matching step however does depend on image content as the presence of gradients determine propagation. The time required to copy the result back to host memory is specifically excluded because it is expected that a streamlined registration system will perform triangulation, point cloud filtering, etc on the GPU too. Table 3 compares the runtime of the sequential method on the aforementioned Xeon CPU, highlighting a performance increase of 3–9 fold.

Table 3. Runtime of the proposed algorithm, averaged over a number of different sequences, compared to the sequential method. All reported times are in milliseconds, with μ being the mean and σ the standard deviation.

Image size		Prepare	Match		Total time	Seq. CPU		Speed up
input	cropped to		μ	σ		μ	σ	
360 x 288	352 x 288	1.1	73.2	11.3	74.3	253.6	8.4	3.4
1920 x 540	1920 x 512	4.9	373.9	45.6	378.8	2879.9	225.3	7.6
1920 x 1080	1920 x 1056	9.5	481.2	79.0	490.7	4447.9	260.4	9.1

4   Discussion and Conclusions

The proposed method is able to perform stereo-matching at interactive frame rates with an accuracy suitable for laparoscopic applications. Contrary to many existing methods, the proposed one does not rely on stereo-rectified images; it performs a 2D search instead of a 1D search along the epipolar line. While this increases processing cost significantly, it increases the number of successfully matched pixels as each seed is free to propagate along image structures in any direction. However, stepping the neighbourhood window N simultaneously for both left and right ensures that matches will not criss-cross (observing a local 2D ordering constraint). Also, ZNCC is a very expensive cost function. However, it was chosen for its robustness against radiometric changes between different views. It was found to be reliable [13] on the Middlebury data set, however, not the top performer. Contrary to a controlled lab environment, minimally invasive surgery exhibits severe radiometric issues due to uncontrollable auto-gain in the camera, non-uniform lighting and inter-tissue reflections. As the algorithm is effectively a variant of winner-takes-all in the match propagation phase and first-come-first-served with respect to multi-threading, its output depends on timing and scheduling details. While this sounds bad from a computational point of view, it has no impact in practice and relaxing a strict no-race-condition requirement allows for significant improvements to execution speed. A particular problem not addressed yet is related to object segmentation: the camera views the abdominal cavity, possibly with many unrelated structures in view. This will be addressed in future work.

Acknowledgements. This publication presents independent research commissioned by the Health Innovation Challenge Fund (HICF-T4-317), a parallel funding partnership between the Wellcome Trust and the Department of Health. The views expressed in this publication are those of the authors and not necessarily those of the Wellcome Trust or the Department of Health. The authors also thank NVIDIA for the kindly donated Quadro K5000 and SDI capture card.

References

1. Peterlík, I., Duriez, C., Cotin, S.: Modeling and real-time simulation of a vascularized liver tissue. In: Ayache, N., Delingette, H., Golland, P., Mori, K. (eds.) MICCAI 2012, Part I. LNCS, vol. 7510, pp. 50–57. Springer, Heidelberg (2012)
2. Pratt, P., Stoyanov, D., Visentini-Scarzanella, M., Yang, G.-Z.: Dynamic guidance for robotic surgery using image-constrained biomechanical models. In: Jiang, T., Navab, N., Pluim, J.P.W., Viergever, M.A. (eds.) MICCAI 2010, Part I. LNCS, vol. 6361, pp. 77–85. Springer, Heidelberg (2010)
3. Haouchine, N., Dequidt, J., Berger, M.O., Cotin, S.: Deformation-based augmented reality for hepatic surgery. In: Medicine Meets Virtual Reality, MMVR 20 (2013)
4. Kingham, T.P., Jayaraman, S., Clements, L.W., Scherer, M.A., Stefansic, J.D., Jarnagin, W.R.: Evolution of image-guided liver surgery: Transition from open to laparoscopic procedures. Journal of Gastrointestinal Surgery 17(7), 1274–1282 (2013)
5. Clements, L.W., Chapman, W.C., Dawant, B.M., Galloway Jr., R.L., Miga, M.I.: Robust surface registration using salient anatomical features for image-guided liver surgery: Algorithm and validation. Medical Physics 35(6), 2528–2540 (2008)
6. Meerbergen, G.V., Vergauwen, M., Pollefeys, M., Gool, L.V.: A hierarchical symmetric stereo algorithm using dynamic programming. International Journal of Computer Vision 47(1-3), 275–285 (2002)
7. Sizintsev, M., Wildes, R.P.: Coarse-to-fine stereo vision with accurate 3D boundaries. Image and Vision Computing 28(3), 352–366 (2010)
8. Chang, P.L., Stoyanov, D., Davison, A.J., Edwards, P.E.: Real-time dense stereo reconstruction using convex optimisation with a cost-volume for image-guided robotic surgery. In: Mori, K., Sakuma, I., Sato, Y., Barillot, C., Navab, N. (eds.) MICCAI 2013, Part I. LNCS, vol. 8149, pp. 42–49. Springer, Heidelberg (2013)
9. Mei, X., Sun, X., Zhou, M., Jiao, S., Wang, H., Zhang, X.: On building an accurate stereo matching system on graphics hardware. In: 2011 IEEE International Conference on Computer Vision Workshops (ICCV Workshops), pp. 467–474 (2011)
10. Richardt, C., Orr, D., Davies, I., Criminisi, A., Dodgson, N.A.: Real-time spatiotemporal stereo matching using the dual-cross-bilateral grid. In: Daniilidis, K., Maragos, P., Paragios, N. (eds.) ECCV 2010, Part III. LNCS, vol. 6313, pp. 510–523. Springer, Heidelberg (2010)
11. Roehl, S., Bodenstedt, S., Suwelack, S., Kenngott, H., Mueller-Stich, B.P., Dillmann, R., Speidel, S.: Dense GPU-enhanced surface reconstruction from stereo endoscopic images for intraoperative registration. Medical Physics 39(3), 1632–1645 (2012)
12. Stoyanov, D., Scarzanella, M.V., Pratt, P., Yang, G.-Z.: Real-time stereo reconstruction in robotically assisted minimally invasive surgery. In: Jiang, T., Navab, N., Pluim, J.P.W., Viergever, M.A. (eds.) MICCAI 2010, Part I. LNCS, vol. 6361, pp. 275–282. Springer, Heidelberg (2010)
13. Hirschmueller, H., Scharstein, D.: Evaluation of stereo matching costs on images with radiometric differences. IEEE Transactions on Pattern Analysis and Machine Intelligence 31(9), 1582–1599 (2008)

Deblurring Multispectral Laparoscopic Images

Geoffrey Jones[1], Neil Clancy[2,3], Simon Arridge[1], Dan Elson[2,3],
and Danail Stoyanov[1]

[1] Centre for Medical Image Computing, Department of Computer Science,
University College London, WC1E 6BT
[2] Hamlyn Centre for Robotic Surgery, Institute of Global Health Innovation,
Imperial College London, SW7 2AZ, UK
[3] Department of Surgery and Cancer, Imperial College London, SW7 2AZ, UK

Abstract. Multispectral imaging is an optical modality that can provide real-time *in vivo* information about tissue characteristics and function through signal sensitivity to chromophores in the tissue. In this paper, we present a deblurring strategy that enables imaging of dynamic tissues at wavelengths where the required acquisition time can cause significant motion blur and obscure the image. We use deconvolution for spatially varying kernels to process multispectral information obtained by using a novel laparoscopic imaging device. The trinocular design of the system allows visible light images provide information about the tissue morphology and motion that we use to construct a per pixel deformation map. We demonstrate that with the proposed method the multispectral image stack can be synthesised into a meaningful signal even in the presence of significant tissue motion. Experiments on synthetic data validate the numerical properties of the method and experiments with *ex vivo* tissue demonstrate the practical potential of the technique.

Keywords: Non-rigid Deblurring, Multispectral Imaging, Surgical Imaging, Surgical Vision.

1 Introduction

Multispectral imaging captures sequential images, band filtered in the frequency domain, that can be used to detect chromophores such as haemoglobin [1,2], melanin and water [3] in order to perform tissue characterisation and functional interrogation of the surgical site. The imaging technique is based on the acquisition of multiple images of a tissue sample at different illumination wavelengths so that a complete spectral response can be built up for each pixel of the sample projection. By modelling the interaction of light and the tissue, the spectral features of interest can be observed and used to infer information about the sample. Such real-time non-contact optical imaging can potentially provide an invaluable clinical tool for intra-operative diagnosis and functional monitoring in a wide variety of applications which require a quantitative knowledge of mesenteric oxygenation. Examples include the diagnosis or mesenteric ischaemia, assessment of the bowel anastomosis to identify the risk of anastomotic dehiscence, bowel

D. Stoyanov et al. (Eds.): IPCAI 2014, LNCS 8498, pp. 216–225, 2014.

ischaemia surgery and transplanted organ viability or visualisation of the bile duct [4].

Multispectral systems for minimally invasive surgery (MIS) are typically based on a single optical channel laparoscope [5] and either rely on switching of the illumination source or rely on an additional scope for visible white light visualisation, a full discussion can be found in [6]. More recently, a system was developed by using a multiple optical channel laparoscope and a liquid crystal tunable filter (LCTF)[4]. This integrated device is practical for clinical use through a single trocar. Additionally the LCTF is capable of achieving a high spectral resolution (<10nm) and can be electronically-controlled, allowing on-demand access to wavelengths of interest. However, the main drawback of LCTFs is their poor transmission properties, which are wavelength-dependent and can require a long exposure time to acquire an image that has sufficient source signal to identify the sample's spectral response. As a result the acquisition of a complete stack of multispectral images may take several hundred milliseconds or longer. This poses a challenge because during surgery physiological motion can deform the tissue and the laparoscope can move causing misalignment of the multispectral data and significant motion blur in certain spectral ranges. In order to provide a correct signal response from the multispectral stack the images need to be processed for removing motion blur and an attractive approach is to use computational deblurring methods.

Image deblurring can recover detail in scenes imaged under motion by using deconvolution as an inverse problem with optional priors. The Richardson Lucy (RL) algorithm[7,8] is one of the most established approaches requiring a known point spread function (PSF). Semi-blind methods incorporate priors [9] however often this makes optimisation non-convex. Blind deblurring using natural image statistics is also possible [10], [11] but a major challenge for *in vivo* multispectral images is the lack of constraints to anatomical structural correspondence. Stochastic deconvolution [12] allows for better correspondence utilising a know spatially varying point spread functions (SVPSF), as well as being able to include arbitrary regularisation without the need for complex optimisation, at the cost of a slower execution time. Multiple camera methods are able recover the information from one or more cameras and use it to formulate the SVPSF in another [13]. This can be achieved using optical flow to estimate a discrete SVPSF to use as a seed for iterative optimisation [14]. The typical suggested extension for deconvolution algorithms to the spatially varying case, is to perform the same technique on a piecewise decomposition of the image into areas of similar motion [15]. This is not practical when a dense *per-pixel* SVPF is required because for frequency domain approaches it introduces a further order of complexity. Extending convolution deblurring methods to utilise an unique per-pixel SVPSF also presents a significant computational challenge and requires excessive memory storage for the individual blur kernels. Therefore, currently there are significant difficulties for existing methods to computationally deblurr images from MIS which contain non-rigid motion and deformation combined with complex reflectance functions.

In this paper, we propose an efficient pixel parallel deblurring technique which can accommodate SVPSF and be implemented taking advantage of modern parallel computing architectures. We demonstrate how this approach can be used to improve the signal in multispectral imaging using a custom trinocular channel laparoscope. To our knowledge, this is the first deblurring technique applied to multispectral surgical imaging and the proposed method further generalises to allow for completely non-rigid scene deformation. We evaluate the numerical performance of the proposed algorithm on synthetic data with known ground truth and we present promising results on *ex vivo* tissue within a controlled laboratory experimental environment.

2   Methods

2.1   Multispectral Trinocular Laparoscope

The multispectral trinocular laparoscope used for this study is shown in Figure 1. The scope delivers colour stereo images at a resolution of 1024×768 pixels using two IDS Imaging, uEye 2230-C cameras. The wide-angle central channel of the scope is routed through a LCTF (Varispec, CRI, Inc) to a monochrome camera (Thorlabs DCU 223M). The LCTF has a spectral range running from 400-720 nm with a resolution of 10 nm. The multispectral camera was synchronised with the LCTF so that a given wavelength range, decomposed into contiguous non-overlapping 10 nm bands, is captured such that each image corresponds to a single band. Due to the low transmission of the LCTF, a long integration time is required for the multispectral camera, making this the speed-limiting element. For the *in vivo* experiment, the integration time and gain were set to 1000ms and 25 respectively for the multispectral camera, and 90 ms and 20 for the stereo cameras.[1] We create an efficient deblurring processing step that runs

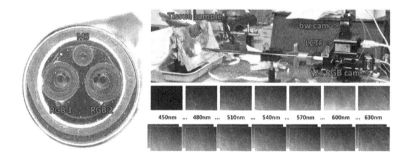

Fig. 1. Clockwise from left. The front of the laporoscope and the three camera multiplex; the experimental configuration; a sample from a typical capture data set for a single multispectral stack, with corresponding stereo RGB.

---

[1] Further details of scope design and configuration are found in [15].

simultaneous with the image capture, operating on each of the multi spectral images utilising scene flow information recovered from the stereo cameras.

2.2   Non-blind Deconvolution

Using a non-blind deconvolution process requires prior knowledge of the deformation to construct the spatially varying blurring function. We obtain scene flow using the white light stereo RGB channels of the trinocular laparoscope, and project this into the image plane of the multispectral camera. Subsequently, our deconvolution method is an extension of the RL algorithm which can be expressed using blurring by convolution [16,17] as follows:

$$I^{(n+1)} = \left\{ \left\{ \frac{B}{I^{(n)} \otimes k} \right\} \otimes \hat{k} \right\} I^{(n)} \tag{1}$$

such that for a 2D PSF k with an index space $\Omega \subseteq \mathbb{R}^{2+}$, the inverse point spread function $\hat{k}$ is

$$\hat{k}(\mathbf{x}) = k(\max(\Omega) - \mathbf{x}), \mathbf{x} \in \Omega.$$

The formulation of Equation 1 can be extended to the spatially varying case by generalising to per-pixel level kernels. However, a standard pixel-wise convolution model for blur will become unstable for SVPSFs as illustrated in Figure 2 and for an extreme case in Figure 3 [18][19]. This stems from the non-symmetrical nature of the *forward* blurring kernel compared to the *inverse* blurring operation. Additionally, there is also a high computational cost for calculating blur kernels at every point in the image. This is particularly restrictive for real-time application and cannot trivially be solved by pre-computing all kernels, as storing them in memory rapidly becomes impractical even for low resolution images. To overcome this limitation, in this study we use a generalisation of the RL algorithm and propose a new non-symmetric blur method that directly utilises the source deformation field via successive re-sampling.

2.3   Generalised Richardson Lucy

The RL algorithm can be expressed as an error metric and an iteration update with the blur model formulation independent of the algorithm. This follows from Equation 1, for which the blur model is the convolution operator and as such is equivalent to the original summation based expression of the RL algorithm. The generalisation is to exchange the convolution model for an alternative equivalent blur model, an appropriate accumulative blur model may be selected to replace the convolution operation[19].

Generalised Richardson Lucy Algorithm

```
1  for observed blurred image B
2    L_est = B
3    for i to i_max
4      # calculate an error image from the current estimate
5      B_est = Blur(L_est)
6      err   = B./Best
7      # accumulate the error to contributor locations
8      err_b = invBlur(err)
9      L_est = err_b.*L_est
```

2.4 Re-sampling Blur

We propose using a blur method that warps a sampling grid, repeatedly re-sampling the grid locations, incrementally deformed by a spatially varying deformation field. The sampling grid is used to accumulate samples from a source image to form the blurred image. The method follows from the PSF generation method of [18] where blur kernels are rendered by drawing line segments of a motion path weighted by the relative time duration the segment corresponds to. Using the same approach we propagate a sampling point s_n through a deformation field D and instead of drawing the trace of this sampling point into a kernel we use it to accumulate successive samples from the source image. To create the blurred image B from input image I, we calculate the value at $b_i \in B$ as

$$b_i = \Delta \sum_{n=0}^{N} I(s_n) \tag{2}$$

where $\Delta = \frac{1}{N}$, and s_n is the sampling position calculated recursively as

$$s_{n+1} = s_n + \Delta t D(s_n) \tag{3}$$

with s_0 initialised as the coordinate location of b_i and t as the length of exposure. B-Spline sampling is used to sample the deformation $D(s_n)$ and input $I(s_n)$ for each location s_n. In order to integrate this blur model with the generalised RL algorithm an inverse blurring function can be expressed by negating the deformation fields. To avoid zigzag drift, as shown in Figure 3 as an artefact of rotational blur, we modify the update for s_n to use a weighted filter over a neighbourhood centred at s_n. So for filter f with indexing space Ω, the update equation for s_n becomes:

$$s_{n+1} = s_n + \sum_{x}^{\Omega} f(x) \Delta t D(s_n + x) \tag{4}$$

In our use case we found that a discretized zero mean Gaussian filter with $\sigma = 0.5$ gave sufficient drift stabilisation for most of our synthetic and experimental test cases. For more extreme deformations it may be appropriate to use more specialised particle filters to better track the sampling locations.

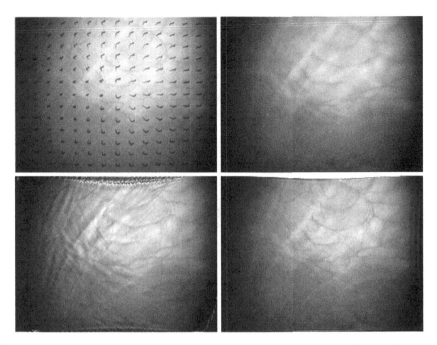

Fig. 2. Left to right top to bottom: ground truth with overlaid realistic deformation field; tissue imaged under simulated spatially varying motion as defined by the deformation field; deblurring using typical [14] spatially varying extension of the Richardson Lucy algorithm; deblurring using our proposed re-sampling blur model method

3   Experiments and Results

3.1   Synthetic

Synthetic data was generated by blurring multispectral images of ex vivo tissue with known deformation fields to assess our proposed method against the standard RL with ground truth. Various deformation fields could then be applied to the images to explore the stability of the algorithm under different simulated conditions. For simulated motion levels representative of physiological motions that are observed in surgery our method performed better than RL as shown in Figure 2. Our results contain fewer artefacts arising from incorrect error accumulation. Additionally, our proposed method performed well even on particularly challenging blur such as large rotations for which standard convolution based RL performs very unstably and our proposed method proved to be robust even for many iterations. The rotational experiment also clearly demonstrates how improving the tracking of the sampling grid translates directly to an improvement in the stability of the algorithm.

We compare the results in the frequency domain (Figure 4) and our deblurred results have a similar frequency profile to that of the ground truth, where as the

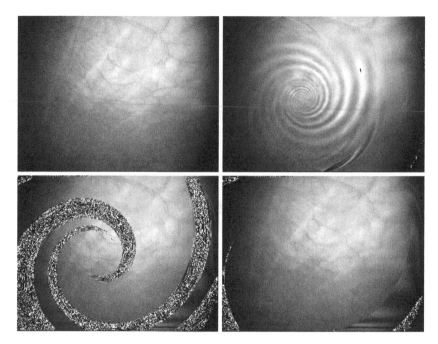

Fig. 3. Comparative stability of different blur models using the Richardson Lucy deconvolution algorithm, on a large synthetic rotational blur. Left to right top to bottom; ground truth; 10 iterations of standard convolution blur model (where inverse blurring is achieved by convolving with the reverse indexed froward kernel) with per-pixel kernels[18]; 500 iterations of deconvolution using re-sampled accumulation at 500 iterations; 500 iterations of deconvolution using Gaussian filtered re-sampled accumulation

blurred data has significantly more weighting to the lower frequencies as expected. Furthermore by looking at how the PSNR for the frequency domain varies, over scale space, we see that the proposed method improves on the standard RL, and blurred results, by recovering finer image structures at the trade off of less large scale accuracy. Frequency domain comparisons were chosen because they would be more sensitive to errors often created by RL deconvolution such as ringing artefacts typically introduced during deblubrring.

3.2 Ex-vivo

To evaluate our method on laboratory data we performed experiments using both a reference macbeth colour chart and *ex vivo* porcine stomach tissue samples. The tissue samples were mounted onto a computer controlled translation stage (Velmex BiSlide) whose motion was programmed using LabView. The trinocular cameras were used to perform synchronized imaging of the samples while the stage was in motion. By positioning the plane of translation non-parallel to the imaging plane of the camera a large spatially varying projective motion could be

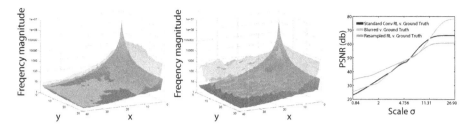

Fig. 4. Left and centre; a comparison of the absolute difference in the frequency domain against ground truth for re sampled blur model and blurred respectively, positive quadrant. Right; a comparison of PSNR across scale space for convolution model deblurring; re-sampled deblurring and input blurred image for reference, illustrating how re-sampled blur model more accurately recovers fine scale details.

generated. The multispectral stacks were registered using the method of [15] and points of interest identified by making reference to the associated RGB camera data, patches around these positions were then extracted from the multi-spectral images.

For the tissue samples, haemoglobin concentration [15], were then calculated at each pixel by minimising

$$\begin{bmatrix} x_{\lambda_0} \\ \vdots \\ x_{\lambda_n} \end{bmatrix} = \begin{bmatrix} \epsilon_{HbO_2}^{\lambda_0} & \epsilon_{Hb}^{\lambda_0} & 1 \\ & \vdots & \\ \epsilon_{HbO_2}^{\lambda_n} & \epsilon_{Hb}^{\lambda_n} & 1 \end{bmatrix} \begin{bmatrix} HbO_2 \\ Hb \\ D \end{bmatrix} \quad (5)$$

where x_λ is the reflectance observed at a given wavelength, $\epsilon_{HbO_2}^\lambda$ and ϵ_{Hb}^λ are respectively the extinction coefficients for oxy and de-oxy haemoglobin [20] respectively. Solving for Hb and HbO_2, allowing for a constant dampening from diffusion D, enables an estimate of the total haemoglobin to be made by summing the oxy and de-oxy components. For the colour chart reconstruction of the spectral response at each pixel was compared to that of a static reference.

We compared the result of reconstructing the total haemoglobin measure for patches without preprocessing against preprocessing by deblurring using our proposed re-sampled blur model. Figure 5 shows two selected feature points observed in the data and compares the results of total haemoglobin reconstruction, that indicates a greater degree of structural cohesion when using deblurring.

For 100 pixels PSFs deblurring our images (1024x768) took approximately 5 minutes, this could be improved by taking advantage of optimised texture sampling routines available on most graphics cards. Memory usage is efficient since deformation is stored as a field instead of per-pixel kernels, allowing for easy GPU implementation. This is important because uncompressed per-pixel floating point 40×40 kernels would require over 6GB for all kernels for a one megapixel image.

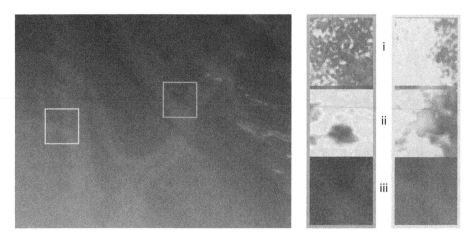

Fig. 5. Total haemoglobin reconstruction at two locations. i) reconstruction performed without prior deblurring, ii) reconstruction with prior deblurring, iii) corresponding RGB information.

4 Discussion

In this study we have shown that incorporating a spatially varying blur model with the generalised RL algorithm provides an accurate and computationally efficient deblurring of multispectral images even with non-uniform blur. Current limitations are that characteristic artefacts the RL approach appear when very hard edges are visible in the image such as near surface vessels but it may possible to dampen the expression of these artefacts [21]. The atomic design of our algorithm allows for implementation on parallel computing architectures and with optimization we believe that near real-time performance is possible which is critical for translating the proposed computational method to practice.

Acknowledgements. We gratefully acknowledge the loan of the laparoscope by Intuitive Surgical, Inc. Funding for this project was provided by ERC grant 242991, The Royal Academy of Engineering/EPSRC Fellowship and the UCL IMPACT scheme.

References

1. Ilias, M.A., Hggblad, E., Anderson, C., Salerud, E.G.: Visible hyperspectral imaging evaluating the cutaneous response to ultraviolet radiation, pp. 644103–644103-12 (2007)
2. Sorg, B.S., Donovan, O., Cao, Y., Dewhirst, M.W., Moeller, B.J.: Hyperspectral imaging of hemoglobin saturation in tumor microvasculature and tumor hypoxia development. Journal of Biomedical Optics 10(4), 044004–044004-11 (2005)
3. Sowa, M.G., Payette, J.R., Hewko, M.D., Mantsch, H.H.: Visible-near infrared multispectral imaging of the rat dorsal skin flap. Journal of Biomedical Optics 4(4), 474–481 (1999)

4. Clancy, N.T., Stoyanov, D., Sauvage, V., James, D., Yang, G.-Z., Elson, D.S.: A triple endoscope system for alignment of multispectral images of moving tissue. Biomedical Optics and 3-D Imaging, BTuD27 (2010)
5. Leitner, R., Biasio, M.D., Arnold, T., Dinh, C.V., Loog, M., Duin, R.P.: Multispectral video endoscopy system for the detection of cancerous tissue. Pattern Recognition Letters 34(1), 85–93 (2013)
6. Stoyanov, D.: Surgical vision. Annals of Biomedical Engineering 40(2), 332–345 (2012), http://dx.doi.org/10.1007/s10439-011-0441-z
7. Richardson, W.H.: Bayesian-based iterative method of image restoration. J. Opt. Soc. Am. 62(1), 55–59 (1972)
8. Lucy, L.: An iterative technique for the rectification of observed distributions. The Astronomical Journal 79, 745 (1974)
9. Dey, N., Blanc-Feraud, L., Zimmer, C., Kam, Z., Olivo-Marin, J.C., Zerubia, J.: A deconvolution method for confocal microscopy with total variation regularization. In: IEEE International Symposium on Biomedical Imaging: Nano to Macro, 2004, vol. 2, pp. 1223–1226 (2004)
10. Fergus, R., Singh, B., Hertzmann, A., Roweis, S.T., Freeman, W.T.: Removing camera shake from a single photograph. ACM Transactions on Graphics (TOG) 25(3), 787–794 (2006)
11. Krishnan, D., Tay, T., Fergus, R.: Blind deconvolution using a normalized sparsity measure. In: 2011 IEEE Conference on Computer Vision and Pattern Recognition (CVPR), pp. 233–240. IEEE (2011)
12. Gregson, J., Heide, F., Hullin, M.B., Rouf, M., Heidrich, W.: Stochastic Deconvolution. In: IEEE Conference on Computer Vision and Pattern Recognition (CVPR) (June 2013) (to appear)
13. Li, F., Yu, J., Chai, J.: A hybrid camera for motion deblurring and depth map super-resolution. In: IEEE Conference on Computer Vision and Pattern Recognition, CVPR 2008, pp. 1–8. IEEE (2008)
14. Tai, Y.-W., Du, H., Brown, M.S., Lin, S.: Correction of spatially varying image and video motion blur using a hybrid camera. IEEE Transactions on Pattern Analysis and Machine Intelligence 32(6), 1012–1028 (2010)
15. Clancy, N.T., Stoyanov, D., James, D.R.C., Marco, A.D., Sauvage, V., Clark, J., Yang, G.Z., Elson, D.S.: Multispectral image alignment using a three channel endoscope in vivo during minimally invasive surgery. Biomed. Opt. Express 3(10), 2567–2578 (2012)
16. Holmes, T.J.: Blind deconvolution of quantum-limited incoherent imagery: maximum-likelihood approach. J. Opt. Soc. Am. A 9(7), 1052–1061 (1992)
17. Fish, D., Brinicombe, A., Pike, E., Walker, J.: Blind deconvolution by means of the richardson–lucy algorithm. JOSA A 12(1), 58–65 (1995)
18. Ben-Ezra, M., Nayar, S.K.: Motion deblurring using hybrid imaging. In: Proceedings of the 2003 IEEE Computer Society Conference on Computer Vision and Pattern Recognition, vol. 1, pp. 1–657. IEEE (2003)
19. Tai, Y., Tan, P., Brown, M.: Richardson-lucy deblurring for scenes under a projective motion path. IEEE Transactions on Pattern Analysis and Machine Intelligence (2009)
20. Prahl, S.A.: Tabulated molar extinction coefficient for hemoglobin in water
21. Yuan, L., Sun, J., Quan, L., Shum, H.-Y.: Progressive inter-scale and intra-scale non-blind image deconvolution. ACM Trans. Graph. 27(3), 74:1–74:10 (2008)

Simulated Field Maps: Toward Improved Susceptibility Artefact Correction in Interventional MRI

Martin Kochan[1], Pankaj Daga[1], Ninon Burgos[1], Mark White[2],
M. Jorge Cardoso[1,3], Laura Mancini[2], Gavin P. Winston[4],
Andrew W. McEvoy[2], John Thornton[2], Tarek Yousry[2], John S. Duncan[4],
Danail Stoyanov[1], and Sébastien Ourselin[1,3]

[1] Centre for Medical Image Computing,
University College London, London, UK
m.kochan.12@ucl.ac.uk
[2] National Hospital for Neurology and Neurosurgery,
UCLH NHS Foundation Trust, London, UK
[3] Dementia Research Centre, Institute of Neurology,
University College London, London, UK
[4] Department of Clinical and Experimental Epilepsy, Institute of Neurology,
University College London, London, UK

Abstract. Intraoperative MRI is a powerful modality for acquiring structural and functional images of the brain to enable precise image-guided neurosurgery. In this paper, we propose a novel method for simulating main magnetic field inhomogeneity maps during intraoperative MRI-guided neurosurgery. Our method relies on an air-tissue segmentation of intraoperative patient specific data, which is used as an input to a subsequent field simulation step. The generated simulation can then be used to enhance the precision of image-guidance. We report results of our method on 12 patient datasets acquired during image-guided neurosurgery for anterior lobe resection for surgical management of focal temporal lobe epilepsy. We find a close agreement between the field inhomogeneity maps acquired as part of the imaging protocol and the simulated field inhomogeneity maps generated by the proposed method.

Keywords: image-guided neurosurgery, interventional MRI, inhomogeneity field map simulation.

1 Introduction

Anterior temporal lobe resection (ATLR) is an effective treatment for refractory temporal lobe epilepsy. However, resective surgery may result in severe complications such as contralateral superior visual field deficit (VFD) that restricts the seizure-free patient from returning to regular activity. Magnetic resonance imaging (MRI) is the preferred modality for imaging soft-tissue brain morphology

D. Stoyanov et al. (Eds.): IPCAI 2014, LNCS 8498, pp. 226–235, 2014.

and function for diagnosis and postoperative follow-up. Additionally, interventional MRI (iMRI) can potentially be used to enhance the precision of pathological tissue resection while minimizing the damage to healthy brain structures. By preserving critical brain tissues, the patients may benefit from improved outcomes and quality of life.

Image-guided neurosurgery for ATLR is an established surgical specialisation but localization accuracy can be adversely affected by intraoperative physiomechanical deformation of the soft tissue, generally referred to as *brain shift*, which can be caused by cerebrospinal fluid (CSF) drainage, tissue retraction, brain swelling and the resection itself [1]. Imaging using iMRI can provide valuable information about the anatomy, which can be used to compensate for brain shift by registering preoperative and intraoperative images. Recently, Daga *et al.* [2] have proposed multimodal co-registration of anatomical T1-weighted MRI images paired with fractional anisotropy maps (DWI-FA) derived from diffusion-weighted imaging (DW-MRI) image sets, as a means of estimating brain shift. This approach takes into account the locations of white matter tracts that are not discernible visually nor on the T1-weighted anatomical scans. However, DW-MRI image sets are acquired using the echo planar imaging (EPI) MRI pulse sequence, which suffers from severe geometric distortion, caused by the very limited acquisition bandwidth of EPI in the phase-encode (PE) dimension of the image. Severe distortion occurs in EPI images even due to small inhomogeneity in the main magnetic field B_0 on the order of several ppm.

The first source of B_0 inhomogeneity is due to hardware constraints and can be reduced (shimmed) to several ppm by means of superconducting shim coils [3]. The second source of B_0 field inhomogeneity is due to perturbation of the magnetic field by non-uniform geometric distribution of magnetic susceptibility in the imaged volume. This inhomogeneity is largest near air-tissue boundaries, such as the sinuses, the petrous part of the temporal bone [4], and the resection cavity itself. The susceptibility-related inhomogeneity is shimmed using a set of room-temperature (RT) shim coils. However, imperfect shimming and higher-order perturbations result in residual inhomogeneity. The distortion of the EPI image associated with this residual inhomogeneity is called the *susceptiblity artefact*. A popular approach to correct for the susceptibility artefact is to acquire the residual inhomogeneity field maps using a specific MR pulse sequence [4]. However, the acquired inhomogeneity field maps differ from the true field maps due to low SNR near air-tissue boundaries (e.g. the resection margin) and due to MR signal dropout (e.g. close to head-holder attachment pins) [5]. In iMRI guided neurosurgery, the diversions from true field maps can adversely affect image guidance accuracy.

In this paper, we propose to simulate a field map from T1-weighted and T2-weighted iMRI images acquired as part of a standard iMRI scanning protocol. Previously, Jenkinson *et al.* [6] demonstrated a perturbation method to calculate a B_0 inhomogeneity field from air-tissue segmentation derived from computed tomography (CT) images. Poynton *et al.* [5] demonstrated that non-surgical T1-weighted images can be segmented into air and tissue classes using a probabilistic

CT atlas, and reported that a subsequent application of the method [6] results in close overall agreement between the acquired and simulated field maps. However, we observe that a probabilistic atlas is not suited to the segmentation of intraoperative iMR images that contain air-filled craniotomy and resection areas of variable shape that depend on the surgery and patient morphology. Instead, we employ an expectation-maximization (EM) based segmentation method informed by priors derived from a synthetic CT image. We compute the synthetic CT from the intraoperative T1-weighted image and a database of MR/CT pair templates. We subsequently feed the air-tissue segmentation into the method [6]. The field map simulation is evaluated by comparison with field maps acquired during iMRI guided ATLR neurosurgery for 12 cases. The proposed method generates field maps in close agreement with the acquired field maps.

This result has the potential to lead to improvements in EPI image correction and image guidance for neurosurgery. Additionally, the proposed method can also be used to correct distortion in historical intraoperative EPI datasets, which did not include field map acquisition as part of the acquisition protocol.

2   Methods

2.1   Field Map in Terms of Voxel Displacement

Let the magnetic field at point x be $B_0 + \Delta B_0(x)$ [T] where B_0 is the homogeneous field and $\Delta B_0(x)$ is the inhomogeneity field map, which can be equivalently expressed as $\gamma \Delta B_0(x)$ [rad/s] or $\frac{\gamma \Delta B_0(x)}{2\pi}$ [Hz]. For the purposes of image correction, one is interested in the millimetre displacement along the phase encode direction that the inhomogeneity causes to an EPI image. The displacement can be calculated based on theory in [4,7]. Consider the acquisition of a single EPI slice with matrix size $N \times N$ and voxel dimensions r_{FE} in the frequency encode (FE) direction and r_{PE} in the phase encode (PE) direction, respectively. The EPI slice is reconstructed by the inverse Fourier transform of the MR signal. In the PE direction, the MR signal sampling rate is $\frac{N}{T_{acq}}$ [Hz], where T_{acq} is the signal acquisition time. The reconstructed image resolution in the PE direction is $\frac{N}{NT_{acq}} = \frac{1}{T_{acq}}$ [Hz/pixel] or T_{acq} [pixel/Hz]. Since the PE gradient is used to encode position along the PE direction, the above offset corresponds to a distortion along the PE direction of size:

$$d_{PE}(x) = \frac{\gamma \Delta B_0(x)}{2\pi} T_{acq} r_{PE} \ . \tag{1}$$

In this study, the EPI image correction itself was only performed for visual confirmation (Figure 2), by converting the field map into a vector displacement/deformation vector field and subsequently resampling the image using cubic spline interpolation [8].

2.2   Field Map Acquisition

Field map acquisition was based on the method introduced in [4], whereby the field map is dependent on phase difference map between the phase components of MR images acquired during two MR signal echoes, separated by echo difference time T_{ED}. The phase difference corresponds to spin phase evolution during T_{ED} but is modulo-2π phase-wrapped due to unknown number of elapsed revolutions. Additionally, the phase difference signal is noisy in low spin-density areas (air and bone) and has low SNR near air-tissue boundaries. Therefore, to recover the inhomogeneity $\gamma \Delta B_0(\boldsymbol{x})$, we used a novel phase-unwrapping algorithm based on a probabilistic model spatially constrained by means of a Markov random field (MRF) formulation, as presented in [8]. We de-meaned the recovered phase difference map, since the recovered phase difference necessarily has an arbitrary constant component.

2.3   Air-Tissue Segmentation

The magnetic susceptibility values for soft tissue ($\approx -9.1 \times 10^{-6}$) and bone ($\approx -11.4 \times 10^{-6}$) are similar, but both are significantly different from that of air ($\approx 0.4 \times 10^{-6}$) [5]. Therefore, we need a binary labelling of the head into tissue and air. For each subject, a segmentation was performed on the sum of the T1- and T2-weighted iMRI image (a pseudo spin density image). In this image, the soft tissues (grey and white matter, the eyes) were grey, CSF and fat tissue were bright, and air and bone were black.

For the air-tissue segmentation, we used a segmentation algorithm based on an expectation-maximization (EM) intensity model spatially regularized using an MRF [9]. Tissue was segmented into three partial volume classes: air, bone and soft tissue (Figure 1, centre right) and later the bone and soft tissue classes were combined into the tissue class. Each class had its associated spatial prior map. The spatial prior maps were calculated from a closed skull synthetic CT. In CT, each of the 3 classes has a unique intensity range and therefore, the CT was intensity-transformed using 2 sigmoid functions that acted as separators to select tissue based on intensity. During the EM segmentation, full MRF strength was chosen to enforce the presence of air in the resection area (as opposed to soft tissue) and of air in the craniotomy area (as opposed to bone).

The closed skull synthetic CT image was constructed from the T1-weighted iMRI image following the method described by Burgos *et al.* [10]. The method relies on a database consisting of 6 pairs of co-registered T1-weighted MR / CT images from healthy subjects. Each MR image from the database was non-rigidly registered to the intraoperative iMRI image so that each CT could be propagated into the iMRI space. The resampled CT images were fused together using a voxel-wise rank-based weighting scheme (Figure 1, centre left).

The intraoperative field of view contains the cranial part of the head, but does not include the head below the nose level. The later field map simulation step (as described in Section 2.4) assumes that no tissue is present outside of the air-tissue segmentation volume that has a significant contribution to the field distribution inside the volume. Therefore, an approximated lower head tissue volume was constructed in a volume inferior to the iMRI (Figure 1, right). To construct the lower head tissue volume, the affine registration from the CT synthesis step was reused to resample the MR templates into the target volume, and the resampled volumes intensity transformed using a sigmoid function and averaged.

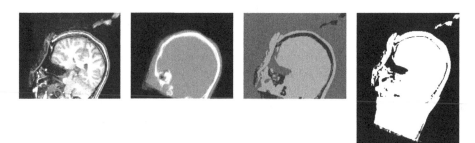

Fig. 1. Air-tissue segmentation. Left: a T1-weighted intraoperative image. The section runs through a plane close to the anatomical coronal plane (head at angle due to intraoperative orientation). Middle left: an accompanying synthetic CT. Middle right: the result of the segmentation (red for air, green for soft-tissue, blue for bone). Right: the final air-tissue segmentation (black for air, white for tissue) with the fitted lower head volume.

2.4 Field Map Estimation

The field map estimation follows from [6] and models the first order perturbations of the main magnetic field. The susceptibility χ can be expanded as $\chi = \chi_0 + \delta\chi_1$, where χ_0 is the magnetic susceptibility of air, δ is the susceptibility difference between air and brain tissue and χ_1 is a binary variable describing the tissue type. The first order perturbations of the z-component of the main magnetic field (B_z^1) can be written in terms of the main magnetic field (B_z^0):

$$B_z^1 = \frac{\chi_1}{3 + \chi_0} B_z^0 - \frac{1}{1 + \chi_0}\left(\left(\frac{\partial^2 G}{\partial z^2}\right) * (\chi_1 B_z^0)\right) \qquad (2)$$

where G is the Green's function $G(x) = (4\pi r)^{-1}$ and $r = \sqrt{x^2 + y^2 + z^2}$. Note that the expression is simplified considerably due to the fact that we only have a non-zero component in the longitudinal axis (z-direction) of the main magnetic field.

The convolution $H(\boldsymbol{x})$ for a single voxel with the resolution (a, b, c) for a constant field along the z-axis is given by:

$$H(\boldsymbol{x}) = \left(\frac{\partial^2 G}{\partial z^2}\right) * (\chi_1 B_z^0) = \sum_{i,j,k\in(-1,1)} (ijk)F\left(x + \frac{ia}{2}, y + \frac{jb}{2}, z + \frac{kc}{2}\right) \qquad (3)$$

where $F(\boldsymbol{x}) = \frac{1}{4\pi}\arctan(\frac{xy}{zr})$.

Due to the linearity of Equation (2), the single voxel solutions can be added together to compute the total field:

$$B_z^1(\boldsymbol{x}) = \sum_{\boldsymbol{x}'} \chi_1 \boldsymbol{x}' H(\boldsymbol{x} - \boldsymbol{x}') \qquad (4)$$

where $\boldsymbol{x}'$ are the voxel locations and $\boldsymbol{x}$ is the point where the field is evaluated. This can be implemented using the 3D Fast Fourier Transform.

Although this approach simulates the field distribution due to the main coil, MRI scanners also contain room-temperature (RT) shim coils, whose purpose is to decrease the inhomogeneity in the imaged volume. The RT shim coils are wound to form magnetic fields that follow first- and second-order spherical harmonics, $S(\boldsymbol{x}) = [x, y, z, z^2 - (x^2 + y^2)/2, xz, yz, x^2 - y^2, 2xy](\boldsymbol{x})$, where $\boldsymbol{x} = \boldsymbol{0}$ at the magnet isocentre [11]. The field in the scanner becomes $B_z^1(\boldsymbol{x}) - S\boldsymbol{\theta}$, where the coefficients $\boldsymbol{\theta} = [\theta_1, \theta_2, \ldots, \theta_8]^T$ are proportional to the currents in the shim coils, which are dynamically optimized by the scanner during image acquisition based on the field in the imaged volume [11]. In this simulation, we approximate the shim currents as a linear combination that minimizes the inhomogeneity field across the field of view, as used in [5]. We perform a least-squares fit of the spherical harmonics to determine $\hat{\boldsymbol{\theta}} = \mathrm{argmin}_{\boldsymbol{\theta}}(B_z^1(\boldsymbol{x}) - S\boldsymbol{\theta})$.

3   Results

The proposed algorithm was validated on 12 datasets that were acquired using interventional MRI during ATLR procedures. Validation was done as part of an audit to assess the usability of simulated field maps in a clinical scenario. The images were acquired using a 1.5T Espree MRI scanner (Siemens, Erlangen, Germany) designed for interventional procedures. The intraoperative protocol included a T1-weighted FLASH image (TR = 5.25 ms, TE = 2.5 ms, flip angle = 15°, 0.547 × 0.547 × 1.25 mm grid of 512 × 512 × 176 voxels) and a T2-weighted turbo spin echo image (TR = 3200 ms, TE = 510 ms, flip angle = 120°, 1.0 × 1.0 × 1.0 mm grid of 256 × 256 × 176 voxels), a DW-MRI dataset of 65 diffusion-weighted images acquired using a single shot EPI sequence with GRAPPA-based parallel imaging (acceleration factor of 2, 2.5 × 2.5 × 2.5 mm grid of 84 × 84 × 49 voxels, readout time 35.52 ms) and a field map acquired using a gradient-recalled echo pulse sequence (2.91667 × 2.91667 × 2.9 mm grid of 72 × 72 × 43 voxels, echo time difference of 4.76 ms).

The DW-MRI dataset for each subject was corrected as per Section 2.1 using the acquired field map and the proposed simulated field map, respectively. An example for a subject is shown in Figure 2.

The most direct validation of the simulated field map would be to compare DWI images corrected using acquired and simulated field maps, respectively, against anatomical landmarks identified on the intraoperative T1-weighted images, which are not affected by the susceptibility artefact (Figure 2). However, due to the low resolution and low signal-to-noise ratio of DW-MRI, the landmarks are challenging to identify reliably and repeatably. Since there is no way of measuring the true field maps *in vivo*, we compared the simulated field maps to the acquired field maps (Figure 3). The field maps were expressed in mm of

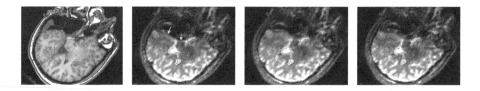

Fig. 2. Detail of correction for the susceptibility artefact. Left: an intraoperative T1-weighted image unaffected by the distortion. The section runs through a plane close to the anatomical axial plane (head at angle due to intraoperative orientation). A brain surface outlined using a surface extractor[2] is shown for reference (red outline). Middle left: an uncorrected "b0" DW-MRI image (an image for which no diffusion gradients are applied). Arrows point at an area of severe susceptibility distortion. Middle right: the "b0" image corrected using the acquired field map. Right: the "b0" image corrected using the simulated field map.

Table 1. Quantification of absolute difference (in mm) between the correction displacement in the phase encode direction as predicted by the proposed simulated field map and the acquired field map, respectively, for the 12 subjects. Only voxels within brain mask are considered. The mean, standard deviation, median, and 90th, 95th and 99th percentile values are reported. The bottom row contains column averages.

Mean (std)	Median	P90	P95	P99
0.86 (1.13)	0.57	1.83	2.64	5.34
1.16 (1.50)	0.68	2.68	3.78	7.15
0.98 (1.37)	0.55	2.30	3.36	6.29
0.89 (1.29)	0.48	2.08	3.03	5.97
1.00 (1.37)	0.63	2.16	3.19	6.24
0.77 (1.03)	0.50	1.60	2.25	4.74
0.93 (1.17)	0.60	1.98	2.80	5.67
0.94 (1.41)	0.49	2.12	3.21	7.06
1.35 (1.84)	0.80	2.94	4.22	9.03
1.06 (1.47)	0.65	2.36	3.33	6.83
1.23 (1.84)	0.60	2.99	4.33	9.50
0.95 (1.39)	0.56	2.10	3.13	6.44
1.01 (1.40)	0.59	2.26	3.27	6.69

displacement along the PE direction, as these are the units significant to the correction. Next, we calculated statistics for the difference between the simulated and acquired field maps. The results for the 12 subjects are reported in Table 1. For most of the brain, there is a close agreement. However, the differences follow a long-tailed distribution, so that in some areas, there are larger disagreements.

---

[2] As included in NiftyView (http://cmic.cs.ucl.ac.uk/home/software)

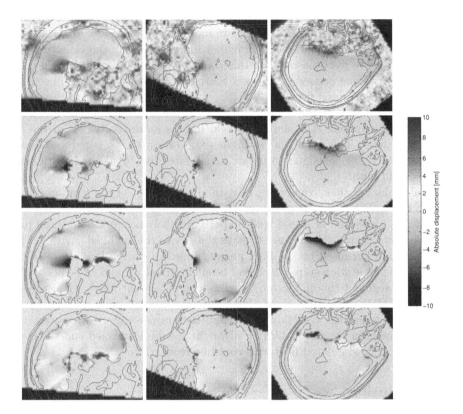

Fig. 3. Field maps expressed as mm of displacement along the phase-encode direction. The view is centered at the resection area of surgery. First row: A phase-wrapped acquired field map for a representative subject, showing a step change in phase value close to the resection margin. Second row: The acquired field map after phase-unwrapping. Only the volume inside the brain mask, as employed by the phase-unwrapping algorithm, is shown. Third row: A corresponding simulated field map (considered only inside the brain mask for fair comparison). Last row: The voxel-wise absolute difference between the simulated and the phase-unwrapped acquired field maps. Left to right: coronal, sagittal and axial sections, not coincident with anatomical planes due to intraoperative orientation of the head.

4   Discussion

Across the subjects, the simulated and acquired field maps on average differ by 1.01 ± 1.40 mm in the brain volume. This is within the voxel size of the DWI dataset (2.5 mm, which is typical for DW-MRI datasets). This number also has to be evaluated with respect to a desired resection accuracy, which is patient and surgeon specific and difficult to define. We believe that 1 mm resection accuracy in areas of low difference is clinically useful. However, since the difference between field maps follows a long-tailed distribution, we attempt to interpret the values of the field maps in areas of more significant difference to deduce where the simulated field maps are more correct, and vice versa.

We observe that the simulated field map is more positive in the vicinity of the resection area. We hypothesize that this could be due to an accumulated error in phase-unwrapping caused by the low SNR in this area and hence due to an underestimated acquired field map.

We observe that near the regions of signal dropout, as visible near the head-holder attachment pins, the simulated field map is more positive than the acquired field map. This is in line with the expectation to see a reduced phase evolution in regions of signal dropout and hence due to an underestimated acquired field map.

We also observe that, conversely, near the petrous part of the temporal bone in both hemispheres and anteriorly in the frontal lobe, the simulated field maps are 2–3 mm above the acquired field maps. This likely occurs because the proposed segmentation method overestimates the size of the air-filled cavities. This overestimation is caused by the high penalty imposed on the bone class in the EM/MRF segmentation step, which had been empirically found to be necessary, to robustly segment the craniotomy area as completely air-filled, when relying on the EM/MRF algorithm alone. Therefore, if it was possible to introduce a method to segment the resection cavity and the craniotomy area robustly, the penalty on bone in the the EM/MRF algorithm could be relaxed and the overestimation of the simulated field map could be reduced.

5   Conclusion

In summary, field map simulation is important for iMRI guided neurosurgery and in this study we have proposed a method that can achieve a close agreement between the simulated and acquired field maps for 12 patients. We suggest that in the future, simulated field maps could be used to regularize the phase-unwrapping of intraoperatively acquired field maps.

While our results are promising, a significant obstacle for intraoperative use of the proposed method is the computational time required to simulate the field map, currently above 20 minutes (Intel Core i5 @ 3.30 GHz). Therefore, a possible future work would be to explore methods to speed up the CT synthesis and field map calculation, for instance using GPU hardware.

Acknowledgements. This work was supported by the UCL Doctoral Training Programme in Medical and Biomedical Imaging studentship funded by the EPSRC. Danail Stoyanov would like to thank for the support of The Royal Academy of Engineering/EPSRC Research Fellowship. Sebastien Ourselin receives funding from the EPSRC (EP/H046410/1, EP/J020990/1, EP/K005278), the MRC (MR/J01107X/1), the EU-FP7 project VPH-DARE@IT (FP7-ICT-2011-9-601055), the NIHR Biomedical Research Unit (Dementia) at UCL and the National Institute for Health Research University College London Hospitals Biomedical Research Centre (NIHR BRC UCLH/UCL High Impact Initiative).

References

1. Nimsky, C., Ganslandt, O., Cerny, S., Hastreiter, P., Greiner, G., Fahlbusch, R.: Quantification of, visualization of, and compensation for brain shift using intraoperative magnetic resonance imaging. Neurosurgery 47(5), 1070–1080 (2000)
2. Daga, P., Winston, G., Modat, M., White, M., Mancini, L., Cardoso, M.J., Symms, M., Stretton, J., McEvoy, A.W., Thornton, J., Micallef, C., Yousry, T., Hawkes, D.J., Duncan, J.S., Ourselin, S.: Accurate Localization of Optic Radiation During Neurosurgery in an Interventional MRI Suite. IEEE Transactions on Medical Imaging 31(4), 882–891 (2012)
3. Clare, S., Evans, J., Jezzard, P.: Requirements for room temperature shimming of the human brain. Magn. Reson. Med. 55, 210–214 (2006)
4. Jezzard, P., Balaban, R.S.: Correction for geometric distortion in echo planar images from b0 field variations. Magn. Reson. Med. 34, 65–73 (1995)
5. Poynton, C., Jenkinson, M., Wells III, W.: Atlas-Based Improved Prediction of Magnetic Field Inhomogeneity for Distortion Correction of EPI Data. In: Yang, G.-Z., Hawkes, D., Rueckert, D., Noble, A., Taylor, C. (eds.) MICCAI 2009, Part II. LNCS, vol. 5762, pp. 951–959. Springer, Heidelberg (2009)
6. Jenkinson, M., Wilson, J.L., Jezzard, P.: Perturbation method for magnetic field calculations of nonconductive objects. Magnetic Resonance in Medicine 52(3), 471–477 (2004)
7. Hutton, C., Bork, A., Josephs, O., Deichmann, R., Ashburner, J., Turner, R.: Image distortion correction in fMRI: A quantitative evaluation. Neuroimage 16(1), 217–240 (2002)
8. Daga, P., Modat, M., Winston, G., White, M., Mancini, L., McEvoy, A.W., Thornton, J., Yousry, T., Duncan, J.S., Ourselin, S.: Susceptibility artefact correction by combining B0 field maps and non-rigid registration using graph cuts. In: SPIE Medical Imaging, International Society for Optics and Photonics, pp. 86690B–86690B (2013)
9. Cardoso, M.J., Clarkson, M.J., Ridgway, G.R., Modat, M., Fox, N.C., Ourselin, S.: Improved Maximum a Posteriori Cortical Segmentation by Iterative Relaxation of Priors. In: Yang, G.-Z., Hawkes, D., Rueckert, D., Noble, A., Taylor, C. (eds.) MICCAI 2009, Part II. LNCS, vol. 5762, pp. 441–449. Springer, Heidelberg (2009)
10. Burgos, N., et al.: Attenuation Correction Synthesis for Hybrid PET-MR Scanners. In: Mori, K., Sakuma, I., Sato, Y., Barillot, C., Navab, N. (eds.) MICCAI 2013, Part I. LNCS, vol. 8149, pp. 147–154. Springer, Heidelberg (2013)
11. Gruetter, R., Boesch, C.: Fast, noniterative shimming of spatially localized signals, In vivo analysis of the magnetic field along axes. Journal of Magnetic Resonance 96(2), 323–334 (1992)

Orientation-Driven Ultrasound Compounding Using Uncertainty Information

Christian Schulte zu Berge[1], Ankur Kapoor[2], and Nassir Navab[1]

[1] Chair for Computer Aided Medical Procedures
Technische Universität München, Munich, Germany
christian.szb@in.tum.de, nassir.navab@tum.de
[2] Imaging and Computer Vision,
Siemens Corporate Technology, Princeton, NJ, USA
ankur.kapoor@siemens.com

Abstract. Compounding 2D ultrasound sweeps into 3D volumes is, due to its cost- and time-efficiency, of great clinical significance in both diagnostic and interventional imaging. However, today's algorithms restrict the sweeps to have homogeneous pressure and a linear trajectory, which limits their use in clinical applications such as breast or musculoskeletal ultrasound where artifacts occur due to soft and uneven surfaces. In this work, we present two techniques to resolve those restrictions by using an orientation-driven approach, first compensating for probe pressure changes and then resolving ambiguities in regions, where multiple ultrasound frames from different acoustic windows overlap. After clustering incoming frames by orientation, we determine the final voxel intensities based on per-pixel uncertainty information. Qualitative and quantitative evaluation of our methods shows that these techniques provide reconstructions of superior quality for ultrasound sweeps of inhomogeneous pressure and twisted trajectories. Furthermore, we propose optimizations in the implementation of these techniques towards real-time applications, interactively updating and refining the reconstructed volume.

1 Introduction

Ultrasound spatial compounding is the reconstruction of 3D volumes from 2D ultrasound sweeps and has the potential to replace or extend current standard clinical procedures for several applications, such as breast cancer diagnosis and musculoskeletal (MSK) applications. Here, X-Ray does not only have the drawback of using ionizing radiation but also shows weak tissue contrast. MR imaging is rather slow, expensive and additionally restricts the patient to be in a position that might not be suited well for diagnostics. In contrast, ultrasound is relatively low-cost, portable, real-time capable and offers good soft tissue contrast.

Recent advances in tracking calibration and compounding algorithms have led to a significant increase in image quality of ultrasound compounding: Current ultrasound probe calibration methods achieve millimeter tracking-accuracy and the various spatial compounding algorithms offer different tradeoffs between algorithm complexity and quality of the compounded volume. As a consequence,

D. Stoyanov et al. (Eds.): IPCAI 2014, LNCS 8498, pp. 236–245, 2014.

ultrasound compounding is making its way into commercial products shaping the term 3D freehand ultrasound.

So far however, the term 3D freehand ultrasound promises more than it actually can deliver, since current methods implicitly assume constraints such as constant probe pressure and/or constant motion of the ultrasound transducer along a linear path. While this may be negligible for applications such as carotid ultrasound where the anatomy is easily accessible, breast and MSK applications have highly curved surfaces requiring reconstruction of twisted sweep trajectories.

Curved sweeps lead to a challenging issue during the spatial compounding process because some of the acquired ultrasound frames may overlap with each other. Due to the dynamics and high complexity of the ultrasound image formation being dependent on incident angle, probe pressure and patient positioning, ultrasound may yield different information (i.e. image intensities) for the same point within the anatomy if scanned from different perspectives or at different times. Our orientation-driven methods handle these ambiguities to result in more accurate 3D reconstructions than current state-of-the art methods.

2   Related Work

In [1] Solberg et al. provide an overview on different 3D ultrasound compounding techniques and identify three different classes of algorithms:

Pixel-based methods traverse the pixels in each 2D ultrasound frame, transform the pixel location into voxel coordinates and write the pixel's intensity information into the initially empty volume. Since multiple pixels might contribute to a single voxel, the final voxel value may be determined by averaging or using the maximum intensity of all contributing pixels.

Voxel-based methods work the other way around by traversing the voxel grid of the target volume and are thus also referred to as backward-warping methods. For each voxel, they compute the corresponding pixels of the nearby ultrasound frames and use a weighting function based on intensity and/or distance to determine the final voxel value. Wein et al. show in [2] that voxel-based methods yield superior quality and smaller computation time than pixel-based methods. Furthermore, backward-warping algorithms can easily be used to compute multi-planar reconstructions (MPR) from the original ultrasound images without computing the reconstructed volume before.

Finally, *function-based methods* estimate the coefficients for a set of locally supported basis functions to approximate the input data. These functions are then evaluated on the voxel grid to reconstruct the compounded volume [3,4]. Klein et al. [5] propose to use radio frequency (RF) data instead of reconstructed B-mode images and a finite mixture model to obtain reconstructions of higher quality and address the view-dependency of ultrasound. While these methods yield 3D ultrasound reconstructions of very high quality, they are currently not feasible for clinical practice due to being computationally expensive.

To compensate for probe pressure changes, Treece et al. use an image-based non-rigid registration technique [6]. By computing the line-wise maximum normalized correlation between two adjacent B-mode images and applying a monotonicity constraint they estimate the deformation in depth introduced by the probe pressure. To avoid drift in the registration they constrain the registration results to the tracking. However, regularization will fail in case of inaccurate calibration of the ultrasound probe, especially in the error-sensitive rotational part.

3   Methods

3.1   Inter-frame Registration and Pressure Compensation

To correct for errors and inaccuracies in the tracking data (e.g. due to inaccurate calibration or patient movement), as well as for artifacts due to probe pressure changes, we propose an orientation-driven inter-frame registration technique:

Similar to Treece et al. [6], we perform an intensity-based registration between adjacent ultrasound frames. Using a simple and thus real-time capable pixel-wise uphill search evaluating the SSD, each ultrasound frame is registered to its surrounding frames independently in terms of in-plane translation and in-plane rotation. However, we perform the regularization by registering each ultrasound frame to a window W of surrounding frames. This ensures to compensate for drift independently of the tracking calibration accuracy.

Since the correlation between two ultrasound frames does not only depend on their proximity but also on their orientation to each other [7], we determine the weights for the frames in W by a combination of a Gaussian kernel of size N and a term C, which describes the orientation-based correlation between two images. For a given reference patch P and equally sized moving patch P' the windowed SSD (wSSD) is given by

$$\text{wSSD}_{P,P',N}(i) = \sum_{\substack{p \in P, \\ p' \in P'}} \sum_{n=-N}^{N} C(i, i+n) \cdot e^{\frac{n^2}{2\sigma^2}} \cdot \left(I_i(p) - I_{i+n}(p')\right)^2 \quad (1)$$

where i is the index of the reference frame and $I_i(p)$ denotes the image intensity of ultrasound frame i at the position p. The correlation term $C(i, j)$ for frames i and j is defined by the cosine distance of their normals n_i, n_j to model the decreasing correlation between frames of increasing orientation difference:

$$C(i, j) := 1 - \frac{2}{\pi} \cdot \text{acos}\left(\frac{n_i \cdot n_j}{\|n_i\|\|n_j\|}\right) \quad (2)$$

To compensate for probe pressure artifacts, our method applies the above inter-frame registration technique not only to a single patch, but to a grid of independent patches of 1cm × 1cm size. Since we expect the deformation to be orthogonal to the skin surface, our model allows free in-plane movement of the patches to be flexible enough to allow both linear and curvilinear probes. After computing the transformation for each patch as above, we set the transformation of the central patch as rigid part and the difference to the other patches as deformation field. The results can be seen in Fig. 1.

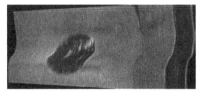
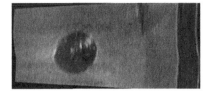

(a) No pressure compensation   (b) With pressure compensation

Fig. 1. Reconstruction of an abdominal phantom scan with probe pressure changes: (a) MPR through the compounded volume without applying our pressure compensation technique; (b) the same MPR through the compounded volume with pressure compensation applied

3.2 Compounding of Non-homogeneous Sweeps

In a tortuous acquisition sweep parts of the ultrasound frames overlap and may show different information for the same anatomy depending on the viewing angle. Here, classical ultrasound compounding techniques with averaging or distance-based weighting fail in correctly reconstructing such regions:

Given a set of ultrasound frames from different angles that all intersect near our target voxel to reconstruct as depicted in Fig. 2. Standard compounding algorithms such as [2] take the closest pixels in each ultrasound frame and determine the final voxel intensity based on a weighting function usually preferring closer pixel over pixels being farther away, hence the closest ultrasound frame has the highest influence. If we now consider a neighbor voxel, the closest frame may have a completely different orientation and thus show different information (due to the view dependency of ultrasound). This yields to artifacts in the compounded volume as depicted in Fig. 3a.

Furthermore, distance-based weighting can lead to incorrect reconstruction since the distance of the frame to the voxel has no correlation with the amount of information present in this pixel (i.e. level of uncertainty/noise). For instance, it may ignore a pixel being farther away but having low uncertainty and instead prefer a high uncertainty pixel (i.e. noise) because it is closer to the voxel.

Our orientation-driven ultrasound compounding technique tackles these issues by exploiting additional uncertainty information using a two-step approach. Our method assumes that for each ultrasound pixel with intensity I_i, we also have an uncertainty value u_i that we later use for weighting the image intensities. While the actual method is independent from it, we use for our implementation the attenuation maps proposed by Karamalis et al. [8]. Even though they model ultrasound physics only to a limited amount, their attenuation maps can be interpreted as uncertainty information.

Clustering of the Ultrasound Sweep by Direction: As a first step, we perform a hierarchical clustering to identify tortuous sweep trajectories and regions of overlapping ultrasound frames. This partitions the ultrasound sweep

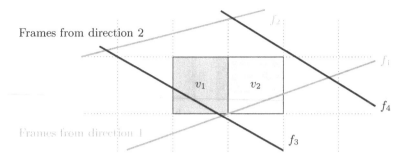

Fig. 2. Illustration of artifacts occurring in distance-weighted compounded regions where multiple ultrasound frames from different angles intersect. The intensity of voxel v_1 will be mainly influenced by the information of frame f_3 while the intensity of neigbour voxel v_2 will be mainly influenced by the information in frame f_1. Since the frames travel through different acoustic windows, the information at this spatial location may significantly differ.

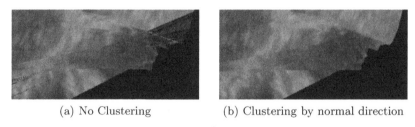

(a) No Clustering   (b) Clustering by normal direction

Fig. 3. Effect on the clustering of ultrasound frames by normal direction: (a) shows a compounding of a twisted ultrasound sweep with artifacts caused by the filtering based on the distance to the voxel. (b) shows a compounding of the same sweep with our clustering technique applied.

trajectory into parts where the frames have homogeneous orientation without requiring us to predefine the number of clusters. We apply an average group linkage algorithm using cosine distance to the normals of the ultrasound frames Eq. (2). This yields a set of sub-sweeps meeting the usual restriction of being contiguous and uniformly oriented.

A backward-warping algorithm then compounds each cluster c into a 3D volume applying our pressure compensation method as discussed in Section 3.1. Since the ultrasound frames of each cluster are guaranteed to have the same orientation and are thus travelling through the same acoustic window, we can safely assume the distributions of uncertainty within the frame to be homogeneous within nearby frames. We compute the intensity for voxel x as

$$I_c(x) = \frac{\sum_{i \in S} I_i \cdot d_i^{-\mu}}{\sum_{i \in S} d_i^{-\mu}} \tag{3}$$

where S is the set of frame pixels close to the compounded voxel x, d_i the Euclidean distance of pixel i to the compounded voxel and $\mu > 1$ a smoothness parameter ensuring that $I_c(x)$ approximates the original data for $d_i \to 0$ [9]. Furthermore, we propagate the uncertainty to the 3D volume using the same weighting:

$$U_c(x) = \frac{\sum_{i \in S} u_i \cdot d_i^{-\mu}}{\sum_{i \in S} d_i^{-\mu}} \tag{4}$$

Uncertainty-Based Fusion of the Compounded Clusters: Since ultrasound image formation is a highly non-linear process and the pixel-based uncertainty values u_i are relative to the image content and thus not necessarily comparable between different frames, we perform the uncertainty-based fusion in a second step to avoid artifacts such as the ones depicted in Fig. 3a. In this second step our method fuses clusters into the final 3D volume based on the propagated uncertainty values. Let C be the set of clusters, then the final intensity I at voxel x is given by

$$I(x) = \frac{\sum_{c \in C} (1 - U_c(x)) I_c(x)}{\sum_{c \in C} 1 - U_c(x)} \tag{5}$$

4   Implementation

Our implementation of orientation-driven ultrasound compounding employs several optimizations to allow real-time applications such as an interactive update and refinement of the compounded volume: The regularized inter-frame registration needs only a limited number of frames lookahead (i.e. size of the regularization window) and can hence be performed on-line as well as the clustering by orientation, which simply starts a new cluster as soon as the cosine distance is beyond the threshold.

Our incremental compounding adapts the two-step compounding of multiple clusters to an in-place algorithm. Instead of reconstructing a separate volume for each cluster, we use a single volume as accumulation buffer. The reconstructed voxels of each cluster can be incrementally added by rewriting equation 5 to a recurrence scheme, to gain a significantly lower complexity and memory footprint: Given the voxel intensity I_{i-1} and uncertainty U_{i-1} of the previous runs and I_c, U_c of the current run, we define the new intensity I_i and uncertainty U_i as:

$$I_i = \frac{U_{i-1} I_{i-1} + (1 - U_c) I_c}{U_{i-1} + (1 - U_c)}, \quad U_i = U_{i-1} + (1 - U_c) \tag{6}$$

The incremental compounding technique is further accelerated by using an intermediate lookup structure for the backward-warping: Each ultrasound frame is sampled into a lower resolution brick structure using a scanline voxelization technique as an efficient sampling method. Similar to scanline rasterization in Computer Graphics, we compute the coordinates of the four corners of the frame,

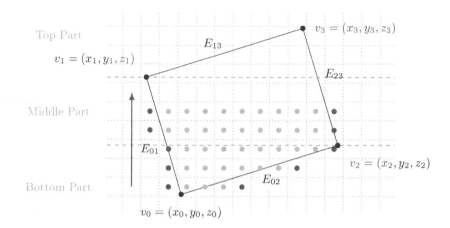

Fig. 4. Illustration of the scanline voxelization scheme (for simplicity in 2D): Starting at the bottom-most scanline around v_0, we compute the left-most and right-most voxel covered by the ultrasound frame. Using the slope of the edges $E_{02} = E_{13}$ and $E_{01} = E_{23}$ we can incrementally compute the start- and end-voxel for the next scanline by simple additions. The increments have to be changed when advancing beyond v_1 resp. v_2 (advancing to middle/top part).

define a scanline axis and sort the corners along the axis. Exploiting the rectangularness of the image, we can compute the increments (i.e. slopes) along the other two axes for one step along the scanline axis. Iterating brick-wise along the scanline axis, we can compute all bricks touched by the frame using simple additions as depicted in Fig. 4. The brick structure can then be used to accelerate the lookup of all ultrasound frames close to a voxel.

5   Evaluation and Results

To evaluate our methods, we used an ACUSON S2000^{TM} ultrasound machine equipped with an Acuson 9L4 linear transducer and Ascension trakSTAR^{TM}2 electromagnetic tracking hardware being calibrated as described in [10].

To confirm the physically correct reconstruction of anatomy, we acquired ultrasound sweeps of an abdominal phantom including a tumor target of spherical shape as depicted in Fig. 1. We computed 50 MPRs of arbitrary orientation through the target and compared the maximum diameter with measurements acquired from CT: The reconstructed ultrasound volume yielded an average target diameter of 14.63 ± 0.48 mm compared to 14.5 ± 0.84 mm in CT. Since the target is positioned relatively close to the surface, it can be scanned from different directions and is prone to deformation, hence being a relevant scenario to evaluate our method.

The effects of our inter-frame registration and pressure compensation technique can be observed in Fig. 1 showing the reconstructions of an ultrasound sweep through the abdominal phantom: Due to the probe pressure changes the

MPR through the reference volume (a) shows deformation of the originally round target. Our techniques restore the original shape, seen in (b) showing the same MPR through the volume compounded with pressure compensation.

Figure 3 shows the effect of our clustering technique when reconstructing a twisted ultrasound sweep of human shoulder. Due to the overlapping frames the baseline compounding in (a) shows artifacts because the closest frames for neighboring voxels may be acquired from different angles. The reconstruction in (b) uses our clustering technique to avoid overlapping frames and the occurring artifacts and additionally exploits uncertainty information when fusing the clusters so that unreliable intensities do not bias the final result.

Table 1. NCC and log-scale SNR in the overlapping region after registering the two compounded volumes of two sweeps with perpendicular trajectories of the same anatomy

	Baseline [2]		Our technique	
	NCC	SNR_{dB}	NCC	SNR_{dB}
Phantom / constant pressure	0.90	19.39	0.94	23.16
Phantom / pressure changes	0.81	13.02	**0.94**	**22.47**
In-vivo leg / constant changes	0.72	9.21	0.76	11.69
In-vivo leg / pressure changes	0.67	8.53	**0.75**	**11.03**

For quantitative evaluation we acquired pairs of overlapping sweeps with perpendicular main trajectory of both phantom and in-vivo data. After compounding the sweeps into separate 3D volumes using our methods, we applied a 3D-3D rigid registration using the tracking data as initialization. Expecting our techniques to yield better matching volumes, we compared their differences in the overlapping region with the baseline method (standard backward-compounding and no pressure compensation as described in [2]). With the average of the two volumes as expected result for a correct reconstruction, we quantify their difference in Normalized Cross-Correlation (NCC) and log-scale Signal to Noise Ratio (SNR_{dB}), for which define the signal as average of the volumes and the noise as RMS of the differences (Table 1). The sweeps with pressure changes show a significant improvement in terms of increase in both NCC and SNR_{dB} when our technique is applied. Furthermore, when comparing constant pressure with pressure changes, our technique shows significantly less drop of the measures. The slight improvements for the sweeps acquired with constant pressure are mainly due to the inter-frame registration correcting for the tracking error. Since the sweeps are acquired with perpendicular trajectories and the volumes therefore show different interpretations of the underlying data, no algorithm yields a perfect match. Furthermore, the in-vivo sweeps are expected to have lower similarity since they show by far less homogeneous anatomy. Figure 5 shows the difference images for the second phantom sweep.

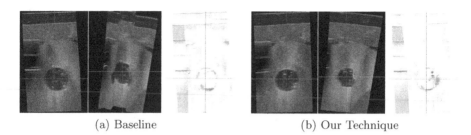

(a) Baseline   (b) Our Technique

Fig. 5. Illustration of our evaluation method: First two images show the MPRs for each perpendicular sweep, the third one shows the squared difference of their intensities after 3D-3D rigid registration. (a) traditional backward-compounding fails to align the different structures; (b) our technique yields alignment of all structures. The quantitative results are shown in Table 1.

6   Discussion and Conclusion

In this work, we presented a novel orientation-driven approach to allow 3D free-hand ultrasound for a broader range of clinical applications. Typical acquisition sweeps in breast or musculoskeletal (MSK) ultrasound have pressure changes, back- and forth or twisting motion, which are not handled well by current state-of-the-art methods yielding artifacts for regions where the frames overlap. We cluster the ultrasound frames based on orientation and proximity and thereby guarantee that no frames in a cluster overlap. We further use per-pixel uncertainty information when fusing the clusters into the compounded volume, which yields more accurate reconstructions in places where we have information from different acoustic windows, because intensities from uncertain regions do not affect reliable intensities. Our method for probe pressure compensation uses a similar inter-frame registration approach as [6] but also incorporates the orientation of the frames to each other and uses a regularization independent from the tracking calibration quality.

Since the evaluation of our methods shows very good results for the reconstruction of non-homogeneous ultrasound sweeps, the question arises why our two-step compounding approach of first clustering by frame orientation and then fusing based on uncertainty information is superior to a classical one-step approach. We assume that the low signal-to-noise ratio of ultrasound, its high view-dependency and thus very limited consistency in time and movement sets the main challenge when compounding non-homogeneous ultrasound sweeps. Our orientation-driven two-step compounding technique introduces an additional interpolation step and thus compensates better for those highly non-linear effects. By exploiting uncertainty information we ensure that this additional interpolation does not impair the final image quality but even improves the result in regions where we have inconsistent image information from different acoustic windows. Also other applications [11] have shown the benefit of this uncertainty based approach to information fusion.

3D freehand ultrasound has a wide band of applications in both diagnostic and interventional imaging. Our work allows high quality reconstructions also in applications such as breast or MSK where soft and uneven surfaces lead to sweeps of non-homogeneous pressure and non-linear trajectory. Our implementation shows optimizations to stream-line our methods to allow real-time applications where the compounded volume gets updated and refined interactively during the acquisition, providing the clinician with direct feedback. Hence, we believe that our orientation-driven methods will have a significant impact in bringing ultrasound compounding further to clinical applications.

References

1. Solberg, O.V., Lindseth, F., Torp, H., Blake, R.E., Hernes, T.A.N.: Freehand 3d ultrasound reconstruction algorithms - a review. Ultrasound in Medicine & Biology 33(7), 991–1009 (2007)
2. Wein, W., Pache, F., Röper, B., Navab, N.: Backward-warping ultrasound reconstruction for improving diagnostic value and registration. In: Larsen, R., Nielsen, M., Sporring, J. (eds.) MICCAI 2006. LNCS, vol. 4191, pp. 750–757. Springer, Heidelberg (2006)
3. Rohling, R., Gee, A., Berman, L.: A comparison of freehand three-dimensional ultrasound reconstruction techniques. Medical Image Analysis 3(4), 339–359 (1999)
4. Sanches, J.M., Marques, J.S.: A multiscale algorithm for three-dimensional freehand ultrasound. Ultrasound in Medicine & Biology 28(8), 1029–1040 (2002)
5. Klein, T., Hansson, M., Navab, N.: Modeling of multi-view 3d freehand radio frequency ultrasound. In: Ayache, N., Delingette, H., Golland, P., Mori, K. (eds.) MICCAI 2012, Part I. LNCS, vol. 7510, pp. 422–429. Springer, Heidelberg (2012)
6. Treece, G., Prager, R., Gee, A., Berman, L.: Correction of probe pressure artifacts in freehand 3d ultrasound. Medical Image Analysis 6(3), 199–214 (2002), Special Issue on Medical Image Computing and Computer-Assisted Intervention 2001
7. Housden, R.J., Gee, A.H., Treece, G.M., Prager, R.W.: Sensorless reconstruction of unconstrained freehand 3d ultrasound data. Ultrasound in Medicine & Biology 33(3), 408–419 (2007)
8. Karamalis, A., Wein, W., Klein, T., Navab, N.: Ultrasound confidence maps using random walks. Medical Image Analysis 16(6), 1101–1112 (2012)
9. Shepard, D.: A two-dimensional interpolation function for irregularly-spaced data. In: Proceedings of the 1968 23rd ACM National Conference, ACM 1968, pp. 517–524. ACM, New York (1968)
10. Wein, W., Khamene, A.: Image-based method for in-vivo freehand ultrasound calibration. In: SPIE Medical Imaging 2008, San Diego (February 2008)
11. Comaniciu, D., Zhou, X.S., Krishnan, S.: Robust real-time myocardial border tracking for echocardiography: an information fusion approach. IEEE Transactions on Medical Imaging 23(7), 849–860 (2004)

2D/3D Catheter-Based Registration for Image Guidance in TACE of Liver Tumors

Pierre Ambrosini[1], Danny Ruijters[2], Adriaan Moelker[3], Wiro J. Niessen[1,4], and Theo van Walsum[1]

[1] Biomedical Imaging Group Rotterdam,
Department of Radiology and Medical Informatics,
Erasmus MC, Rotterdam, The Netherlands
`p.ambrosini@erasmusmc.nl`
[2] Philips Healthcare, Interventional X-ray Innovation, Best, The Netherlands
[3] Department of Radiology, Erasmus MC, Rotterdam, The Netherlands
[4] Imaging Science and Technology, Faculty of Applied Sciences,
Delft University of Technology, Delft, The Netherlands

Abstract. Image fusion of liver 2D X-ray images and pre or peri-operative 3D reconstructions can add valuable contextual information during image guided interventions. Such image fusion requires 2D/3D registration. In abdominal interventions, such as TACE of liver tumors, the initial alignment may be invalidated by e.g. breathing motion. We present a method that maintains the alignment between 3D Rotational Angiography (3DRA) and 2D X-ray, using the catheter position. To this end, we use the catheter in the 2D X-ray and the blood vessels in the 3DRA, then fuse 2D/3D using the knowledge that the catheter is inside the vessels. The registration is performed in two steps: First, we use a shape constraint to determine the most likely catheter positions inside the blood vessel tree. Next, we perform a rigid registration and take the best transformation over all previous selected catheter positions. The method is evaluated on phantom, clinical and simulated data.

Keywords: 2D/3D, Rigid, Catheter, Registration, Guidance, X-ray, Fluoroscopy, 3DRA, Abdominal, TACE, Liver, Breathing, Compensation.

1 Introduction

Minimally invasive procedures are more and more common in medical intervention. They enable procedures with minimal trauma for the patient. Image guidance is essential for minimally invasive procedures. However, common interventional modalities, such as intra-operative 2D X-ray imaging and 2D/3D ultrasound have limitations: X-ray imaging using ionizing radiation is a projection technique, and requires contrast agent to visualize vasculature. Ultrasound imaging is operator-dependent, and hard to interprete. Integration of information from 3D (pre or peri-operative) modalities to improve the image guidance may therefore be a useful strategy in minimally invasive interventions. This requires fusion of the intra-operative images with the pre or peri-operative images,

D. Stoyanov et al. (Eds.): IPCAI 2014, LNCS 8498, pp. 246–255, 2014.

which is often performed using image registration. After an initial alignment of the 3D image to the interventional situation, patient motion or breathing may invalidate the alignment. The purpose of our work is to develop and evaluate a method to maintain this alignment in TACE procedures.

Transcatheter Arterial ChemoEmbolization (TACE) is a minimal invasive procedure to treat liver cancer (mostly Hepatocellular Carcinoma). In these procedures, a catheter is navigated towards a tumor via the femoral and hepatic artery, after which chemotherapeutic agents are injected. Currently, the interventionist guides the catheter using single plane 2D X-ray (fluoroscopy), mainly visualizing only the catheter (Fig. 1). Frequently, angiographies (2D X-ray imaging with contrast agent injection) are acquired to visualize the arteries. CTA is used pre-operatively to visualize the tumors and feedings arteries. The navigation of the catheter using only 2D fluoroscopy is hampered by the inability to continuously visualize the arterial tree.

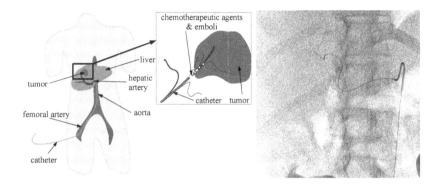

Fig. 1. (left) TACE overview. (right) Fluoroscopy example.

Fusion of the tumor and arterial tree from CTA (or from 3DRA) may greatly facilitate the navigation of the catheter to the tumor. There have been many reports on 2D/3D registration approaches to integrate 3D information in X-ray guided interventions. These approaches were described for example for abdominal [1–3], cardiac [4, 5] and neuro-vascular [6] cases (see [7, 8] for a thorough review). Most methods proposed for abdominal applications perform 2D/3D registration with single plane or bi-plane 2D intra-operative angiography and 3D pre-operative CTA [1–3]. [9] developped a semi-automatic respiratory motion tracking method using a small part of the catheter. In [6, 9], peri-operative 3DRA was used instead of pre-operative CTA, to register with 2D X-ray images using the calibrated geometry of the C-arm. Thus, the initial alignment is accurate and based only on the C-arm position, which is known.

Our method is also based on this initial alignment. However in abdominal intervention, breathing, patient and table motion lead to misalignments. We propose a novel approach for maintaining the registration and thus a spatially

aligned roadmap. Such an approach may facilitate catheter navigation and reduce contrast agent use during intervention. Unlike most methods, 2D angiographies are not required and registration is performed for each frame independently
and fully automatically. Our method uses the centerlines of the arterial tree that
are extracted from a 3DRA image (acquired at the start of the intervention),
and the complete cathether shape/position from the single plane fluoroscopic
images. The registration uses the projection of the 3D blood vessel tree with
the extracted 2D catheter shape (Fig. 2). In this work, we focus on keeping the
2D/3D alignment up-to-date. Both the arterial tree extraction (which is relatively easy given the high contrast in the 3DRA), and the real-time catheter
detection, which may still be challenging [10] are not discussed here.

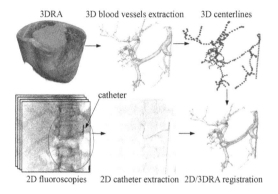

Fig. 2. Global overview

2   Methods

The registration method consists of two stages. The first stage uses a shape
constraint to rank the potential vessels in the blood vessel tree to locate the
most likely position of the catheter. The second stage aligns the catheter in 2D
with the potential vessels that result from the previous stage. In the following,
we give definitions, followed by the details of each stage.

2.1   Definitions

We define the following coordinate systems (CS) for our setup in the intervention
room:

- CS_w, the world 3D CS, located at the iso-center of the C-arm, and oriented
  along the C-arm in its default position
- $CS_{detector}$, the detector 3D CS (X-ray image plane)
- CS_{fluoro}, is the 2D CS of the fluoroscopic image
- CS_{3DRA}, 3D CS of the 3DRA

Accordingly, the following coordinate transforms are defined:

- $T_{\text{detector}\leftarrow\text{w}}$, transform matrix from the world 3D CS to the detector 3D CS
- T_{proj}, cone-beam projection matrix from CS_{detector} to CS_{fluoro}
- $T_{\text{w}\leftarrow\text{3DRA}}$, transform matrix from the 3DRA 3D CS to the world 3D CS
- T_{motion}, transform matrix of the breathing and the patient motion in the world 3D CS, CS_{w}

$T_{\text{detector}\leftarrow\text{w}}$ and T_{proj} are assumed to be known for the X-ray images because of the known geometry and orientation of the C-arm. $T_{\text{w}\leftarrow\text{3DRA}}$ is the identity because the 3D acquisition is around the iso-center of the C-arm. T_{motion} will be the result of our registration.

It then follows that a 3D point in the 3DRA, $p_{\text{CS}_{\text{3DRA}}}$, can be projected on CS_{fluoro} using the following equation (in homogeneous coordinates):

$$p_{\text{CS}_{\text{fluoro}}} = T_{\text{proj}}.T_{\text{detector}\leftarrow\text{w}}.T_{\text{motion}}.T_{\text{w}\leftarrow\text{3DRA}}.p_{\text{CS}_{\text{3DRA}}} \qquad (1)$$

The catheter is defined as an ordered set of N points:

$$C_{\text{2D}} = \{c_1, c_2, ...c_i, ..., c_N\}$$

where $c_i \in \mathbb{R}^2$ is a 2D point at the center of the catheter in CS_{fluoro}. Note that c_1 is the tip of the catheter.

The blood vessel tree extracted from 3DRA is represented as a directed tree:

$$G_{\text{3D}} = (V, E)$$

where V is the set of 3D points of the centerlines in CS_{3DRA} and E the set of directed edges between points.

2.2 Vessel Selection Based on Shape Similarity

Given the complexity of the blood vessel tree, we first select the most likely matching vessels for registration. To achieve this, we rank all possible vessels of G_{3D}. One vessel is a set of points starting from any location in the tree G_{3D} to its root. The ranking is based on shape similarity between the 2D catheter and the 2D projection of the 3D blood vessel path; we use the following metric for the shape similarity S:

$$S = \int_0^l \overrightarrow{C}_{\text{2D}}(u).\overrightarrow{f}(S_{\text{3D}}(u))\mathrm{d}u \qquad (2)$$

where l is the length of the 2D catheter, S_{3D} is one vessel from G_{3D} and f is the 2D projection $f = T_{\text{proj}}.T_{\text{detector}\leftarrow\text{w}}.T_{\text{w}\leftarrow\text{3DRA}}$.

This shape similarity metric integrates the 'alignment' of both structures (based on the dot-product of their direction vectors). The resulting value is in the range $[0, 1]$, and a high value implies a good match. This metric is not robust to large rotational motions, as those will change the orientation. As we are focusing on correcting for breathing motion, we expect the rotational motion to be small, and thus this metric should be sufficient. After computing the shape similarity for all possible vessels, the K best ranking vessels are used in the subsequent registration.

2.3   Rigid 2D/3D Registration with Forward Projection

To match the 2D catheter with the vessels, we need to find the rigid transform T_{motion} in CS_{w} that yields the best match with the 2D catheter in CS_{fluoro}. We decompose the transformation as follows:

$$T_{\text{motion}} = T_{\text{w}\leftarrow\text{detector}}.T_{\text{translation}}.T_{\text{detector}\leftarrow\text{w}}.T_{\text{rotation}}$$

where T_{rotation} is a rotation matrix with three unknowns (Euler angles, α, β and γ) and $T_{\text{translation}}$ is a translation matrix with three unknowns (x, y, z), where the translations are aligned with CS_{detector}. A translation along the projection axis in CS_{detector} will only have a very minor effect in the projection. We therefore exclude z from the registration parameters, leaving us with a five degrees of freedom transformation.

The distance metric we use is based on the distances in CS_{fluoro}. It is the sum of the minimal distance between each point of the catheter and any point of the current 3D selected vessel:

$$Dist(c, S, t) = \min_{s \in S} ||c - f(s,t)|| \tag{3}$$

where $c \in \mathbb{R}^2$, S is a vessel, t is a rigid transformation matrix and $f(s,t) = T_{\text{proj}}.T_{\text{detector}\leftarrow\text{w}}.t.T_{\text{w}\leftarrow\text{3DRA}}.s$.

The final transformation is the one with the smallest cumulative distance metric.

$$T_{\text{motion}} = \arg\min_{t \in T} \sum_{c \in C_{\text{2D}}} Dist(c, S_{\text{3D}}^{\text{sel}}, t) \tag{4}$$

where T is the set of possible rigid transformation matrices and $S_{\text{3D}}^{\text{sel}}$ is one of the K best ranking selected vessels from G.

We apply a brute force search for the optimum over the five unknowns search space, which is feasible as the search space is small in case of breathing motion. The registration is performed among the K selected vessels and we keep the one with the smallest distance metric.

3   Experiments and Results

To evaluate the accuracy and the robustness of our method, we propose three experiments: one on phantom data, one with clinical data and the last one with clinical data and simulated catheter positions (therefore with a ground truth).

3.1   Parameters

We set the intervals of our brute force search to ± 50 mm (with 0.2 mm step) for x and y and $\pm 7°$ (with 0.05° step) for α, β and γ. These intervals are sufficiently large to capture breathing motion. K is set to 5. The computation time is less than one minute for each frame.

3.2   Phantom Acquisition

In the first experiment, we evaluate the method in the context of ideal data. To this end, we used two rigid phantoms (Fig. 3): a heart phantom with coronary arteries and one made of copper wire. We acquired 3DRA images of these phantoms and subsequently we acquired fluoroscopic images: 10 and 21 images for the heart and copper phantom, respectively. Each image has a different C-arm angle either in propeller or in roll positions. The intervention table and the phantoms were fixed, thus the relation between the 3DRA and the fluoroscopy is given by the positioning information of the C-arm system. Next, we registered the X-ray images to the 3DRA. In order to provide an impression of the registration accuracy, for each frame, the median of the remaining distances (Eq. 3) is presented in Fig. 3 : $Dist(c, S_{3D}^{best}, T_{motion})$ for each $c \in C_{2D}$ where S_{3D}^{best} is the best registered vessel from the K best ranking selected vessels. As we do not use calibrated angles of the C-arm, we observe an offset before the registration. The offset is much larger with the second phantom. This is caused by different C-arm motions (roll and propeller) during 3DRA and fluoroscopy acquisition.

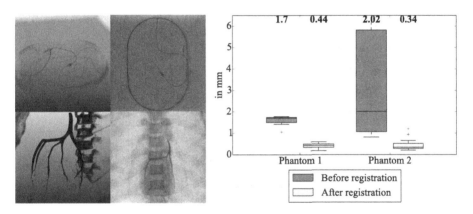

Fig. 3. (left) 3DRAs and fluoroscopies of both phantoms. (right) Medians of the distances between 2D catheter points and 2D projected 3D vessels points, for every segmented frames.

3.3   Clinical Data

In the next experiment we evaluate the performance of the method with clinical data. To this end, we retrospectively acquired image data from 13 TACE procedures. For each TACE procedure, we have one 3DRA acquired during the inhalation phase when the catheter is in the left or right hepatic artery and several (from 1 to 15) X-ray sequences. In total, we acquired 101 X-ray sequences. In each sequence, we segmented the catheter manually in three frames: one in inhale, one in exhale and one in-between. We applied our registration approach on each of these 303 frames, using the C-arm information and the initial position of the 3DRA. We report the median of the distances between the catheter points and the best vessel points (Eq. 3), and also visually inspected the results.

Figure 4 shows the results of the registration on clinical data. In all except two cases, the median of the distances, for each patient, is below 1 mm. In the case of one patient, the 3DRA image is of low quality, and parts of the vasculature are missing, especially the hepatic and aorta. For the other patient with a larger median distance, the 3DRA acquisition was not correctly centered on the liver, so part of the hepatic and aorta are not in the 3DRA. We obtained the following medians of the average of the distances (Eq. 3): 1.35 mm, 1.45 mm and 1.78 mm for 'inhale', 'in-between' and 'exhale', respectively. Unlike medians in Fig. 4, averages point out differences between the breathing states. The medians of the average of the distances close to the tip (10% of the catheter) are: 1.46 mm, 1.59 mm and 1.54 mm. When we visually checked the registrations, in 71% of the cases, the correct vessel was registered (Fig. 5). In the other cases, the registration was incorrect: 58% due to 3DRA misacquisition and 20% due to large catheter deformation.

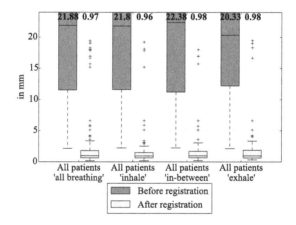

Fig. 4. Medians of the distances between 2D catheter points and 2D projected 3D vessels points, for every segmented frames

3.4   Clinical Data with a Simulated Catheter

Finally, we used the same clinical images to generate synthetic data for which we have a ground truth. We used all clinically acquired 3DRAs, but instead of using fluoroscopies and a manually segmented catheter, we annotated an artificial catheter in the 3DRA vasculature (using the registered vessel from previous results of clinical data) and then project it as 2D curve onto the fluoroscopic image, using the C-arm settings. To achieve this, we used the set of frames at inhale (101 images). Additionally, we simulated the stretching behaviour of the catheter by applying a Gaussian kernel smoothing on the 3D annotated catheter curve

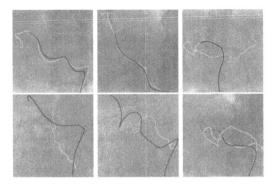

Fig. 5. Registration of the catheter (red) and the best registered vessel (green). (top) Successful registrations. (bottom) Missed registrations. (bottom-left) 3D arterial tree segmentation misses too many vessels (aorta and hepatic artery). (bottom-middle) 3D arterial tree misses the aorta. (bottom-right) The distance metric does not take into account the vessel continuity.

Table 1. Parameter randomizations of the simulations

	Slight	Moderate	Large
Translation x (in mm)	[-30, 30]	[-30, 30]	[-30, 30]
Translation y (in mm)	[-20, 20]	[-40, -20]∪[20, 40]	[-50, -40]∪[40, 50]
Translation z (in mm)	[-30, 30]	[-30, 30]	[-30, 30]
Rotation α, β, γ (in °)	[-6, 6]	[-6, 6]	[-6, 6]
Catheter smoothing σ	[1, 5]	[5, 10]	[10, 15]

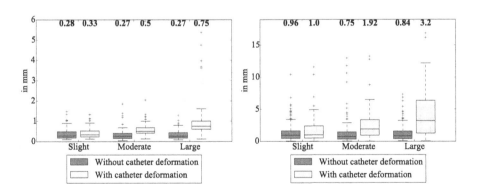

Fig. 6. (left) Medians of the distances between 2D catheter points and 2D projected 3D vessels points, for every segmented frames, after registration. (right) Distance between the real tip and the registered tip after registration.

and we applied different random translations and rotations for the transformation T_{motion}. We performed three simulations (slight, moderate and large) of breathing and deformations (Table 1). Breathing is done along the axis y.

Table 2. Percentage of tips inside the registered vessel

No catheter deformation			With catheter deformation		
Slight	Moderate	Large	Slight	Moderate	Large
88%	89%	92%	82%	89%	81%

As we know the exact position of the catheter, we can compute the distance between the real 2D catheter position and the 2D catheter position obtained by applying the registration result T_{motion}, and for the tip as well. Figure 6 shows these distances. We also report whether the registered vessel contains the catheter (Table 2).

4   Discussion

We presented and evaluated a method that is able to maintain alignment of liver vascular roadmaps in the presence of patient breathing, using a vessel selection and rigid registration approach. We evaluated the method on phantom, clinical and simulated data. The median distances between catheter and vessel centerlines are below 1 mm for most cases. For the simulated data, the median of the tip position accuracy is below 2 mm, except when the catheter has a large deformation. Most of the registrations have small (< 1 mm) median distances, which demonstrates that the approach we propose is feasible. In addition, the third experiment, where the catheter does not exactly match the vasculature, demonstrated that the method is robust to deformations and relatively large displacements. However, the last experiment also demonstrated that a large deformation may lead to incorrect vessel selection. Furthermore, this experiment indicated that registration distance below 1 mm does not imply a tip position below 1 mm. Failure in accurate registration for the real patient data was often caused by insufficient quality (missing vessels) of the 3DRA data. This underlines the need of adequate imaging for our proposed approach.

Based on these results, we are considering several improvements. Firstly, adding temporal and contextual knowledge may reduce large misregistrations caused by incorrect vessel selections. Indeed, a catheter is more likely to be in the vessel that was used in previous registrations, especially in the case of slight catheter movement. Secondly, during the procedure, as the tip position is more important than the proximal part of the catheter, more weighting the registration result close to the tip may be relevant to improve the accuracy of the roadmap near the tip. Utilizing temporal information may also be beneficial here. Also, a real-time method should be achieved with advanced optimizers, the use of GPU and also by downsampling the catheter and blood vessel resolution. Lastly, in the future, we plan to investigate non-rigid registration as well, to address those cases where the rigid registration fails to completely capture the breathing effects. It should yield better accuracy in case of deformation caused by catheter stiffness and breathing.

To conclude, we presented a method that allows performing continuous registration of a 3D vascular roadmap to 2D fluoroscopic images, based on the extracted vascular tree and the catheter position. We evaluated the feasibility of our approach on phantom, clinical and simulated data, demonstrating an overall median registration error less than 1 mm.

Acknowledgement. This research is funded by Philips Healthcare, Best, The Netherlands.

References

1. Groher, M., Zikic, D., Navab, N.: Deformable 2D-3D registration of vascular structures in a one view scenario. IEEE Transactions on Medical Imaging 28(6), 847–860 (2009)
2. Rivest-Henault, D., Sundar, H., Cheriet, M.: Nonrigid 2D/3D registration of coronary artery models with live fluoroscopy for guidance of cardiac interventions. IEEE Transactions on Medical Imaging 31(8), 1557–1572 (2012)
3. Jomier, J., Bullitt, E., Van Horn, M., Pathak, C., Aylward, S.R.: 3D/2D model-to-image registration applied to TIPS surgery. In: Larsen, R., Nielsen, M., Sporring, J. (eds.) MICCAI 2006. LNCS, vol. 4191, pp. 662–669. Springer, Heidelberg (2006)
4. Ma, Y., King, A., Gogin, N., Gijsbers, G., Rinaldi, C., Gill, J., Razavi, R., Rhode, K.: Clinical evaluation of respiratory motion compensation for anatomical roadmap guided cardiac electrophysiology procedures. IEEE Transactions on Biomedical Engineering 59(1), 122–131 (2012)
5. Metz, C., et al.: Alignment of 4d coronary cta with monoplane x-ray angiography. In: Linte, C.A., Moore, J.T., Chen, E.C.S., Holmes III, D.R., et al. (eds.) AE-CAI 2011. LNCS, vol. 7264, pp. 106–116. Springer, Heidelberg (2012)
6. Ruijters, D., Homan, R., Mielekamp, P., van de Haar, P., Babic, D.: Validation of 3d multimodality roadmapping in interventional neuroradiology. Physics in Medicine and Biology 56(16), 5335–5354 (2011)
7. Markelj, P., Tomaževič, D., Likar, B., Pernuš, F.: A review of 3D/2D registration methods for image-guided interventions. Medical Image Analysis 16(3), 642–661 (2012)
8. Liao, R., Zhang, L., Sun, Y., Miao, S., Chefd'hotel, C.: A review of recent advances in registration techniques applied to minimally invasive therapy. IEEE Transactions on Multimedia 15(5), 983–1000 (2013)
9. Atasoy, S., Groher, M., Zikic, D., Glocker, B., Waggershauser, T., Pfister, M., Navab, N.: Real-time respiratory motion tracking: roadmap correction for hepatic artery catheterizations. In: Proc. SPIE 6918, Medical Imaging 2008: Visualization, Image-guided Procedures, and Modeling, p. 691815 (March 20, 2008)
10. Heibel, H., Glocker, B., Groher, M., Pfister, M., Navab, N.: Interventional tool tracking using discrete optimization. IEEE Transactions on Medical Imaging 32(3), 544–555 (2013)

Filter-Based Speckle Tracking for Freehand Prostate Biopsy: Theory, *ex vivo* and *in vivo* Results

Narges Afsham[1], Siavash Khallaghi[1], Mohammad Najafi[1], Lindsay Machan[2],
Silvia D. Chang[2], Larry Goldenberg[3], Peter Black[3],
Robert N. Rohling[1,4], and Purang Abolmaesumi[1]

[1] Dept. of ECE, University of British Columbia, Vancouver, BC, Canada
[2] Dept. of Radiology, University of British Columbia, Vancouver, BC, Canada
[3] Dept. of Urologic Sciences, University of British Columbia, Vancouver, BC, Canada
[4] Dept. of Mechanical Engineering, University of British Columbia,
Vancouver, BC, Canada

Abstract. In conventional prostate biopsy for cancer diagnosis, the 2D
nature of ultrasound (US) guidance limits targeting accuracy and does
not allow a 3D record of core locations. Several research groups are investigating the use of an electromagnetically tracked US transducer to
reconstruct a volumetric scan. Unfortunately, the tracking measurements
contain significant errors that affect spatial accuracy. We propose a new
filter-based framework of speckle tracking for enchantment of prostate
volume reconstruction based on speckle/noise extraction and provide its
theoretical basis. A gamma multiplicative noise model is considered and
a probability patch-based non-local means (PPB-NLM) filter is used for
the task of speckle extraction. The spatial variation of the beam profile is also incorporated using a linear regression model of the beam.
Validation tests are first performed on tissue samples obtained *ex vivo*
using a linear motor stage and an optical tracker as gold standards. Further validation is performed on the gastrocnemius muscle *in vivo*. We
then demonstrate the performance of the tracking system on prostate
scans obtained *in vivo*. The results show that the proposed approach produces visually continuous anatomical boundaries in reconstructed 3D US
volumes of the prostate.

Keywords: Sensorless freehand ultrasound, prostate biopsy, speckle
tracking.

1 Introduction

Prostate Cancer (PCa) is the second most prevalent cancer and the third cause of
cancer mortality in North American men [1, 2]. The current clinical standard for
PCa diagnosis is histological analysis of Transrectal Ultrasound (TRUS) guided
biopsy samples. The 2D nature of the conventional biopsy limits targeting accuracy and does not allow a 3D record of core locations. To alleviate this issue,

D. Stoyanov et al. (Eds.): IPCAI 2014, LNCS 8498, pp. 256–265, 2014.

several groups have proposed 3D targeted biopsy, where the biopsy targets and extracted cores are recorded in the space of a TRUS volume acquired prior to the start of the procedure [3–5]. TRUS volume reconstruction is generally accurate using a 3D TRUS transducer [3]; however, such transducers are not part of a typical standard-of-care. When a 3D TRUS volume is reconstructed from a swept 2D TRUS, the best results have been reported with a sophisticated mechanical stabilizer [4]. The simplest, least expensive solution that is closest to the current standard-of-care, is to use a magnetically tracked, freehand 2D TRUS transducer (Fig. 1a) [5, 6]. In our experience with such magnetically tracked TRUS transducers, we still observe significant spatial reconstruction errors, due to a combination of tracking inaccuracy from proximal metal objects such as the bed, calibration inaccuracy, and shifts in organ position. We propose to supplement magnetic tracking with speckle tracking, thereby taking advantage of the speckle pattern within the anatomy to create a more geometrically correct volume.

Conventional speckle tracking has been previously used to increase the reliability and accuracy of electromagnetic tracking [7] and to improve the result of multi-modal 3D US to CT registrations of spine [8]. However, the rarity of Fully Developed Speckle (FDS) in real tissue is among the major causes of inaccuracy in conventional speckle tracking methods. The fundamental basis of most correlation-based speckle tracking holds true only for non-coherent speckle, known as FDS. The rarity of such patterns reduces the accuracy of the elevation displacement estimation. Previous methods addressed this issue by using a heuristic approach for correction of coherency [9] and learning the pattern of decorrelation for real tissues [10]. To overcome the limitations of heuristic and learning-based approaches, we previously proposed a generalized closed-form formulation for the correlation of the non-coherent part of every patch in the [11]. In spite of promising results, the computational cost of our previous approach hinders its clinical applications. Using the same processing hardware as [11], the proposed method performs about three times faster. It is also possible to increase the speed more by a block-wise implementation of PPB-NLM filter. Moreover, EM estimations of PDFs as used in [11] are prone to local minima; however, NLM filters have shown superior results in noise estimation.

In this work, we propose a novel method of speckle tracking based on noise extraction by means of a denoising filter. The first advantage of the filter-based approach is the rapid processing of the image using a pre-defined speckle model. Another advantage is to use full and partially developed speckle information extracted throughout the entire image, which reduces drift in pose transform calculations. A third advantage is that our our filter-based approach is designed to work with both RF data and B-mode US images, which expands the range of systems and clinical applications. We incorporate this speckle tracking method into 3D TRUS reconstruction by using the magnetic tracking information of freehand 2D TRUS images as the initial guess. We demonstrate that such integration of the two tracking technologies can reduce some of the visible misalignment errors in the reconstructed prostate volume.

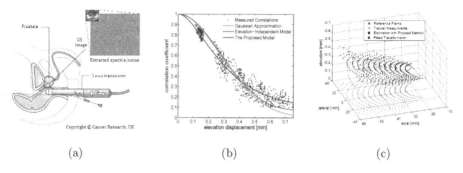

(a)   (b)   (c)

Fig. 1. Image acquisition and speckle tracking framework. (a) Speckle extraction from the US image (b) Elevation displacement estimation. In this figure we demonstrate the correlation curve by which the elevation distance is estimated given a measured noise. The different fitted ρ models on the measured correlation coefficients of US noise for the prostate data are shown. (c) Transform estimation. The scattered points show the 3D position of patch centers in the reference frame (red) and the adjacent frame.

2   Methods

If we consider speckle/noise extraction as the estimation of the space-varying parameters of noise, given the noise model, the separation of the coherent and non-coherent parts of US is equivalent to denoising. Several US denoising filters have been introduced in the literature [12]. Here, we require a method of denoising that is spatially local and incorporates the statistical noise model. Hence, we use a probabilistic patch-based generalization of the non-local means filter to estimate the space-varying parameters the speckle/noise [13] (Fig. 1a). We also use a position dependent beam profile in the calculation of correlation coefficient to improve the accuracy of speckle tracking [11] (Fig. 1b).

2.1   Beam Profile Modeling for Speckle Tracking

US 2D registration-based speckle matching and the cross correlation of US RF signals have shown their ability to measure the in-plane displacement [14]. The main challenge for 3D US speckle tracking is the estimation of out-of-plane displacement. The finite width of the US beam profile creates overlapping resolution cells for two adjacent US patches along the elevation direction, which is used to estimate the out-of-plane displacement. The amount of this overlap contributes to the correlation value of speckle patterns in two consecutive US frames. Based on linear systems theory, the resulting autocorrelation of the echo signal as a function of displacement can be written as:

$$R(\Delta X) = R_m(\Delta X) * g(-\Delta X) * g^*(\Delta X). \tag{1}$$

where R_m is the autocorrelation function of the physical variation in the scatterer field of the medium and ΔX is the 3D translation vector. g is the Point

Spread Function (PSF) of the transducer and g^* is the complex conjugate of g. Theoretically, the scatterer field of FDS has a delta correlation function. As a result, the correlation value of two FDS patches is only related to the convolution of two PSFs. It is conventional to use the Gaussian approximation for the correlation coefficient; however it is shown that the closed-form Pearson's correlation coefficient equals [11] (Fig. 1b):

$$\rho = \frac{3\sigma^2}{2}\left(\frac{1 - sinc(\frac{2\Delta y}{\sigma})}{(\pi\Delta y)^2}\right), \tag{2}$$

where Δy is the elevation displacement and σ is the resolution cell width of the US beam. To compensate for the spatial changes of beam profile, we modelled σ as a linear regression of the position parameters and the elevation displacement:

$$\sigma = \sigma_0 + ar + b\theta + c\Delta y, \tag{3}$$

where r is the radius and θ is the angle in the polar coordinate of a curvilinear probe that we used *in vivo*. The resolution cell width increases along the axial direction, r, which is responsible for the lower resolution at the lower parts of the US image. The US profile is almost constant in the lateral direction, θ. Δy dependency compensates the deviation of correlation curve from the theoretical function [11]. We used Levenberg-Marquart algorithm to solve Δy.

2.2   Speckle Extraction

In the Goodman's speckle noise model, the US signal is considered as the multiplication of the square root of the desired signal (Z) and the noise (N):

$$A = \sqrt{N}\sqrt{Z}. \tag{4}$$

The noise part, can be modeled as an L-look FDS noise following the gamma distribution with the scale parameter of $\frac{1}{L}$ and the shape parameter of L:

$$p_N(n) = \frac{L^L}{\Gamma(L)}n^{L-1}e^{-nL}, \tag{5}$$

where $\Gamma()$ is the Gamma function.

Under the gamma distribution assumption, $\sqrt{N}$ follows Nakagami distribution with shape parameter L and unit spread parameter. Using the closed-form formula of the nth order moment of the multiplication of two independent Nakagami random variables, we may derive the mean (μ_m) and the autocorrelation function (R_m) of two closely positioned frames as follows:

$$\mu_m = \mu_{\sqrt{Z}}\underbrace{\left(\frac{\Gamma(L + \frac{1}{2})}{\Gamma(L + 1)}\right)\left(\frac{1}{L}\right)^{0.5}}_{a}, \tag{6}$$

$$R_m(\Delta y) = <Z><\sqrt{N_1 N_2}> = \begin{cases} \mu_z & : \Delta y = 0 \\ a^2\mu_z & : \Delta y \neq 0 \end{cases}, \tag{7}$$

where $<>$ represents the expected value of the random variable and $\mu_{\sqrt{Z}}$ is the average of the desired signal square root.

By rewriting $R_m(\Delta y)$ as $\mu_Z\left[(1-a^2)\delta(\Delta y)+a^2\right]$, using (6) and (7), and following the same calculation presented in [11], after some arithmetic:

$$\rho = \frac{\mu_Z(1-a^2)\sigma(\frac{1-sinc(\frac{2\Delta y}{\sigma})}{(\pi\Delta y)^2}) + a^2\sigma_{\sqrt{z}}^2}{\mu_Z(1-a^2)\frac{2}{3\sigma} + a^2\sigma_{\sqrt{z}}^2}, \tag{8}$$

where μ_Z and $\sigma_{\sqrt{z}}$ are the mean and standard deviation of the desired signal Z.

The desired signal Z, is the intended output of any denoising filter. For the purpose of speckle tracking, a method of denoising is of interest that considers the distribution of the uncorrelated noise in its model and it is capable of space-varying noise estimation. A probability-based NLM filter, which outperforms other state-of-the-art denoising algorithms [13], serves the purpose best.

In the NLM denoising approach, the desired signal Z is estimated based on the weighted average of the neighboring pixels [12]:

$$\hat{Z}_s = \frac{\sum_t w(s,t)A_t^2}{\sum_t w(s,t)}. \tag{9}$$

where $\hat{Z}$ is the estimated signal, and s, t indicate the location of the two neighboring patches.

The definition of the weights is the key in the success of NLM filters. Since the posterior distribution of the US amplitude, A, in (4) has a closed-form (10), a Bayesian approach can be followed to derive the Weighted Maximum Likelihood Estimation (WMLE) of Z.

$$p(A|Z) = \frac{2L^L}{\Gamma(L)Z^L}A^{2L}e^{-\frac{LA^2}{Z}}. \tag{10}$$

In the case of L-look FDS noise the WMLE of the weights can be found iteratively as follows [13]:

$$w(s,t)^i = exp(\sum_k (\frac{1}{\tilde{h}}log(\frac{A_{s,k}}{A_{t,k}} - \frac{A_{t,k}}{A_{s,k}}) + \frac{L}{T}\frac{|\hat{Z}_{s,k}^{i-1} - \hat{Z}_{t,k}^{i-1}|^2}{\hat{Z}_{s,k}^{i-1}\hat{Z}_{t,k}^{i-1}})), \tag{11}$$

where $\hat{h} = \frac{h}{2L-1}$ and h, T can be considered as dual parameters to balance the trade-off between the noise extraction and the fidelity of the estimate.

2.3 Transform Estimation

Theoretically, by having the out-of-plane distances of at least three corresponding points between two frames, it is possible to solve for the three degrees of freedom of the out-of-plane motion, i.e. elevation displacement, tilt, and yaw angles. The sign of the elevation displacement is determined by the electromagnetic tracker in this work; however, approaches proposed in [15] and [16] can be followed to solve for direction ambiguity. We first determine the in-plane motion between pairs of patches by performing a sub-pixel cross correlation-based registration. Then to solve for the correspondent elevation displacement of each pair, the Pearson's correlation coefficient of the extracted noise, ρ, is measured using the following formulation (Note that given ρ, the out-of-plane displacement, Δ_y, is determined using (2)):

$$\rho = \frac{\sum_i (I_s(i) - \bar{I}_s) \sum_i (I_k(i) - \bar{I}_k)}{\sqrt{\sum_i (I_s(i) - \bar{I}_s)^2 \sum_i (I_k(i) - \bar{I}_k)^2}}, \tag{12}$$

where I is the intensity of the pixels and $\bar{I}$ is the average intensity over the patch. In the experiments, 364 overlapping patches of size 6×8 mm with ≈ 3000 pixels in each patch were used. We used unit quaternions to estimate the 3D rigid body transformation (Fig. 1c). The transformation is first estimated using all the patches. The patches with the center point residual error of more than 0.5 mm were considered as outliers and discarded, and the transformation is calculated again. It is possible to find the transformation between any given frame and the first frame (^1T_n) by multiplying the transformations from the consecutive pairs of frames as in (13). Therefore, the whole volume can be constructed relative to the first frame:

$$^1T_n = {}^1T_2 {}^2T_3 \ldots {}^{n-1}T_n. \tag{13}$$

3   Experiments and Results

In a one-time calibration step, the sigma function parameters were estimated from turkey, chicken and beef tissue samples *in vitro*. The tissues were placed on a linear motion stage and were moved in 0.1 mm steps relative to the transducer. Three subsets of 40 frames were captured for each sample type. Sigma function parameters were estimated using the known elevation distance between the parallel frames and they were averaged (intra-tissue) for each sample type. To access the tissue independency, the coefficient of variation is calculated over

Table 1. Accumulated drift and RMS error in the out-of-plane parameters compared to tracker over 100 frames

		Patient1	Patient2	Patient3
Midpoint (mm)	Drift	-3.2	4.8	0.8
	RMS	1.93	2.96	1.1
Tilt (degree)	Drift	2	0.1	6.6
	RMS	1.28	1.11	4.7
Yaw (degree)	Drift	2.95	1.1	1.2
	RMS	0.73	0.39	0.75

Table 2. Sigma variations at different depths

	Mean	STD
Top	0.58	0.11
Middle	0.71	0.07
Bottom	0.90	0.06

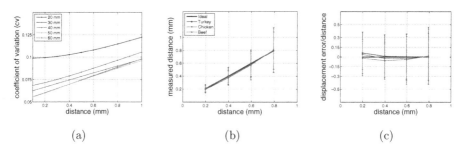

Fig. 2. (a) CV plot of the sigma parameter. Inter-tissue measurements for (b) the elevation distance estimation and (c) the ratio of displacement error.

different axial and elevation distances. The overall variation is less than %12 over tissue types and the variation is smaller around axial focus (30 mm), as expected (Fig. 2a). Table. 2 shows the total sigma variations for different tissue types at three different depths of 1, 3, and 6 cm for an elevation displacement of 0.5 mm. Small variations confirm the tissue independency of the method. In the subsequent experiments, the inter-tissue average of the sigma parameters are used for the *in vivo* speckle tracking.

The accumulative elevation distance and the measured elevation error over the true value of displacement are shown in Fig. 2b, 2c. Since it is possible to use the information all over the image in the proposed method, the drift is minimal. The changes of the beam profile that are not captured in the model cause relatively larger Standard Deviations (STD). One way to decrease the error STD is to limit the range of estimation to the focal zone [11].

A practical factor that affects the elevation displacement estimation is the presence of out-of-plane rotation, i.e. tilt and yaw. In our *in vivo* experiments, the relative out-of-plane rotations were less than 0.5° and hence, the influence of that on the decorrelation is likely small. However, to evaluate the performance of the proposed method, we performed a set of experiments on beef tissue samples similar to [17] with relative tilt and yaw angles of 1°. To avoid sign ambiguity, elevation distances more than 0.3 mm are considered. Fig. 3a, 3b show the results. For the yaw rotation the drift is negligible for smaller distances, but tilt rotation causes underestimation in the elevation measurements. The results agree with previous research [17]. A freehand feasibility experiment was first performed on human gastrocnemius muscle, where the tracking information was obtained from an optical tracker as gold standard. The mean and variation of the estimations are smaller for smaller displacements. However, the aggregation of the displacements all over the image will reduce the transform estimation error. Weighted aggregation based on the displacement reliability estimation is the subject of future research (Fig. 3c).

Prostate B-mode images were acquired during freehand TRUS-guided prostate biopsy sessions. An EC9-5 endocavity transducer (Ultrasonix Corp., Richmond, Canada) with a built-in electromagnetic sensor was used. A reference electromagnetic sensor was placed close to the pelvic bone, which provided the patient

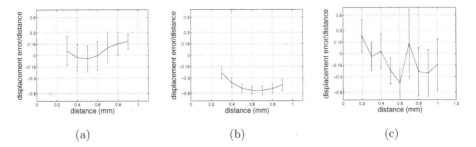

      (a)   (b)   (c)

Fig. 3. The ratio of the measured displacement error to the true elevation separation for (a) 1° yaw and (b) 1° tilt rotation on beef tissue (c) freehand *in vivo* human gastrocnemius muscle

coordinate system. In this paper, three patients have been processed out of 11 patients scanned to date. For each patient, we analyzed 100 consecutive B-mode images obtained while the transducer was moved freehand in a transverse sweep from apex to base. The approximate size of the prostate region covered by this sweep is half of the prostate length.

We used the initial information of the magnetic tracker for the first frame in the sweep, and calculated the relative transformation of the rest of the frames based on the proposed speckle tracking approach. The errors in the estimation of the out-of-plane parameters (tilt, yaw and midpoint elevation displacement), were measured and compared to the electromagnetic tracker over the entire sweep (Table 1). The error drift shows that our proposed approach generally follows the magnetic tracking transformation even after 100 frames.

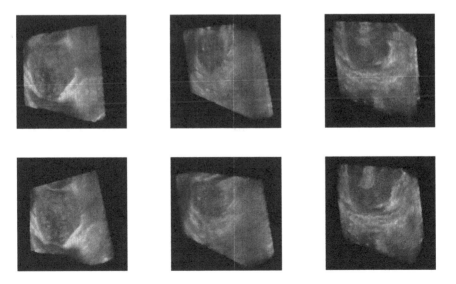

Fig. 4. Reconstructed volumes over 100 frames from smoothed magnetic tracker data (top row) and the proposed approach (bottom row) for three patients

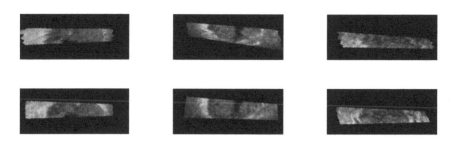

Fig. 5. Coronal reslice of the reconstructed volumes from smoothed magnetic tracker data (top row) and the proposed approach (bottom row)

To reduce the impact of drift on the overall 3D reconstruction accuracy, while taking advantage of the speckle tracking information, we updated the transformation obtained using the speckle tracking with the magnetic tracker information every 25 frames, and smoothed the transformation parameters in quaternion space by an averaging window of size 5. A volume was then reconstructed from the acquired transforms. Fig. 4 and 5 show the reconstructed volumes using magnetic tracking, where the transformations were smoothed with a low-pass filter, and the volumes obtained with our proposed combination of speckle tracking and magnetic tracking. Comparison of the reconstructed volumes show smooth boundaries and less visual discontinuity with our proposed method.

4   Discussion and Conclusion

In this work, a novel method of speckle tracking based on denoising is proposed and its theoretical basis is provided. A probability-based NLM filter is used to extract speckle information from the US image enabling B-mode speckle tracking. Using the extracted speckle, it is possible to estimate the out-of-plane displacement for any given patch in the image with very low drift. A closed-form regression model is used for the correlation function to approximate the deviations of beam profile more accurately. We validate the approach using *ex vivo* data, and *in vivo* data from three patients who underwent prostate biopsy. 3D TRUS volumes were reconstructed from the prostate of those patients. When compared to the magnetic tracker, results show visual improvement in the reconstructed boundaries of the prostate. Future work will focus on the integration of this approach with a targeted prostate biopsy system.

References

1. American Cancer Society, "Cancer facts and figures". ACS, Atlanta (2013)
2. Canadian Cancer Societys Advisory Committee on Cancer Statistics, "Canadian cancer statistics. Canadian Cancer Society, Toronto (2013)
3. Baumann, M., Mozer, P., Daanen, V., Troccaz, J.: Prostate biopsy tracking with deformation estimation. Medical Image Analysis 16(3), 562–576 (2012)

4. Bax, J., Cool, D., Gardi, L., Knight, K., Smith, D., Montreuil, J., Sherebrin, S., Romagnoli, C., Fenster, A.: Mechanically assisted 3D ultrasound guided prostate biopsy system. Medical Physics 35(12), 5397–5410 (2008)
5. Xu, S., Kruecker, J., Turkbey, B., Glossop, N., Singh, A.K., Choyke, P., Pinto, P., Wood, B.J.: Real-time MRI-TRUS fusion for guidance of targeted prostate biopsies
6. Cool, D., Sherebrin, S., Izawa, J., Chin, J., Fenster, A.: Design and evaluation of a 3D TRUS prostate biopsy system. Med. Phys. 35(10), 4695–4707 (2008)
7. Lang, A., Mousavi, P., Fichtinger, G., Abolmaesumi, P.: Fusion of electromagnetic tracking with speckle-tracked 3d freehand ultrasound using an unscented kalman filter. In: Proc. of SPIE (2009)
8. Lang, A., Mousavi, P., Gill, S., Fichtinger, G., Abolmaesumi, P.: Multi-modal registration of speckle-tracked freehand 3D ultrasound to ct in the lumbar spine. MIA 16(3), 675–686 (2012)
9. Gee, A.H., James Housden, R., Hassenpflug, P., Treece, G.M., Prager, R.W.: Sensorless freehand 3D ultrasound in real tissue: Speckle decorrelation without fully developed speckle. MIA 10, 137–149 (2006)
10. Laporte, C., Arbel, T.: Learning to estimate out-of-plane motion in ultrasound imagery of real tissue. MIA 15, 202–213 (2011)
11. Afsham, N., Najafi, M., Abolmaesumi, P., Rohling, R.: A generalized correlation-based model for out-of-plane motion estimation in freehand ultrasound. IEEE TMI (2013)
12. Buades, A., Coll, B., Morel, J.-M.: A review of image denoising algorithms, with a new one. Multiscale Modeling & Simulation 4(2), 490–530 (2005)
13. Deledalle, C.-A., Denis, L., Tupin, F.: Iterative weighted maximum likelihood denoising with probabilistic patch-based weights. IEEE TIP 18(12), 2661–2672 (2009)
14. Housden, R.J., Gee, A.H., Treece, G.M., Prager, R.W.: Subsample interpolation strategies for sensorless freehand 3D US. UMB 32(12), 1897–1904 (2006)
15. Laporte, C., Arbel, T.: Combinatorial and probabilistic fusion of noisy correlation measurements for untracked freehand 3-D ultrasound. IEEE TMI 27(7), 984–994 (2008)
16. Housden, R.J., Gee, A.H., Treece, G.M., Prager, R.W.: Sensorless reconstruction of unconstrained freehand 3D us. UMB 33, 408–419 (2007)
17. Housden, R.J., Gee, A.H., Prager, R.W., Treece, G.M.: Rotational motion in sensorless freehand three-dimensional ultrasound. Ultrasonics 48, 412–422 (2008)

Efficient Tissue Discrimination during Surgical Interventions Using Hyperspectral Imaging

Dorra Nouri[1], Yves Lucas[1], and Sylvie Treuillet[2]

[1] Laboratoire PRISME, IUT Bourges, Université d'Orléans, France
{dorra.nouri,yves.lucas}@univ-orleans.fr
[2] Laboratoire PRISME, Polytech' Orléans, Université d'Orléans, France
{sylvie.treuillet}@univ-orleans.fr

Abstract. A new hyperspectral imaging system has been designed for integration in the operating room to detect anatomical tissues hardly noticed by the surgeon's naked eye. This LCTF-based spectral imaging system is operative over visible and near infrared range (400-1100 nm). After spectral calibration and spatial registration, the tricky process consists in reducing the huge amount of acquired data and removing redundancy without losing valuable information. Band transformation and selection methods are applied on both labeled and unlabeled tissues to extract relevant information to be displayed on surgeon's RGB monitor. Visualization processing involving global and local contrast enhancement is then performed. To provide a reference for evaluation, surgeon's perception of the scene is also simulated based on retina cell spectral responses. Experiments on pig ureter hyperspectral datasets reveal that band selection methods are the most effective on this type of intervention, providing sharp interpretation and accurate visualization of the biological tissues.

Keywords: Hyperspectral imaging, dimensionality reduction, visualization, contrast enhancement, operating room, surgical intervention.

1   Introduction

Hyperspectral imaging (HSI) consists of hundreds of images taken in narrow and adjacent spectral bands. Stacked into three-dimensional hyperspectral (HS) data cubes, they provide both spectral and spatial information of the imaged scene. In the last decades, HSI was involved in remote sensing but its efficiency is now experimented successfully in many emerging applications fields. Recently, HS are involved in medical applications [1– 4]. Although rich spatial and spectral information is provided by the HS sensors, processing of this huge amount of data may be troublesome and leads to high computational cost. Dimensionality reduction is a crucial step in HS data analysis in order to alleviate the computational burden, to avoid the dimensionality curse and to reduce the redundant and correlated information without losing valuable details that are needed for further processing like classification, target detection, visualization, etc.

There are numerous dimensionality reduction techniques that can be classified into two main categories: the band transformation also called feature extraction methods

D. Stoyanov et al. (Eds.): IPCAI 2014, LNCS 8498, pp. 266–275, 2014.
© Springer International Publishing Switzerland 2014

and the band selection methods. Band transformation techniques project the original HS information onto a space of lower dimension so that a new transformed and reduced data set is generated. While, band selection methods select the relevant range of wavelengths to obtain a subset data from the initial HS information.

In previous works, both of these methodologies are used to reduce the dimensionality of the HS data cube. Band transformation techniques can be either linear methods [5] including Principal Component Analysis (PCA) [6], Independent Component Analysis (ICA) [7] and projection pursuit [8] or non linear methods [9] including Locally Linear Embedding (LLE) [10] and Isomap [11]. A comparative study of these techniques was carried out in [12] and concluded that PCA outperforms the other methods in different investigated tasks. Several other studies focused on band selection methods [13, 14]. Band selection methods can be roughly categorized into three groups, i.e. statistics techniques [15, 16], information-based methods [17, 18] and signal processing techniques [19, 20]. Sometimes the dimensionality reduction is performed by changing the space representation through derivative [14] or wavelet transform [21]. One drawback of the band transformation approach is the loss of some important and critical information that could be compromised and distorted since the data are transformed. However they are less time-consuming methods compared to band selection methods. Both methods can be carried out depending on the specific pointed applications of the HSI.

In this paper, we transposed HSI band selection and band transformation methods commonly used in remote sensing to the medical field in order to detect some vital anatomical and hardly noticeable tissues that must be not damaged like the ureter. Our purpose is to enhance the surgeon's visualization when operating. Consequently, the HS data cube processing should be fast enough synthesized and resumed graphically on a RGB screen. The remainder of this paper is organized as follow. In section 2, we begin by describing the HSI prototype used for data acquisition. Then, the performed band selection and band transformation methods are detailed and the visualization enhancements are described in section 3. In the next section, the performance of the dimensionality reduction methods are compared and evaluated. Finally, the experimental results are presented and discussed.

2   Data Acquisition

Prior to this study, a HSI prototype was developed. It is operative in the visible (VIS) and short-wavelength near infrared (SNIR) spectral ranges (400-1100 nm). The acquisition of HS images is based on liquid crystal tunable filters (LCTF). The HSI prototype consists of an illumination system, a spectral imager and a computer with data acquisition software. The illumination system consists of focused and powerful halogen lighting. The spectral imager is composed of two LCTFs with programmable bandwidth (Varispec, CRI VIS-10-20 and SNIR-7-20): the VIS LCTF operates in 400-720 nm and the SNIR one operates in 650-1100 nm, a high sensibility monochromatic CCD camera (Lumenera LM165) and a 35 mm focal length lens. After HS system hardware integration, software was developed to control the camera and the LCTFs allowing an automatic HS image sequence acquisition. The 141 bands (1392 x 1040 pixels) of the HS data cube were acquired in nearly 2 min. For next surgical operation on patients, this duration will certainly be reduced after finding the best relevant three wavelengths.

Designing a HS system is a complicating process of selecting optical, electronic and mechanical elements. Thus, a spatial and spectral calibration steps are necessary to characterize the overall system performance and each of its components [22]. The true spectral reflectance values were calculated for each pixel location in the HS images. The spectral reflectance value is defined as the ratio of the reflected light power and the illuminating light power per unit area of the object surface [23]. However, when taking into account the exposure time corresponding at each wavelength λ and the dark current of the sensor element at each exposure time, the spectral reflectance value is computed using the equation (1).

$$R(\lambda) = s(\lambda) \times \frac{t_W}{t_I} \times \frac{I(\lambda, t_I) - D(\lambda, t_I)}{W(\lambda, t_W) - D(\lambda, t_W)} \qquad (1)$$

Where R is the scene spectral reflectance image, I is the raw image, D is the dark current image, W is the white reference image and s is the spectral reflectance value of the spatially homogeneous standard reflectance target which is accurately known through manufacturer data sheet. The respective t_W and t_I are the exposure time applied for standard reflectance target and raw image.

Our main objective is to acquire HS images in the context of surgical interventions in order to discriminate between different tissues and to explore some anatomical structures. After consulting a panel of surgeons, the ureter detection problem has been found to occur in frequent interventions, so that HIS could provide valuable display enhancement and pig has been selected as a model for the first preclinical experimentations.

3   Hyperspectral Data Processing

3.1   Dimensionality Reduction

The dimensionality reduction aims to reduce the huge amount of acquired data and the redundancy between the spectral bands without losing valuable information. In this paper, band transformation and band selection methods performance has been compared, without and then with *a priori*, knowledge on tissues in the scene contents. A rigid affine registration between HS images acquired in visible and in near infrared spectral ranges was initially performed. The shift noticed in the images was occurred because of LCTF module interchanging and the animal's breathing.

- **Without Knowledge on Tissues**
Band transformation method: PCA [6] is one of the most popular and very frequently used techniques for dimensionality reduction. This method performs an orthogonal linear transformation and projects the original data to a lower dimensional space of uncorrelated attributes called Principal Components (PC) based on the bands covariance matrix. The generated outputs of PCA are eigenvalues and a set of vectors of coefficients, one for each new dimension. The eigenvalues represent the degree of variance represented by each PC. They also indicate the amount of valuable information in the new dimension. The coefficients denote the influence of the original

dimensions regarding to the new one. Generally, the first few PCs contain the most valuable information. However, the higher-order ones would be expected to include little variance. Therefore, the first few PCs are expected to represent the global variability in the image scene.

Band selection methods: Statistic methods aim to preserve the maximum variability (information) in the image. They are based on second-order statistics such as correlation and variance which are used to investigate redundancy between HS images. They used to assign spectral bands according to their information content. The Optimum Index Factor (OIF) [24] method aims to select the best three bands combination according to their respective variance and correlation allowing to visualize maximum details in a HS cube. OIF method was used for remote sensing applications [15, 16, 25]. In fact, the highest values of OIF correspond to the three bands combination with the most information content. It is defined in equation (2).The Sheffield index (SI) [26] criterion is another band selection method that measures the contained information in bands combination. It is defined as the covariance matrix determinant of the selected subset (equation (3)).

$$OIF = Max \left[\frac{\sum_{i=1}^{n} \sigma(i)}{\sum_{j=1}^{n} |\rho(j)|} \right] \qquad (2)$$

$$SI = |M_{3x3}| \qquad (3)$$

Where n is the total number of bands, σ_i is the variance of the ith band, ρ_j is the correlation coefficient of the jth band and M is the covariance matrix.

- **With Knowledge on Tissues**

Band transformation method: Knowing the spectral signatures of the ureter and its bounding tissues (equation 1), a supervised PCA was carried out. Unlike PCA stated earlier, PCA $_{Sup}$ was applied only on a region of interest containing the target tissue instead of the whole scene. The first three PCs were extracted and mapped to generate the resulting RGB image.

Band selection method: the spectral signatures of ureter and its surrounding tissue were extracted and plotted (Fig. 1). The band selection was performed in the spectral range of the spectrum where the gap between spectral signatures was maximized. The spectral bands were ranked according to their reflectance gap values. The first three bands were selected to construct the resulting RGB image. This method is referred for us Ref $_{Gap.}$

3.2   Visualization Enhancement

Visualization of the huge data acquired in HSI is not a straightforward issue. Actually, the information content was reduced using the dimensionality reduction approach and the generated RGB image must be displayed on standard screens in order to have consistent meanings with the human visual perception system. First of all, the CMF-based True Color, as opposed to the *false color* or *pseudocolor* image, was created from the Color Matching Functions (CMF) which model the tri-stimulus human perception of colors. The resulting image represents an approximation of how the human eye would ideally visualize the corresponding scene. We used this image as a reference image (Fig.1 middle).

Two contrast enhancement approaches were carried out on the resulting RGB image: a global contrast enhancement approach and a local one. The first approach was performed by adjusting image intensity values. This approach mapped the intensity values in the grayscale image to new values such that 1% of data is saturated at low and high intensities of the input image. We used *imadjust* and *stretchlim* algorithms from Matlab library (MathWorks Inc.) in order to automatically find limits to contrast stretching image. The second approach aimed to locally enhance contrast. It is based on the Contrast-Limited Adaptive Histogram Equalization (CLAHE) method, a more advanced version of histogram equalization. Rather than on the entire image, CLAHE operates on small regions in the image, called tiles, making the assumption that the image varies significantly over its spatial extent. Each tile's contrast is enhanced, so that the histogram of the output region approximately matches the histogram shape of a uniform distribution. The neighboring tiles are then combined using bilinear interpolation to eliminate artificially induced boundaries [27]. CLAHE was applied to the resulting RGB images in both CIELAB and HSV color spaces.

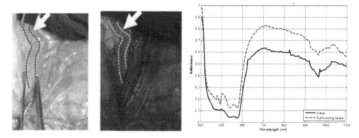

Fig. 1. Left: RGB image acquired by a standard digital camera. Middle: simulated CMF-based True Color image. The ureter is shown by yellow dashed lines and arrow and two surgical clips. Right: spectral signature of the ureter (solid line) and its surrounding tissue (dashed line).

4   Evaluations and Experimental Results

4.1   Entropy, Correlation and Naturalness Measures

The intrinsic properties of the dimensionality reduction methods mentioned above were evaluated using entropy, correlation, and natural rendering measures in order to denote the overall quality of the resulting RGB image.

The entropy, defined in equation (4), was computed to characterize the information content of all pixels of each RGB components. Hence, entropy measures the abundance of information contained in the image. The normalized correlation metric is a statistical measure that was estimated to denote quantitatively the similarity between images. The average correlation coefficient (ACC) between the resulting three RGB channels was calculated using the equation (5). The Natural Rendering (NR) of the resulting RGB image is evaluated and compared with the simulated true color image which is used as a ground truth for naturalness. We used the mutual information computed independently over the three components of the CIELAB color space as in equation (6). The NR metric was also used in [28].

$$H(X) = -\sum_x p(x)\log p(x) \tag{4}$$

$$ACC = \frac{1}{3}\cdot\sum_{i=1}^{3}|\rho_i| \tag{5}$$

$$NR = MI_L + \frac{MI_a + MI_b}{2} \tag{6}$$

Where p(x) is the probability of pixel value x. ρ_i is the pair-wise correlation coefficient between the resulting RGB bands. MI_L, MI_a, MI_b are the mutual information in the L*, a* and b* dimensions respectively.

Table 1 shows the entropies of each RGB components. It is obvious that the entropy that reveals the information contents is larger for the band selection methods comparing to band transformation methods. For instance, the mean value of the entropies for Ref $_{Gap}$ method is 7.203 while it is 3.583 for PCA $_{Sup}$ method. However, Ref $_{Gap}$ method had the highest correlation coefficient (ACC = 0.881) which explains the nearly grey-level image generated (Fig.2). Obviously, Band transformation methods such as PCA provide the lowest correlated bands (ACC = 0.037) since the RGB image is created from the first three PCs that must be linearly uncorrelated. It is worth mentioning that the average mean of entropy and the ACC values were respectively 6.001 and 0.31 for the true color image. Moreover, it can be noticed from Table 1 that band selection methods had the best natural rendering rate compared to band transformation methods. This indicator emphasizes the easy interpretation of the resulting RGB images inasmuch as they provide the closest natural effect as well as the CMF-based true color image which refers to the human perception (Fig. 2).

Table 1. Entropy, average correlation coefficient and natural rendering measures

	Entropy			*ACC*	*NR*
	Band 1	**Band 2**	**Band 3**		
OIF	5.561	6.995	7.265	0.306	9.227
SI	6.875	7.194	6.928	0.606	8.393
PCA	5.729	4.693	5.839	0.037	7.748
PCA *Sup*	3.520	3.419	3.810	0.362	8.035
Ref *Gap*	7.239	7.273	7.097	0.881	8.446

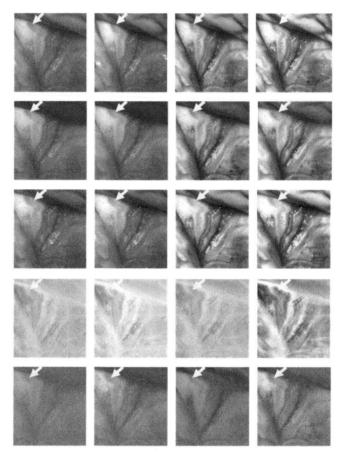

Fig. 2. Resulting RGB images of the surgical scene. The ureter is shown by yellow arrow. From top to bottom: **SI**, **OIF**, **Ref** $_{Gap}$, **PCA**, **PCA** $_{Sup}$. From left to right: Before contrast enhancement, global contrast enhancement, local contrast enhancement in HSV space, local contrast enhancement in CIELAB space.

4.2   Contrast Measure

The contrast was measured in a region of interest containing the ureter and its surroundings in CIELAB color space. It was evaluated after performing an edge detection approach using Sobel edge detector. This method aims to reveal the features in the image at which the intensity changes sharply, so that it characterizes specific features and relevant information in the scene. The contrast value of the true color image is 29.695. It is noteworthy from Table 2 that the contrast enhancement results in better image visualization for all the tested methods, since the ureter and its surroundings contrast values had increased after performing a contrast enhancement. Certainly, local contrast enhancement using CLAHE method had achieved higher contrast values compared with global contrast enhancement using histogram stretching. This is

Table 2. Global and local contrast measures

	Before contrast	*Global contrast*	*Local contrast*	
			HSV	**CIELAB**
OIF	24.597	25.895	51.826	52.711
SI	29.246	39.826	47.545	57.425
PCA	12.772	13.805	10.115	27.937
PCA Sup	12.162	18.559	21.033	29.808
Ref Gap	28.113	30.883	53.571	56.360

due to the partitioning of the image into small tiles which improved specific and meaningful features in the resulting RGB image. There is no doubt that carrying out local contrast enhancement in CIELAB was more efficient than in HSV color spaces since the former is a perceptually uniform space relative to human vision. Promising results for band selection methods are also shown especially for SI method in which the contrast value was increased nearly twice compared to the contrast value in the true color image that should perceive the surgeon's naked eye.

5   Discussion and Conclusion

HSI is an emerging technology recently introduced in medical applications inasmuch as it provides a powerful tool for noninvasive tissue analysis. In this paper, we have investigated HSI in order to enhance surgeon's visual skills in operating room when dealing with some hardly noticeable tissues such as ureter. Two different categories of dimensionality reduction methods were initially performed. Then, comparative performance evaluation was carried out in order to assess information level, independence and natural rendering of the resulting RGB image bands.

Experimental results reveal that band selection methods provide higher information content compared with band transformation methods but lower correlation may be observed between transformed bands. In order to grade these methods on a single scale, we suggested evaluating their efficiency on the resulting tissue detection capability, measured by several contrast indicators which provide an acceptable trade-off to compute contrast enhancement. Consequently, band selection methods will be definitively preferred, especially SI method which preserves maximum information, obtains the highest contrast values and outperforms for natural rendering based on the true color image visualized by the surgeon's naked eye. A convenient reason to rely on band selection methods in this medical context is also the better preservation of the physical meaning of the structures which simplifies scene interpretation. Otherwise the surgeon may be easily confused by this new imaging modality, especially with false color display. More accurate contrast measure will be performed on the image perceived by the eye instead of the displayed one. Another interesting conclusion from this preclinical study is that the best three wavelengths selected to discriminate ureter from bounding tissues are situated in the near infrared spectral range (625 nm, 700 nm, 995 nm). This strengthens our intention to explore farther infrared spectral range (900 – 1700 nm) with an InGaAs camera. Further promising investigations will also focus on advanced band selection methods to alleviate the computational burden.

Acknowledgments. The authors would like to thank the French Conseil Régional Centre, and Ministère de l'Industrie, the European fund for regional development (FEDER) and the French OSéO for their financial support through the smart electricity cluster S2E2.

References

1. Nouri, D., Lucas, Y., Treuillet, S., Jolivot, R., Marzani, F.: Colour and multispectral imaging for wound healing evaluation in the context of a comparative preclinical study. In: Proc. SPIE, pp. 866910–866923 (2013)
2. Akbari, H., Halig, L.V., Schuster, D.M., Osunkoya, A., Master, V., Nieh, P.T., Chen, G.Z., Fei, B.: Hyperspectral imaging and quantitative analysis for prostate cancer detection. J. Biomed. Opt. 17, 76005–76010 (2012)
3. Panasyuk, S.V., Yang, S., Faller, D.V., Ngo, D., Lew, R.A., Freeman, J.E., Rogers, A.E.: Medical hyperspectral imaging to facilitate residual tumor identification during surgery. Cancer Biol. Ther. 6, 439–446 (2007)
4. Zuzak, K.J., Naik, S.C., Alexandrakis, G., Hawkins, D., Behbehani, K., Livingston, E.: Intraoperative bile duct visualization using near-infrared hyperspectral video imaging. Am. J. Surg. 195, 491–497 (2008)
5. Jimenez-Rodriguez, L.O., Arzuaga-Cruz, E., Velez-Reyes, M.: Unsupervised Linear Feature-Extraction Methods and Their Effects in the Classification of High-Dimensional Data. IEEE Trans. Geosci. Remote Sens. 45, 469–483 (2007)
6. Lucini, M.M., Frery, A.C.: Robust Principal Components for Hyperspectral Data Analysis. In: Kamel, M., Campilho, A. (eds.) ICIAR 2009. LNCS, vol. 5627, pp. 126–135. Springer, Heidelberg (2009)
7. Chiang, S.-S., Chang, C.-I., Ginsberg, I.W.: Unsupervised hyperspectral image analysis using independent component analysis. In: IGARSS, pp. 3136–3138. IEEE (2000)
8. Malpica, J.A., Rejas, J.G., Alonso, M.C.: A projection pursuit algorithm for anomaly detection in hyperspectral imagery. Pattern Recognit. 41, 3313–3327 (2008)
9. Chen, Y., Crawford, M.M., Ghosh, J.: Applying nonlinear manifold learning to hyperspectral data for land cover classification. In: Proceedings of the IEEE International IGARSS, pp. 4311–4314 (2005)
10. Han, T.H.T., Goodenough, D.G.: Nonlinear feature extraction of hyperspectral data based on locally linear embedding (LLE). In: Proceedings of the IEEE IGARSS, pp. 1237–1240 (2005)
11. Luo, X., Jiang, M.-F.: A new dimensionality analysis algorithm for hyperspectral imagery. In: 2011 Int. Conf. Comput. Sci. Serv. Syst., pp. 1952–1956 (2011)
12. Burgers, K.: A Comparative Analysis of Dimension Reduction Algorithms on Hyperspectral Data (2009)
13. Bajcsy, P., Groves, P.: Methodology For Hyperspectral Band Selection. Photogramm. Eng. Remote Sens. J. 70, 793–802 (2004)

14. Bajwa, S.G., Bajcsy, P., Groves, P., Tian, L.F.: Hyperspectral image data mining for band selection in agricultural applications. Trans. ASAE 47, 895–907 (2004)
15. Beauchemin, M., Fung, K.B.: On statistical band selection for image visualization. Photogramm. Eng. Remote Sensing 67, 571–574 (2001)
16. Miao, X., Gong, P., Swope, S., Pu, R.L., Carruthers, R., Anderson, G.L.: Detection of yellow starthistle through band selection and feature extraction from hyperspectral imagery. Photogramm. Eng. Remote Sensing 73, 1005–1015 (2007)
17. Sarhrouni, E., Hammouch, A., Aboutajdine, D.: Dimensionality Reduction and Classification feature using Mutual Information applied to Hyperspectral Images: A Filter strategy based algorithm. Appl. Math. Sci. 6, 5085–5095 (2012)
18. Martinez-Uso, A., Pla, F., Sotoca, J.M., Garcia-Sevilla, P.: Clustering-Based Hyperspectral Band Selection Using Information Measures. IEEE Trans. Geosci. Remote Sens. 45, 4158–4171 (2007)
19. Demir, B., Celebi, A., Erturk, S.: A Low-Complexity Approach for the Color Display of Hyperspectral Remote-Sensing Images Using One-Bit-Transform-Based Band Selection. IEEE Trans. Geosci. Remote Sensing 47, 97–105 (2009)
20. Chang, C.I., Wang, S.: Constrained Band Selection for Hyperspectral Imagery. IEEE Trans. Geosci. Remote Sens. 44, 1575–1585 (2006)
21. Kaewpijit, S., Moigne, J., Le, E.-G.T.: Automatic reduction of hyperspectral imagery using wavelet spectral analysis. IEEE Trans. Geosci. Remote Sens. 41, 863–871 (2003)
22. Nouri, D., Lucas, Y., Treuillet, S.: Calibration and test of a hyperspectral imaging prototype for intra-operative surgical assistance. In: Proc. SPIE, pp. 86760P–86760P-9 (2013)
23. Klein, M.E., Aalderink, B.J., Padoan, R., de Bruin, G., Steemers, T.A.G.: Quantitative Hyperspectral Reflectance Imaging. Sensors 8, 5576–5618 (2008)
24. Chavez, P.S., Berlin, G.L., Sower, L.B.: Statistical method for selecting Landsat MSS ratio. J. Appl. Photogr. Eng. 8, 23–30 (1982)
25. Qaid, A.M., Basavarajappa, H.: Application of optimum index factor technique to landsat-7 data for geological mapping of north east of Hajjah, Yemen. Am. J. Sci. Res. 3, 84–91 (2008)
26. Sheffield, C.: Selecting band combinations from multispectral data. Photogramm. Eng. Remote Sensing 51, 681–687 (1985)
27. Zuiderveld, K.: Contrast Limited Adaptive Histograph Equalization. In: Heckbert, P.S. (ed.) Graphics Gems IV, pp. 474–485. Academic Press Professional, Inc., San Diego (1994)
28. Le Moan, S., Mansouri, A., Hardeberg, J., Voisin, Y.: Visualization of spectral images: A comparative study. In: GCIS Proceeding, pp. 1–4. Gjovik, Norvège (2011)

Mousavi, Parvin   108
Müller-Stich, Beat Peter   158

Nagpal, Simrin   108
Najafi, Mohammad   256
Navab, Nassir   68, 100, 148, 178, 236
Niessen, Wiro J.   78, 246
Nolte, L.   128
Nouranian, Saman   90
Nouri, Dorra   266
Nowell, M.   118

Okur, Aslı   148
Osborn, Jill   90, 108
Ourselin, Sébastien   1, 118, 226

Padoy, Nicolas   168, 186
Pauly, Olivier   178
Peter, Loïc   148
Peterlik, Igor   196
Poignet, Philippe   21, 31

Rasoulian, Abtin   90, 108
Regar, Evelyn   78
Richmon, Jeremy D.   41
Rodionov, R.   118
Rohling, Robert N.   90, 108, 256
Ruijters, Danny   246

Sánchez, Alonso   21, 31
Schneider, Armin   148
Schumann, S.   128
Sojoudi, Samira   90

Sorger, Jonathan   41
Speidel, Stefanie   158
Stauder, Ralf   148
Stoyanov, Danail   1, 11, 206, 216, 226

Taylor, Russell H.   41
Thaller, Peter   100
Thompson, Stephen   1, 206
Thornton, John   226
Totz, Johannes   206
Treuillet, Sylvie   266
Twinanda, Andru P.   186

Ungi, Tamas   108

van Soest, Gijs   78
van Walsum, Theo   78, 246
Vedula, S. Swaroop   138

Wehner, T.   118
Weidert, Simon   100, 178
Wekerle, Anna-Laura   158
White, Mark   226
Winston, Gavin P.   226

Yousry, Tarek   226

Zahnd, Guillaume   78
Zemiti, Nabil   21, 31
Zheng, G.   128
Zombori, G.   118
Zuluaga, M.A.   118

Author Index

Abolmaesumi, Purang   90, 108, 256
Afsham, Narges   256
Allan, Max   1
Ambrosini, Pierre   246
Arridge, Simon   216
Azizian, Mahdi   41

Balestra, S.   128
Berge, Christian Schulte zu   236
Black, Peter   256
Borschneck, Dan P.   108
Burgos, Ninon   226

Cardoso, M. Jorge   226
Champion, Benjamin   61
Chang, Ping-Lin   11
Chang, Silvia D.   256
Chen, Chi Chiung Grace   138
Clancy, Neil   216
Clarkson, Matthew J.   1, 118, 206
Cotin, Stéphane   196
Courtecuisse, Hadrien   196

Daga, Pankaj   226
Davidson, Brian R.   206
Davison, Andrew J.   11
De Mathelin, Michel   168, 186
Despinoy, Fabien   21
Diehl, B.   118
Dillmann, Rüdiger   158
Diotte, Benoît   178
Diotte, Benoit   100
Duncan, John S.   118, 226
Duriez, Christian   196

Edwards, Philip "Eddie"   11
Elson, Dan   216
Esposito, Marco   100
Euler, Ekkehard   100, 178

Fallavollita, Pascal   100, 178
Feussner, Hubertus   148

Gangi, Afshin   168
Gärtner, Fabian   158

Gijsen, Frank   78
Goldenberg, Larry   256
Graña, Adrián   31
Gurusamy, Kurinchi   206

Habert, Séverine   178
Hacihaliloglu, Ilker   108
Hager, Gregory D.   138
Handa, Ankur   11
Hawkes, David J.   1, 61, 206
Hennersperger, Christoph   68
Heverhagen, J.   128

Jannin, Pierre   21
Jones, Geoffrey   216

Kadkhodamohammadi, Abdolrahim   168
Kapoor, Ankur   236
Karamalis, Athanasios   68
Karanasos, Antonios   78
Katić, Darko   158
Kelly, John D.   1
Kenngott, Hannes   158
Khallaghi, Siavash   256
Kochan, Martin   226
Kranzfelder, Michael   148

Lessoway, Victoria A.   90, 108
Liu, Wen P.   41
Londei, Roberto   100
Lucas, Yves   266

Machan, Lindsay   256
Malpani, Anand   138
Mancini, Laura   226
Marescaux, Jacques   186
Martin, James   61
Masamune, Ken   51
McClelland, Jamie   61
McEvoy, Andrew W.   118, 226
Micallef, C.   118
Miki, Kohei   51
Miserochi, A.   118
Moelker, Adriaan   246